# X TROOP

# X TROOP

## The Secret Jewish Commandos
## of World War Two

—

## Leah Garrett

*Houghton Mifflin Harcourt*

BOSTON   NEW YORK

2021

For information about permission to reproduce selections from this book, write to trade.permissions@hmhco.com or to Permissions, Houghton Mifflin Harcourt Publishing Company, 3 Park Avenue, 19th Floor, New York, New York 10016.

"The Sweet Life" by Peter Masters reprinted by permission
of the Masters Family Collection.

Jacket photo: Group photo of X Troopers, with Geoff Broadman (center) holding tommy gun. Used by permission.

hmhbooks.com

*Library of Congress Cataloging-in-Publication Data*
Names: Garrett, Leah, 1966– author.
Title: X troop : the secret Jewish commandos of World War II / Leah Garrett.
Other titles: Jewish commandos of World War II
Description: Boston : Houghton Mifflin Harcourt, 2021. | Includes bibliographical references and index.
Identifiers: LCCN 2020044747 (print) | LCCN 2020044748 (ebook) |
ISBN 9780358172031 (hardcover) | ISBN 9780358533306 |
ISBN 9780358533399 | ISBN 9780358177425 (ebook)
Subjects: LCSH: Great Britain. Combined Operations Command. Commando, 10th. No. 3 Troop — Biography. | World War, 1939–1945 — Commando operations — Great Britain. | World War, 1939–1945 — Campaigns — Europe. | World War, 1939–1945 — Secret service — Great Britain — Biography. | Masters, Peter, 1922–2005. | Gans, Manfred. | Anson, Colin Edward, 1922–2016.
Classification: LCC D794.5 .G37 2021 (print) | LCC D794.5 (ebook) |
DDC 940.54/86410923924 — dc23
LC record available at https://lccn.loc.gov/2020044747
LC ebook record available at https://lccn.loc.gov/2020044748

Book design by Chloe Foster

Printed in the United States of America
1 2021

THIS BOOK IS DEDICATED TO THE EXTRAORDINARY

MEN OF X TROOP & THEIR FAMILIES

# Contents

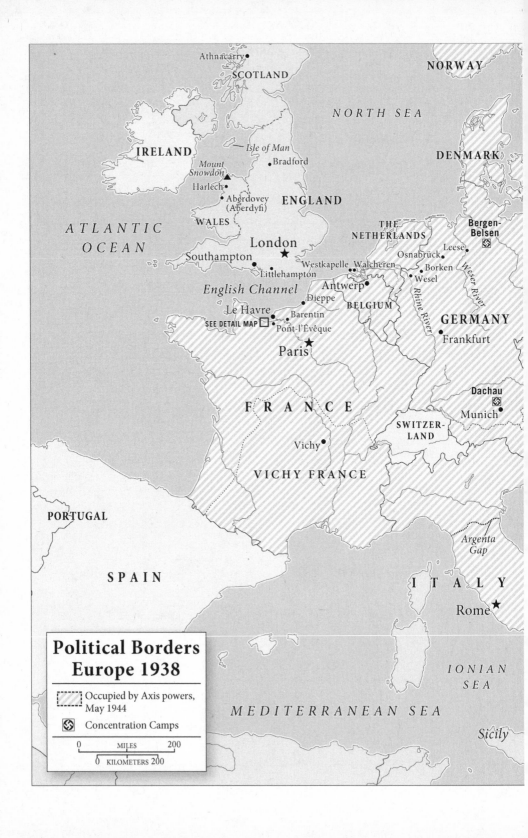

Athnacarry•

SCOTLAND

NORWAY

NORTH SEA

Isle of Man

IRELAND

Mount
Snowdon▲

Harlech•

Aberdovey
(Aberdyfi)•

WALES

•Bradford

ENGLAND

DENMARK

THE
NETHERLANDS

Bergen-
Belsen ⊗

Osnabrück•
•Leese

London ★

Southampton•

•Littlehampton

Westkapelle• •Walcheren
Antwerp•

•Borken
•Wesel

ATLANTIC
OCEAN

English Channel

•Dieppe

BELGIUM

Weser River

GERMANY

Le Havre•
SEE DETAIL MAP ☐•
•Barentin
•Pont-l'Évêque

Rhine River

•Frankfurt

Paris ★

F R A N C E

SWITZER-
LAND

Dachau
⊗
•Munich

Vichy•

PORTUGAL

VICHY FRANCE

Argenta
Gap

SPAIN

I T A L Y

Rome ★

IONIAN
SEA

MEDITERRANEAN SEA

Sicily

## Political Borders
## Europe 1938

```
┊┊┊┊  Occupied by Axis powers,
      May 1944
```

⊗   Concentration Camps

0 ——— MILES ——— 200

0 — KILOMETERS 200

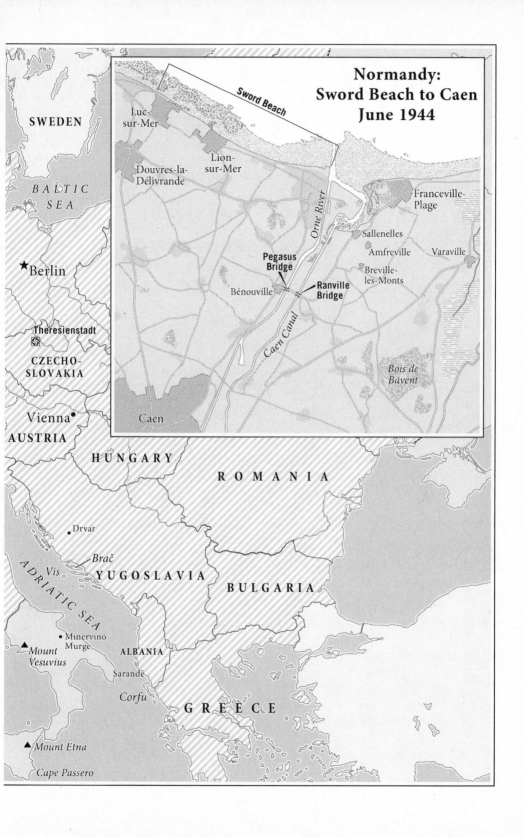

SWEDEN

BALTIC
SEA

★Berlin

Theresienstadt

CZECHO-
SLOVAKIA

Vienna•

AUSTRIA

HUNGARY

ROMANIA

• Drvar

Brač

Vis     YUGOSLAVIA

BULGARIA

ADRIATIC SEA

• Minervino
Murge

▲ Mount     ALBANIA
Vesuvius

Sarandë

Corfu

GREECE

▲ Mount Etna

Cape Passero

## Normandy:
## Sword Beach to Caen
## June 1944

Sword Beach

Luc-
sur-Mer

Lion-
sur-Mer

Douvres-la-
Délivrande

Orne River

Franceville-
Plage

Sallenelles

Amfreville     Varaville

Breville-
les-Monts

Pegasus
Bridge

Ranville
Bridge

Bénouville

Caen Canal

Bois de
Bavent

Caen

# Prologue

LIEUTENANT GEORGE LANE is in big trouble. His waterlogged Sten gun has jammed, and bullets from German rifles and MP40s are flying all around him. He is hiding in the surf next to beach obstacles made of thin iron girders. The Nazis are shooting blindly into the darkness while Lane and Captain Roy Wooldridge, an expert in mines, desperately seek cover. It's May 17, 1944, Ault, northern France, two hours after midnight, three weeks before D-Day.

Something has spooked the Germans, and Lane doesn't know whether they have been discovered and the mission compromised, or the bored guards are now simply letting off steam. He does know that if they are taken prisoner, it will mean almost certain death. Adolf Hitler's 1942 Kommandobefehl edict states that all captured Allied commandos are to be summarily executed.

The two men lie as still as possible on the beach, and after ten minutes the shooting stops. The British officers find their concealed rubber dinghy, which is miraculously unpunctured. They jump in, push into the waves, and start paddling out to sea, hoping to make it back to the motor torpedo boat from which they deployed.

They begin to think that they might just make it back from this mission, but after rowing frantically for twenty minutes, they are spotted by a German E-boat. A blinding spotlight turns on them, and a 37 mm flak cannon and machine guns are pointed at their torsos. "Hände hoch, Tommy!" a Kriegsmarine lieutenant shouts.

Lane and Wooldridge have no choice but to surrender. Lane is thinking more about torture than the Kommandobefehl and summary execution. "The Gestapo make everyone talk," he has been told.

Lane is not worried about giving up any details about D-Day. As a lowly lieutenant he's not privy to such operational information. He is concerned that the Germans will crack his cover story. And if they crack that, they might find out about his brother soldiers and their secret unit: X Troop.

The E-boat takes them ashore. Still in soaking-wet clothes, the prisoners are driven to a command post and put in two separate basement cells for a long, cold, hungry night. Desperate to escape from a likely firing squad, Lane manages to pick his door's lock with a piece of metal ripped from a floor pipe. As he steps out into the dark corridor, a guard yells at him to get back into his cell.

The next morning Lane and Wooldridge are driven to a village in the French countryside. They are wearing blindfolds, but Lane's has been fitted poorly and he is able to make a mental map of his bearings. They arrive at a place on the Seine River called Château de La Roche-Guyon, which has been turned into a Wehrmacht headquarters for Field Marshal Erwin Rommel. Rommel has chosen this spot because it lies neatly at the boundary between his two armies.

The British officers are separated. A German captain offers Lane something to drink and tells him that he should tidy himself up.

Lane asks why.

"Because you're going to be interrogated by someone important," the German explains.

Lane washes his face, cleans his fingernails, and is led into a study.

There is a man at the fireplace with his back to him. He turns. Lane is stunned to discover that it is Field Marshal Rommel himself. Lane instinctively gives him the salute due a superior officer. It's an odd moment. Lane, like all the members of X Troop, is a fanatical anti-Nazi. His unit of Jewish commandos has been mostly recruited from German and Austrian escapees of the Nazi regime. This ragtag group includes a semiprofessional boxer; an Olympic water polo player; a previously Orthodox Jew obsessed with science; and painters, poets, athletes, and musicians. By this stage of the war, the summer of 1944, most of their relatives who weren't able to escape have been murdered in the death camps. To protect themselves and any family members still alive, the men in X Troop have all taken on fake English names and identities. Lieutenant George Lane himself is Lanyi György from Budapest, pretending to be a Welsh infantry officer. He's lived in England for the past eight years; his English isn't bad, but his Welsh accent is terrible.

"You realize that you are in a very tricky situation here, Lieutenant Lane?" Field Marshal Rommel says through an interpreter.

"I don't think so. I happen to be a POW — there's nothing tricky about that," Lane responds.

"Well, my people seem to think that you are a common saboteur," Rommel says.

"If the field marshal believed I was a common saboteur then I don't think he would have invited me for tea," Lane replies.

"So you think this is a polite invitation?"

"Indeed I do and I'm greatly honored by it," Lane answers, to a smile from the field marshal. The ice has been broken.

Rommel's adjutant pours the tea.

"So how is my friend General Montgomery?" Rommel asks.

"Unfortunately I don't know him personally, but as you know he's preparing the invasion, so I imagine you'll see him very soon," Lane says.

Rommel asks Lane where he thinks the invasion might be. Lane explains that he is only a junior officer who is not privy to any of the invasion plans.

Rommel nods. "Of course what you don't realize is that the greatest tragedy today is that you British and we Germans are not fighting side by side against the real enemy, Russia."

Lane knows he should keep his mouth shut, but he can't help himself and he says, "Sir, how can the British and Germans fight side by side considering what we know about what the Nazis are doing to the Jews? No Englishman could ever tolerate such a thing."

"Well, that's a political argument, and as a soldier you shouldn't be interested in politics at all," Rommel answers curtly.

"I'm sorry, sir, but it's very important to us English," replies the Jewish refugee from Budapest.

The conversation peters out. A side door opens and an officer leads Lane away. Lane wonders what Captain Wooldridge will say during his interrogation. He's furious with himself, knowing that he should have stuck to name, rank, and serial number, but he hadn't expected to see Field Marshal Rommel himself.

Lane is given a bite to eat and later that afternoon is handed over to the Wehrmacht — not, he is relieved to find, the Gestapo or the SS.

He is transferred to a prisoner of war camp, where he is released into the general population of POWs. His Welsh cover story doesn't survive one day in the camp, and the English prisoners assume he is a stooge. He finds the camp's Allied commanding officer and explains to him that he isn't George Lane.

"Who the devil are you, then?" the commanding officer demands.

"I'm a member of X Troop."

"And what the blazes is that?"

"Sit down, sir," Lane says, "and I will explain everything."

# X TROOP

# Introduction

AT THE NADIR of World War Two, in Britain's darkest hour, a group of Jewish refugees from Germany, Austria, and Hungary volunteered for a top secret mission to fight as commandos on the front lines against the Nazis. Determined to wreak havoc on Hitler's regime, the eighty-seven men of No. 10 (Inter-Allied) Commando, 3 Troop — better known as X Troop — saw the war as personal. They played a crucial role in the D-Day landings and killed, captured, and interrogated their way across occupied Europe all the way into the heart of the Third Reich.

*X Troop: The Secret Jewish Commandos of World War Two* tells this virtually unknown story for the very first time in book form. To uncover the history of this remarkable unit, I declassified long-sealed, top secret British military records; read the breathless heat-of-the-battle official war diaries; and discovered a trove of startling new materials from the families of the X Troopers. I also conducted interviews with still living commandos and the wives and children of a number of X Troopers. It is a tale that needed telling. This group of highly trained soldiers gained a fearsome reputation, and they found themselves fighting in France, Sicily, mainland Italy, Greece, Yugoslavia, Albania, the Netherlands, and Belgium. When the war was over and most of their comrades were going home, these extraordinary men went hunting for Nazis in the rubble of Hitler's Europe.

As Britain in 1942 sought to claw its way back from the brink of defeat and contemplated the daunting prospect of invading the Nazi-occupied European continent, British military planners determined they would need one weapon that was not yet in their arsenal: highly intelligent, highly motivated, German-speaking commandos. They would use these men to infiltrate behind enemy lines, interrogate prisoners on the spot, and help guide the Allied dagger into the heart of the Third Reich. To fill this role, the British conceived of X Troop, a unique commando force with an unusual combination of skills that usually don't go together: advanced fighting techniques and counterintelligence training. These men had to be special. They had to be heart and head. They had to be both brains and brawn.

Only one group fit the bill: the German-speaking Jewish refugees who had been arriving in Britain since Hitler's rise to power. Most of these "enemy aliens" came to England without their parents on Kindertransport trains or as part of religious missions. Many had lost their families, their homes, their whole worlds to the Nazis. They became one of Britain's most important secret commando units, referred to by Miriam Rothschild, the famous spouse of one particularly storied X Trooper, as a "suicide squad." The anger and hunger for revenge of these commandos was palpable.

Many were brilliant young men, sons of diplomats and scientists, but initially the British didn't trust them because they were German, Austrian, or Hungarian. So they put them in detention camps, often in appalling conditions. Eventually, though, the men were selected or volunteered for unspecified "hazardous duty," which they were told would entail extremely dangerous work that involved taking the fight directly to the Nazis. Every man offered a place in X Troop accepted the mission.

In order to operate behind enemy lines they had to shed their previous lives as refugees and take on new British identities. If they were recognized as Jews, they would be killed instantly and the Gestapo would hunt down their families if they were still alive. Each volunteer was given a few minutes to pick a new British persona, then they had to destroy any connection with their old selves, burning letters from home and throwing out any belongings with their names on them. For those killed in battle this change would remain permanent, and many would be buried under their nom de guerre and a marble cross.

Once they had their new names and identities, the X Troopers underwent tough commando training in Wales and Scotland. They spent days and nights hiking over mountains with full packs, and practiced beach assaults, live ammo drills, rock climbing, parachuting, and demolition work.

When their training was completed, the X Troopers became the very tip of the Allied spear, using their advanced fighting techniques to capture enemy soldiers and then immediately interrogate them rather than wasting valuable time bringing them back to headquarters. *Where are the mines laid? How many soldiers are in your formation? What units are they from? Where is your headquarters? What weapons are being used?* This information was used to make crucial battlefield decisions in the next minutes, hours, and days.

During their service the X Troopers worked with some of the most eccentric, brilliant characters of World War Two: Lord Lovat of the Special Service Brigade, Queen Victoria's great-grandson Lord Mountbatten, Field Marshal Bernard Montgomery, and the famous Captain "Mad Jack" Churchill. They proved their worth again and again. And even after the war was over and the unit was formally disbanded, the X Troopers were central to the denazification campaign: routing out hidden party members (almost capturing the head of the SS, Heinrich Himmler), uncovering sensitive intelligence, and gathering evidence for the Nuremberg trials. At least eighty-seven volunteers passed through the ranks of this elite unit, and half of them would be killed, wounded, or disappear without a trace. Collectively, the survivors and the fallen alike would contribute to the Allied war effort in a way that defies the imagination and that still has not received due credit.

• • •

Each member of X Troop has an exceptional biography, a tale of loss and redemption, of agency stolen and reclaimed. In the words of the commando Peter Masters, "Shocked by history, desperate, and in danger, we were threatened by Hitler . . . the creator of hell on earth, and we fought for the chance to counter those seemingly insurmountable odds." Some of the men were more blunt about their motivations. One of Peter's comrades later said, "Frankly I was looking forward to all the killing."

In this book I focus on three of these men in particular: Peter Masters (birth name: Peter Arany), Manfred Gans (nom de guerre: Fred Gray), and Colin Anson (birth name: Claus Ascher), whose stories are typical of the others'. I also look in some detail at the men who fought under the names George Lane, Ian Harris, Tony Firth, Maurice Latimer, Geoff Broadman, Ron Gilbert, and Paul Streeten.

As of 2021 several military and intelligence files relating to X Troop still remain classified. The book you are reading is my attempt to provide the most comprehensive account of X Troop to date. Until these secret files are fully available to the public, however, the history of this unit will remain somewhat cloaked in shadows — much like the commandos themselves. The X Troopers' aliases also present a challenge to any historian, especially one who aims to tell their individual stories from beginning to end. Many of the men chose to keep their cover identities after the war, living out their lives under the names not of the refugees they had been, but of the soldiers they had become. For the sake of clarity and to honor the decisions of these veterans, I have used the names they chose, rather than the names they were born with. This also reflects a broader truth about this remarkable group of soldiers: after enduring unspeakable abuse at the hands of a genocidal, totalitarian state, the X Troopers became masters of their own fate, winning a personal victory. Their story is a remarkable testament to the human ability to face the most extreme challenges while staying focused on a higher goal: in this case, to right a world that had gone terribly awry.

# EXILE

IN SEPTEMBER 1937 the young man who would become Colin Anson sat with his father at a beer hall in Römerberg Square, Frankfurt. Römerberg is a picturesque medieval site of an ancient trade fair and a famous Christmas market. It was also the place where, in more recent history, Nazi students had conducted a book burning. Marching with lit torches and yelling anti-Jewish slurs, thousands of Hitler supporters made a huge pyre of the works of Sigmund Freud, Walter Benjamin, Franz Kafka, Karl Marx, even Jack London — anyone deemed an enemy of the Nazi ethos.

Nevertheless, on this beautiful fall evening Colin — who at the time was still going by his birth name, Claus Ascher — felt relatively safe sitting with his father, Curt Ascher, as their Alsatian dog, Lorna, lay at their feet. In fact Colin felt a bit of a thrill. He was only fifteen years old, and it was exciting for him to enter the grown-up world of the Bierhalle. This particular beer hall was crowded with men seated at long communal tables who were trying to get some serious drinking done. At the Aschers' table two men were talking loudly about the Spanish Civil War and were boasting about the triumphs of the Nazi Condor Legion and the retreat of the Republicans there.

Colin noticed that his father was getting red in the face and his knuckles were tightening around his stein of foaming Weissbier.

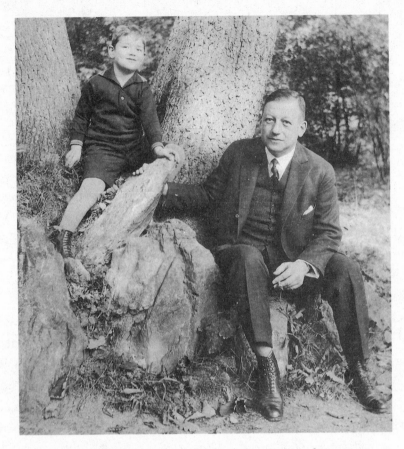

*Young Colin Anson with his father, Curt Ascher*

"Please be careful," Colin whispered.

"I've kept my mouth shut too long," Curt muttered.

"You don't have to say anything to them. We can just finish our drinks and go home," Colin insisted.

But to the boy's horror, his father leaned over and interrupted the two men: "The Nazis are helping General Franco against a democratically elected government!"

The men stopped talking and turned to look at him. The packed beer hall became quiet just like in one of the American Westerns that were so popular in Germany at the time. Conversations stopped mid-sentence,

glasses were lowered, and in an instant the only sound was Lorna thump-
ing her tail against the sawdust-covered floor.

Colin looked nervously at the other men sitting around the table. The
Nazi regime had fostered a shadow state of secret police and paid inform-
ers who were keen to turn people in either for the sake of the Reich or just
to get some easy money. The beer hall today seemed to be filled with a fair
number of German American tourists. In Colin's experience the German
Americans were often the most pro-Nazi of all, awed by the Führer, the
parades, the uniforms. They frequented the beer halls not only because
they were so stereotypically German, but also because their idol, Adolf
Hitler, had attempted to overthrow the government of Bavaria during his
notorious Beer Hall Putsch of 1923. It was one of those Americans who,
just then, yelled something supportive of the Nazis, in heavily accented
German.

Curt was dismissive of the foreigner. "You don't understand anything!"
he replied. "You need to look under the surface of things to where all this
is heading."

A young man whom Colin hadn't noticed before got up and left the hall
in a hurry. The uneasy silence descended again. Colin looked down at his
shaking hands and at his plate of food, a half-eaten sausage with mustard
and sauerkraut.

These were extremely dangerous times to speak out, but Curt Ascher was
furious with the Nazis. He was Jewish but had always considered himself
an extremely patriotic German, in love with German culture. Later Colin
would say of his father that he was "first and foremost a German, his Jewish
background secondary." Curt had served bravely and proudly for the German
Empire in World War One and had nearly died from a skull fracture at the
Battle of the Somme, which had left shrapnel permanently embedded in his
head. The rise of the Nazis had shaken him, and he was desperate to stop
a regime that he sensed was bringing catastrophe to his beloved country.

While his father and the American tourist squared off, the door of the
beer hall opened and the young man who had run out returned with a
police officer. The officer immediately placed Curt under arrest. Colin's

law-abiding father, who prided himself on being a good citizen, stood up shakily. Shocked and humiliated, he followed the policeman outside, leaving behind his walking stick, dog, and frightened son.

The chat and music resumed. Colin sat there, shipwrecked, stunned, not touching his food nor drinking his beer. No one spoke to the boy with the cherubic face under a wheat field of blond hair. Time passed. The minutes turned into an hour and Colin remained there, too scared to move or leave and hoping desperately that his father would come back. Eventually another police officer arrived, paid the bill, and told Colin to come along with him. Colin took Lorna by the leash, grabbed his father's walking stick, and left the beer hall. "How could your father say such things? Doesn't he know how dangerous it is to talk like that nowadays?" the policeman whispered.

Colin followed the officer to the police station where his father was being held. He went to embrace the old man, but rather than hugging him Curt shoved several letters into his son's hands and told him to go home immediately. A despondent Colin left the station and ran home to his mother, Mathilde, and told her what had happened. They burned the letters, which turned out to be compromising political pleas to other potential dissidents.

Just weeks later, on October 2, 1937, Colin's father was transported to Dachau concentration camp outside Munich. The camp, opened in 1933, was originally set up to house around five thousand political prisoners. Life there was brutal. With overcrowding, no heat, and little food, hunger and disease were rife, and death by "natural causes" was alarmingly common.

Less than two weeks after Curt was taken there, on October 15, a Gestapo officer showed up at the family home to tell Mathilde and Colin that Curt had died of "circulation failure."

"My father's ashes were then posted to us in an urn through regular mail," Colin would later recall. "We even had to pay the postage." Along with the urn they received Curt's "two little leather-bound pocket editions of Proust."

For Colin, fifteen at the time, the death of his father was the defining moment of his life. He had always idolized Curt and saw him as a role model of the type of man he wanted to be. The rise of the Nazis had upended everything Colin had believed about himself and his family. Before their takeover of Germany, Colin had been baptized and was a practicing Protestant, attending church regularly. Colin's mother was Christian, his father was highly assimilated, and as with many Jewish and mixed families in Germany at the time, the Aschers raised their child in such a way that he was unaware of his Jewish roots. At first young Colin had found the arrival of the Nazis exciting; like many German children, he was swept away by the grand spectacle and the sense of belonging to something greater than himself. The Nazis' anti-Jewish rhetoric was of no concern to him. Why would he care since he was a good Protestant boy? Also, by nature, Colin was a conformist, who liked to follow the rules. It would have been uncomfortable and potentially dangerous for him to question or oppose the new regime.

For Curt Ascher, however, watching his son's easy embrace of the Nazi regime was deeply troubling. One fateful afternoon a few years before Curt's deportation to Dachau, he called his son to the table, sat him down, and told him that he was Jewish, which meant Colin was half Jewish. Curt had previously protected his son from this knowledge, but now he felt it was crucial to tell him. Colin's views of the Nazis changed almost immediately: the Nazis were talking about him and his family; *they* were the supposed rats and traitors who were destroying Germany!

At school Colin had already been a regular victim of bullies because he had been skipped a grade, which meant that he was smaller than the other boys and an easy target. When he refused to join the Hitler Youth, the bullying intensified and the teachers began to join in as well. The situation became so bad that his parents sent him to a different school that had some Jewish teachers, but then those teachers were dismissed and replaced by Nazis. With the situation rapidly worsening for the Jews of Frankfurt, many began trying to get out. Colin's father, however, had refused to even consider this. He would say, "I'm German, I'm born here, I fought for this country, and I'll die here."

One afternoon all the children at Colin's new school were sent to a rally commemorating the opening of the autobahn connecting Frankfurt to Darmstadt. This was one of many pro-Nazi events the students had to participate in, although this one was unique because Adolf Hitler himself would be there. The stretched Mercedes with a swastika mounted on the front pulled up in front of Colin's school group. As Hitler appeared in his suit and full-length leather trench coat, the crowd, including school-children and mothers with their babies, began screaming and crying and reaching out to touch their idol. They surged forward and Colin was pushed right up against the door of Hitler's car. It was a surreal moment. With the Führer just centimeters away from him, young Colin found him-self unimpressed. "Here was one of the most powerful leaders in Europe, but to me he seemed like a peasant in a Sunday suit."

After Curt's death daily life had become much harder for Colin and his mother. There was no money for school fees, so Colin went to work in an asbestos factory. And then came Kristallnacht, the Night of Broken Glass, the devastating anti-Jewish pogroms of November 9–10, 1938. Throughout Germany, Austria, and the Sudetenland, Jewish businesses, synagogues, and cultural centers were destroyed, with broken glass, a symbol of the mass hatred, covering the streets. Tens of thousands of Jews were arrested and sent to concentration camps, most notably Dachau and Buchenwald, while the Jewish community was charged 10 billion reichsmarks for the destruction the Nazis themselves had wrought against them.

In Frankfurt the beautiful Westend synagogue, where Colin had lately taken cello lessons and participated in cultural life, was defaced and se-verely damaged by fire. Those Jews who had been holding out hope could now, like the biblical hero Daniel, read the writing on the wall. Colin's Christian mother began to devote all her energy to getting her son out of the country. However, the Nazis were doing everything they could to make life impossible for the Jews, and it was becoming more and more difficult to leave. As surrounding countries began limiting the number of Jewish refugees they would admit, the situation became fraught for Colin. He was not only a full Jew under the Nuremberg Laws, but he was also the son of a dissident. Sooner or later he would be arrested.

Colin's mother got him on a waiting list of children to be transported to the United States, but he was given the desperately high number of 24,132, which meant it would be nearly impossible for him to leave. His mother then turned to the British Society of Friends (the Quakers), who had been help-ing Jews in Nazi-occupied Europe. They agreed to take her boy to Britain.

On February 6, 1939, sixteen-year-old Colin arrived at the Frankfurt train station to board a Kindertransport train to Britain. He and his mother had already said their final goodbyes at their apartment so as not to make a scene. He carried a small suitcase that contained things he thought he might need in chilly, rainy England: a blanket, a jacket, a pair of pants, a sweater, two shirts, a pair of long underwear, two pairs of regular underwear, thirty handkerchiefs, a shaving cup, a shoeshine set, a clothes brush, two ties, a pair of shoelaces, a flashlight, a map, photographs, and a case containing pencils, a pencil sharpener, pens, and erasers. These contents suggested a middle-class teenager intent on presenting himself as best he could, but the flashlight and map perhaps imply a slightly ominous frisson.

One can imagine Colin at the Frankfurt Bahnhof, stoically clutching his suitcase, trying to be tough like his father, and making his way to the group of children being chaperoned by a kind gentleman named Mr. Blashke. Colin was the oldest one in the group, and he likely felt he had to keep it together for the sake of the younger children. Together they boarded a train headed to Holland, where they would catch a boat to England. They set off without difficulty, but when the train arrived in Emmerich, on the Dutch border, the engine stopped. SS guards wearing intimidating black uniforms with swastika armbands entered the carriage. "Out! Get out of this train now," they yelled at Mr. Blashke and his terrified charges.

The boys and girls, many of them quite young and small, rushed out of the carriage and jumped onto the siding, landing in painful heaps on the ground. Ankles were sprained, knees were bloodied. The SS began rum-maging through their suitcases and dumping the contents onto the siding, confiscating valuables and then slashing up the cases.

"None of you can leave! You are all staying here! You're not going any-where!" the SS officers shouted.

The traumatized children watched in terror as the wheels of the train ever so slowly began to turn.

"Get back on, Jews!" the SS men shouted.

It had all been some kind of humiliating joke. The children frantically grabbed whatever they could of their strewn possessions. They helped each other back onto the train as the SS guards laughed.

A few moments later Mr. Blashke came into Colin's compartment. "We are on Dutch soil," he exclaimed happily in German. Colin felt faint: "[It] was a bit like a diver coming up too quickly and suffering the bends when the pressure is suddenly released. It was an amazing feeling to be free and gradually we began to breathe and realize that it was over. Nazi Germany was behind us."

Less than a year earlier and some 450 miles southeast of Colin Anson's hometown of Frankfurt, an excited sixteen-year-old was riding his bike through the cobbled streets of Vienna, headed to the Prater soccer stadium in the city's Leopoldstadt district. That day one of the most famous games in the history of the sport was going to be played there, and Peter Masters — or Peter Arany, as he was then called — was determined not to miss it, despite all that had happened recently in his troubled homeland of Austria.

It was three weeks after the Anschluss, Germany's annexation of Austria on March 12, 1938. But Peter, a soccer-crazy Jewish teen, had decided that even at great personal risk he needed to attend the match taking place that afternoon between Germany and Austria. The Austrian national team, dubbed the Wunderteam, had recently qualified for the 1938 World Cup, and Peter was obsessed with them. Today's contest was intended to be the final game between the German and Austrian national teams. It would be a celebration of Austria returning to the Reich, after which the Austrian team would be merged into the weaker German one, in advance of going to the World Cup.

The Praterstadion was the largest, most important stadium in Vienna, and the air was electric with anticipation. Huge swastikas were draped over the field, men in black uniforms mingled with the crowd, and Nazi officials filled the viewing box. Peter entered along with the throngs of other excited fans and found his way to a spot in the stands.

Before the game a Nazi official gave a speech about Greater Germany and the Reich. All of a sudden the men, women, and children around Peter were lifting their right arms in the Sieg Heil. Peter knew it was against Nazi law for him, as a Jew, to give the salute. What was he to do? If he did not raise his arm, he would be a recognizable traitor. He stood there for a moment in terror and then he reached into his pocket and pulled out his binoculars: he couldn't do the Sieg Heil because he was engrossed in watching the players. This particular crisis was averted.

The players took the field, among them the Austrian team's dazzling center forward, Matthias Sindelar, "the Mozart of Football." For the first hour of the ninety-minute game, the far superior "Ostmark" dominated. They did not, however, allow themselves to score because they knew there would be repercussions if they humiliated the German national team. Then, at seventy minutes, unable to hold himself back, Sindelar, a Catholic who had always been friends with Jews (including those who had been kicked off the Austrian team after the Anschluss), flicked a rebound from the German goalkeeper into the bottom right-hand corner of the net. The crowd erupted. They weren't supposed to, but they couldn't help themselves. Peter was delighted. One of his heroes was sticking it to the Nazis.

Then Sindelar and his teammates decided to put on a show, running rings around the flat-footed German defenders. Nazi officials watched in disbelief as minutes later Sindelar passed to Karl Szestak, who thumped the ball into the German goal from forty-five yards. At full time a delirious crowd chanted: "Österreich! Österreich! Österreich!" The Germans were defeated. The Nazi officials looked shocked. An exhilarated Peter Masters rode his bike through Vienna to the apartment he shared with his divorced mom, Clara, and his older sister, Eva. It was to be his last pure moment of joy for a long time.

Life in Vienna was increasingly grim. Hitler, an Austrian himself, had been pressing for the unification of Germany and Austria since he came to power in 1933. The beginning of the end for the Jews of Vienna came when the Austrian chancellor, Kurt von Schuschnigg, who was opposed to unification, called a plebiscite. Hitler, worried that the plebiscite would go against the Germans, announced his intention to annex Austria. Realizing that neither France nor Britain would come to his aid, Schuschnigg resigned, and on March 12, 1938, the Wehrmacht marched unopposed over the Austrian frontier. Most Austrians came out into the streets to welcome the German soldiers, and they were greeted with hugs and flowers. Hitler immediately appointed a new Nazi government, and the next day the Anschluss was declared. Hitler began a tour of his home country starting at Linz and ending in Vienna. He also ordered his own fait accompli plebiscite on whether Austrians supported the unification of the two countries.

Peter's Jewish family was not allowed to vote in the plebiscite, but the family cook, Paula, decided to participate. She brought young Peter along with her to the local polling station. When they entered, a man wearing a swastika armband told her that it was pointless to enter the booth. "You should just cast your vote in front of me since you are probably going to vote yes," he said to her.

Paula responded, "I think I'd like to go to the booth."

The official put an ominous X next to her name. Paula took Peter's hand, led him into the booth, and shut the curtain. Peter looked at the ballot she held in her hand. "Do you wish Austria to be incorporated into the German Reich?" was written at the top, as Peter later recalled, and below it were two circles, one labeled "yes" and the other labeled "no." The first circle, in favor of unification, "was as big as a large silver coin," while the circle against unification "was the size of a shirt-button" with "the word 'no' so tiny that it was barely visible." Peter watched as Paula marked her vote against the unification of Austria and Germany. The official vote was, unsurprisingly, 99.73 percent in favor of the Anschluss.

While these acts of defiance by Paula and Matthias Sindelar were extremely brave, they were also extremely rare. The vast majority of Austrians supported the Nazis, and hundreds of thousands attended Hitler's Vienna homecoming on March 15, when he gave an impassioned speech in Heldenplatz Square to a rapturous crowd. Austrian Jews were just under 10 percent of the population, and like Peter's immediate family most lived in Vienna, were middle-class, and were highly assimilated. Peter's grandparents, however, remained practicing Jews, who made sure he attended synagogue regularly and had a Bar Mitzvah.

Before the arrival of the Nazis, Peter's life was good. A handsome, dark-haired, willowy young man with a dimpled chin, contagious smile, and cheeky sense of humor, he was a born artist. Living in Vienna was perfect for him: he loved art and enjoyed visiting the Albertina and Kunsthisto-risches Museums. His family were jewelers and fashion designers, cultured and appreciative of music and art, like many Viennese Jews. In Austria there was no reason to expect that things were going to change soon. Before the Anschluss there had been some instances of anti-Semitism, but mostly these had been rooted in Catholic beliefs about "Jesus killers" rather than in the racial propaganda of the Nazis.

With the German takeover in March 1938, however, life in Austria changed overnight. In one of many shocking incidents Jews were rounded up and marched through the streets of Vienna in front of leering crowds, then forced to use toothbrushes to scrub graffiti off buildings written in support of the fallen Austrian chancellor, Schuschnigg. Jewish businesses were ransacked, cultural figures publicly humiliated, dissidents arrested and turned over to the Gestapo. His aunt Ida's millinery shop, the Modellhaus Ydelle, where his mother worked full-time with her sister, was confiscated by the Nazis. A month later Ida left for London to take a job managing the millinery section of a Jewish-owned department store on Oxford Street.

Peter's beloved Vienna, the city of his dreams and the home of the art and music he so loved, had become a dystopian landscape where he was no longer safe. A likable, easygoing person, Peter was shocked to find that the state utterly despised him simply because he was born Jewish. At school the Jewish children were separated from the others in classes, and they felt unwelcome in their own country. An avid member of the Boy Scouts, Peter loved their camping trips and survival training. After the Anschluss a number of Boy Scout leaders were arrested, and the peace-loving organization was banned as the Hitler Youth sought to reign supreme among the country's teenagers.

Peter's sister, Eva, now eighteen, pleaded with her mother to let her run away to Italy with a friend. Clara refused, saying they would all leave

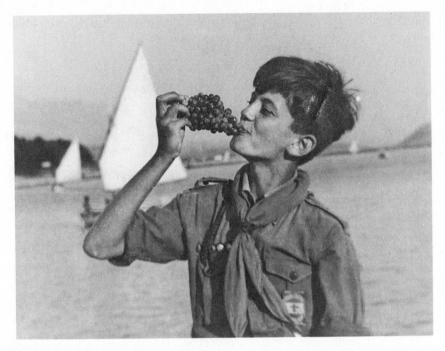

*Peter Masters as a Boy Scout*

together when the time was right. Peter's father, Rudolf, managed to escape to Switzerland.

One beautiful warm morning at this time, Peter and his friend Janek were taking a stroll through Hamerlingpark in the 8th district. The boys found themselves surrounded by members of the Hitler Youth, who started attacking them. They were saved by a sympathetic worker wielding a metal pipe who told the Nazis, "Next time, pick on somebody your own size."

Life had become a nightmare for Peter and his family. The Hitler Youth knew where this Jewish teenager lived, and every time the doorbell rang the family was terrified it was the SS coming to arrest them. Peter was harassed constantly on his bike, and at night his mother received calls every hour ordering them to report to the police. When their cook, Paula, told them she had spotted a Gestapo car outside, they knew they had to leave *now*. Aunt Ida, through begging and cajoling, had managed to get work visas in Britain for all of them (as well as nine additional relatives). But how would they get there, and what would happen to Peter's cherished grandfather, who steadfastly refused to leave?

Arnold Metzger, Peter's maternal grandfather, had been the person most responsible for Peter's connection to Judaism. Arnold had taken him to the local synagogue for his Bar Mitzvah training and led their Passover services in Hebrew. His home was where the family gathered on Friday nights for the sabbath meal. Now in his late seventies, he had been a deeply respected and important goldsmith and silversmith who made jewelry for the Hapsburgs. But Arnold refused to leave Vienna with the others, not wanting to be a burden to them.

Peter, Clara, and Eva said their heartbreaking goodbyes to him and left their apartment late on August 21, 1938, to catch the midnight train to Munich, the heart of Nazi Germany. From there they would head to France, where they would catch a boat to England and use their work permits to join Aunt Ida.

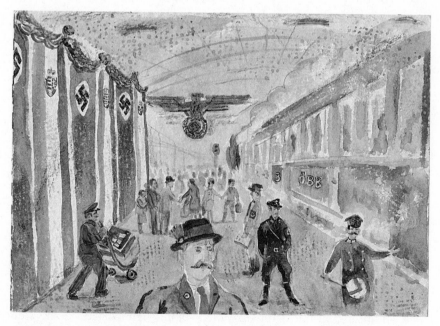

*Peter Masters's painting of the Munich train station during their escape from Austria*

In Munich every inch of the train station was draped with Nazi flags and propaganda about Jews and communists. Peter's family managed to keep a low profile until they boarded a train bound for France.

As the train approached the German border, two Nazi officials entered the car to check their passports. A Frenchman let them pretend they were part of his extended family and all seemed well, but just as the Nazis were about to leave the carriage, one of them turned to the other and muttered, "I think this is one Frenchman and a bunch of Jews trying to escape."

The other officer shrugged and ignored him. As the train passed into France, Peter's mother opened a bottle of cognac she had hidden away for just this moment. The three Austrians and the Frenchman all toasted their survival. The family later made it to Calais and then to England, leaving behind a continent over which the storm clouds had been gathering for years.

It was a late spring Saturday afternoon in April 1935, and Manfred Gans had just turned thirteen years old. His large, beautiful house was packed with friends and family who were there to hear his Bar Mitzvah speech. Manfred lived in Borken, in the northwest of Germany near the border with the Netherlands. It was a picturesque, medieval town of eight thousand or so, surrounded by a moat and walls. Most of the population was Catholic, rural, and poor, although there were about twenty-five Jewish families. Manfred's family was Orthodox and one of the most prominent in town. They lived in one of Borken's finest homes, three stories tall with porticoes and gardens.

The Gans party had just returned from the synagogue, where Manfred had read from the day's Torah section, as well as the haftorah on the Prophets. All of this was done in Hebrew, which wasn't difficult for Manfred, as he had been studying the language in his Jewish day school since kindergarten. No expense had been spared to make the Bar Mitzvah a wonderful event for the large number of guests, and despite the dangerous times they were living in, everyone was determined to enjoy themselves.

A good-looking boy with wavy dark blond hair parted on the side, Manfred began his Bar Mitzvah speech, called the d'var Torah. Typically

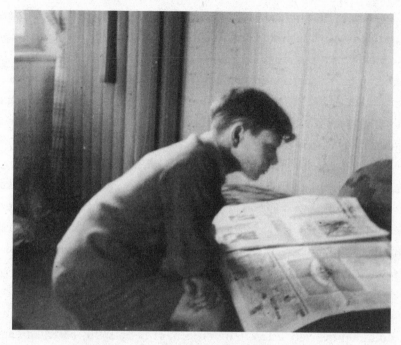

*Manfred Gans at the time of his Bar Mitzvah, 1935*

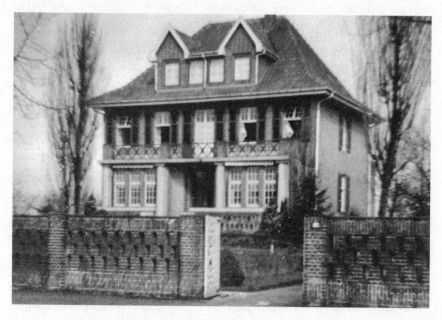

*Manfred Gans's home, Borken, Germany*

these talks were apolitical explorations of the lessons to be learned in the week's Torah portion. But Manfred's speech was different. It went something like this: "The Nazis are calling us the enemy. To them we are vermin, less than human, cheaters and swindlers. They are accusing us of all possible evils. What they don't understand is that our religion, our Torah, does not allow this. Our Torah and the Jewish books teach us to be ethical and forthright. That is who we really are. The Nazis are completely wrong about us."

Manfred's parents, Moritz and Else, looked on with a mixture of horror and resignation. Manfred had always been a fighter and had always spoken his mind. The assembled audience, however, was mortified. It was one thing to talk like this in front of a totally Jewish audience, but it was entirely different to do it in a room where non-Jewish staff were present. If word of this got back to the Gestapo . . .

When Manfred finished his speech, he felt a great sense of relief at having spoken his beliefs out loud. Perhaps because the servants were too busy cleaning up to really listen to his speech, or because his parents treated them well, or just because this was another moment in which Manfred was extremely lucky, there were no immediate repercussions from his words that day.

Manfred's anger was rooted in the injustices meted out against his family, who had, until the rise of Hitler, been leaders of the community. Moritz — whose own father, Karl Gans, was Dutch — had fought bravely and lost a leg for the Germans in World War One. After the war Moritz became a wealthy merchant, selling all sorts of goods, from textiles to vacuum cleaners, in his business, M & E Gans, which he ran in equal partnership with his wife, Else Frankel. Well liked, diplomatic, and persuasive (like his son), Moritz was elected as a Social Democrat to the town council, becoming its first Jewish member ever. He was also president of the League for War Injured, War Orphans, and War Widows, which helped scores of struggling veterans and their families. Their three sons, Gershon, Manfred, and Theo, were extremely close to each other and devoted to their parents. Although they were Orthodox Jews, they were also modern Germans, and family discussions tended to be about literature, music, and films.

Before Hitler became chancellor, Manfred was used to anti-Semitic teasing, and in response to these verbal attacks he used a series of witty rebuttals. Time and again Manfred was asked if he wanted to fight, and often Manfred would say yes. Big for his age, confident, and intimidating, Manfred knew that few would actually take him on. But everything changed for the Jews of Germany on January 30, 1933, when Hitler was appointed chancellor. The mayor of Borken, a friend of the family, was sent to be "reeducated" at a concentration camp and was replaced by a Nazi. Moritz was forced out of his position on the council and as head of the veterans aid group. In all spheres of public life Jews were being harassed and ostracized. Their businesses were boycotted, and they couldn't work in the civil service or at universities or medical establishments. They endured myriad, constant, and treacherous acts of cruelty, from bullying at school and work to summary arrest.

Storm troopers appeared in front of Jewish-owned businesses to block the public from entering. Jews were banned from cinemas, pools, and sporting events. Manfred and his friends managed to sneak into the pool but avoided the other places they loved. At school Manfred and the other Jewish students were frequently singled out, and his biology teacher, Dr. Damen, soon showed up in class with a swastika armband. He began to teach the "science of the races," attempting to prove that Jews were subhuman. The Hitler Youth grew in popularity. Whenever students met their teachers outside of school, they were required to do the Sieg Heil.

Things Manfred used to take for granted, like hiking in the nearby woods, now became extremely dangerous. On one occasion a thug smacked him in the face with a baton, which led to a fight. He was often ambushed or had stones thrown at him. When confronted one-on-one Manfred would usually fight back, but when outnumbered he knew to run. At home Gershon was constantly begging his parents to let him leave to join one of their uncles in Palestine. In 1936, when Gershon was sixteen, his parents finally relented and permitted him to emigrate, with the idea that the rest of the family might eventually join him.

The overwhelming anti-Semitism only seemed to make Manfred stronger. "We had absolutely no identity crisis," he later wrote. "That, I think, is the advantage of having grown up as an Orthodox Jew." Manfred, his brothers, and the other Jewish families of Borken started studying Hebrew nearly every afternoon, attending Zionist groups, and learning more about Judaism. They also started training in practical skills such as carpentry and farming, as potential means of survival in an uncertain future.

Amid this turmoil, Manfred began a romance with a Jewish girl from Berlin, Anita Lamm, whose father was close friends with Moritz. Increasingly worried for the family's safety, Moritz managed to locate extremely hard-to-find ship tickets from France to America and helped them with visas so they could escape from Paris. When Anita's family came through Borken en route to France, Manfred and Anita shared their first kiss. The pair would stay in touch for a time by exchanging letters.

In the summer of 1938, when Manfred was sixteen, his parents understood that things were only going to get worse and decided that he should go to England. For Manfred, an independent and energetic youth, the prospect of going abroad was exciting. Always an optimist, he later wrote that he relished "the thought of new adventures and the thought of a free society where I would be able to talk to anybody and everyone."

On a Friday in July, Manfred said goodbye to his mother and younger brother, Theo, and crossed the Dutch border with his father. They went to their cousin's home in Winterswijk, where they spent the sabbath. Manfred spoke fluent Dutch and on Sunday traveled by himself to the Hook of Holland, where he caught the night boat to England. It was so thrilling he didn't sleep; instead he passed the time practicing his English with some girls he met. Though happy to leave Germany, Manfred wondered if he would ever again see "the beautiful fields, forests, flatlands, mountains, towns and villages where I had grown up. Perhaps the Hitler Reich would last for generations and I would never be allowed to return home."

In fact, of all the millions of Jews who were displaced from their homes by the Nazis, perhaps none of them were to have a homecoming quite as dramatic as Manfred Gans.

# BEHIND THE WIRE

IN THE FINAL months of peace in Europe, refugees from Germany and Austria — most of them Jewish — streamed into England seeking sanctuary. At first the country seemed to be a safe haven from the anti-Semitic terror on the other side of the Channel.

As Colin Anson and the traumatized Kindertransport refugees disembarked in Harwich, they initially found themselves well taken care of. The Quakers who had organized their escape met them with food and tea and put the exhausted children on a train to London, where they would stay temporarily before being sent to different locations. After all they had been through, the English train ride was exciting. It seemed to move faster than the German ones, the seats were much more comfortable, and the windows were plastered with ads for cigarettes. Most important, their fellow passengers were smiling at them and being kind, rather than looking at them angrily as the Germans had. Although only allowed into the country on a transit visa, Colin nevertheless felt that he was, perhaps, finally safe.

After two days in London, Colin was sent to his new home, the Wallingford Farm Training Colony of the Christian Service Union. Two hundred refugee children and orphans from all over Europe were there to receive agricultural training in the hope that they would become useful members of society rather than unemployable burdens on the state. Although the rules were strict and some infractions were met with caning, it was overall a pleasant place to be. Colin was an obedient young man who did not like to make a fuss, and he was therefore chosen as head boy for the refugee children. His main work was gardening, and he received good reviews for being "honest, willing and obliging." He would stay on the farm until the end of 1940, when he was eighteen and could legally volunteer for military service.

Traveling alone, sixteen-year-old Manfred Gans had ridden the ferry from the Hook of Holland to Harwich, arriving in England in July 1938. In Harwich he managed to catch a train to Liverpool Street station in London. His overwhelming impression on arriving in the British capital was one of relief. "Now I am truly free!" he would recall thinking. "I can walk the streets and can talk to anyone without fear of being arrested." His parents had arranged for him to stay with the Jacobses, a Jewish family in North London. At the station's platform he was met by Mrs. Jacobs, a thin, neat woman. She gave Manfred a warm greeting in German, and to his surprise she helped him carry his suitcase down the stairs to the Tube. Manfred was not used to this, and the moment would stay with him for his entire life. Manfred and Mrs. Jacobs took the Circle Line and the Northern Line to Manfred's new home in Golders Green, London. The Jacobses were Orthodox Jews, and Manfred quickly felt at home with them.

Things were looking up for Manfred, but not for his parents back on the continent. The situation in Germany had become febrile, and the rest of Europe seemed poised to follow suit. After Germany's annexation of Austria in March of 1938, Hitler had turned his sights on the Sudetenland, in Czechoslovakia, where there was a large community of Germans who supposedly wanted to be incorporated into the Third Reich. With a second world war possibly looming, a hasty conference was convened in Munich with Hitler, British prime minister Neville Chamberlain, French premier Édouard Daladier, and Italian dictator Benito Mussolini. The Czechs were not invited. The subsequent Munich Agreement, signed on September 30,

1938, stated that France would rip up its treaty with the Czechs and would not intervene if Hitler marched into the Sudetenland. In return for this, Hitler promised that it would be the last territory he would annex.

Upon returning to England Chamberlain was hailed as a national hero by adoring crowds at Heston Aerodrome. In a speech that became famous for its unintentional irony, he declared that he had brought "peace for our time," while waving around a piece of paper that contained the signature and promises of the German Führer. But of course the British prime minister had achieved no such thing, and within months the Germans marched into Prague, occupying all of Czechoslovakia before turning their attention to Poland. Chamberlain might have been surprised by this perfidy on the part of the Nazis, but young Manfred certainly was not.

In the midst of these rising tensions, Manfred registered with the police and was given a temporary visa to remain in the country. Powerless to do much else, he consumed the British newspapers, which were full of the talk of war. Always seeking to increase his knowledge so that he could be better prepared for what lay ahead, Manfred borrowed Hitler's book *Mein Kampf* from the library. It told him everything he needed to know. Hitler could not have been clearer: he was intent on destroying the Jews and wiping them from the face of the earth. While much of the right-wing press had been urging compromise, Manfred learned from *Mein Kampf* that no appeasement could stop Hitler from continuing his advance.

While the gears of war were slowly churning, Manfred was busy trying to get an education in order to pursue his plans for becoming an engineer. He attended a tutorial college to study for his high school exams and found a supportive community among fellow Orthodox Jews. During this time he became his most observant, attending classes in the synagogue, eating only kosher foods, and following the Jewish laws. Tired of living off his father's money, he decided that he needed to find a job, and with the help of a refugee group he moved to Manchester to seek work.

Spring turned to an uneasy summer, and Hitler's ambitions continued to go unchecked. On September 1, 1939, after a number of "border incidents," Germany invaded Poland. Neville Chamberlain, who had promised the British people that he had secured peace, demanded that the Germans withdraw or a state of war would exist between the two countries. Germany did not back down, and two days later, on September 3, 1939, France and Britain declared war on the Third Reich.

Manfred, along with 70,000 other UK residents from Germany and Austria, was overnight turned from a refugee into an "enemy alien." Even though he and 55,000 others in this group were actually Jews who despised the Nazis, that did not seem to matter to the British civil service. They were a "fifth column" who could wage war on the British homeland; as such they were potential enemies who needed to be dealt with. Some of the popular newspapers, which already had a tradition of anti-immigrant sentiment, took up the call with hysterical reports on this internal menace.

By September 28 tribunals were set up around the country to classify the more than 70,000 "enemy aliens" into the appropriate categories. Group A was the greatest potential menace, with around six hundred persons who were immediately interned, as compared with Group C, 64,200 people categorized as "friendly enemy aliens." The majority of German and Austrian Jews, including Manfred, were placed in Group C, which meant that they were a potential but not imminent danger.

Manfred, like countless others, kept his head down and hoped he would fly under the radar. He remained set on his plans to study to become an engineer and decided he would only take a job that furthered that aim, even though unemployment rates were high. In Manchester he boarded with a Jewish couple, Leo and Luise Wislicki, and got a job as a machine fitter. At the same time that he was building a new life in England, his old one seemed to be disintegrating. The mother of Anita Lamm, Manfred's childhood sweetheart, ended their correspondence because she felt that her daughter was too young to be in love and she did not see any possibility that the two would ever be united. Manfred threw himself into his work, "driving myself like the blazes," he later recalled. He finally passed his high school exams in January of 1940 and immediately began studying for an engineering degree at the University of Manchester's night school. Manfred was earning his keep and following his dreams; he even had a solid German bike that his parents had shipped to England.

Meanwhile in Europe, Hitler was triumphant. France and Britain were in no position to honor their pledge to liberate Poland, which had now been occupied by Germany and Joseph Stalin's Soviet Union. In the spring of 1940 German panzer divisions began massing on the French border, and on May 10 the attack on the west began. Germany invaded Holland and Belgium. Neville Chamberlain soon resigned and Winston Churchill became prime minister. Churchill, however, could do nothing to stop the advance of the panzers, and the Nazis had control of the Low Countries within four days.

Manfred read the papers and desperately tried to get news of his grandmother and his parents, Moritz and Else, who he believed were now in Holland. He did not yet know that the Dutch Resistance had managed to place the three of them on a farm on an island in Friesland—an area that had already been "cleared" of Jews and where, for the time being at least, the Nazis were no longer looking. Manfred's older brother, Gershon, was still in Palestine; his younger brother, Theo, had fled to England himself earlier that year, and he and Manfred saw each other frequently. It was a great comfort to Manfred to have at least one family member with him in this strange country, which was soon to grow markedly more inhospitable.

After work one afternoon during the summer of 1940, Manfred found two policemen waiting for him at home. "Sorry, you have to pack up," he was informed. "You're being interned." Manfred knew that any protest would be futile. He stored what he could, packed the largest suitcase he could find with his engineering books and clothes, and gave his notice at the factory.

Manfred, like thousands of other Jewish exiles, was placed formally under arrest and was about to be thrust into one of the least known and darkest chapters in Britain's modern history. The good life was officially over for those who had escaped to Britain in the belief that they would be safe there. The irony was that the anti-Nazi, pro-refugee Winston Churchill had instigated this internment with his order to "collar the lot of them."

Manfred was taken to the police station, registered, and then shipped to the place that would be his home for the coming weeks: the infamous Warth Mills Camp, in Bury, Greater Manchester. Warth Mills was a filthy old cotton mill and was considered to be one of the very worst British internment camps. The lucky remained there only a few days for processing, while the unlucky, like Manfred, were there for weeks.

Thousands of internees were housed at Warth Mills. While they were mostly German Jewish refugees, there was also a group of German Jesuit priests, as well as a contingent of captured Nazi soldiers loyal to Hitler. The floors and walls were filthy with grease and mold and pitted with decay. The windows were broken. The rats were unafraid of the internees and made their nights a particular hell, especially since the prisoners slept on the ground on thin mattresses filled with straw. When it rained, water poured in through the roof and flooded up from the sewers. The former factory had no tables or chairs and no electric lights. The internees ate their meals standing up or on their filthy cots. The food was sparse and poor. Buckets served as toilets.

Manfred, still a teenager, fell in with a group of Orthodox Jews. They kept kosher the best they could by eating nothing but canned vegetables and fish. They prayed three times a day. This helped them endure the filth, the stench of urine, and the rats. As was Manfred's way, he tried to make the best of it. Though the fate of his parents and grandmother weighed heavily on his mind, he spent his time talking about Jewish topics with his fellow internees. He took informal lessons in the Torah and Jewish law from displaced rabbis and despite the conditions tried to keep up his exercise regime.

After enduring this nightmare for nearly a month, on July 27, 1940, young Manfred was transferred to a new camp, Prees Heath, outside Shrewsbury. Originally an army camp for British recruits, it became a home for thousands of enemy aliens. It was a marked improvement over Warth Mills. Here the Orthodox Jews were given their own tents with their own cooking areas. Soon the internees started organizing lectures, sports competitions, and cabaret performances. But there was never enough food, especially for the Orthodox Jews, who could not eat the meat provided. Manfred became skinnier and skinnier. His exercise routine ceased because he became, as he later recalled, "quite weak because of the lack of food."

The days and nights were so rainy at Prees Heath that the tents soon became unlivable. On August 27 Manfred was transferred for the final time to the main internment camp for enemy aliens, the Hutchinson Camp, on the Isle of Man. The Isle of Man was a popular summer destination for British holidayers, but with the war underway and tourism on hold, the Manx Chamber of Commerce saw internment camps as an alternate source of jobs and funds. Barbed wire fences were erected along a series of sequestered homes and boardinghouses overlooking the Irish Sea. In total, there were about 14,000 internees in different camps on the small, egg-shaped island; the Hutchinson Camp housed more than 2,900 male residents. Again the Jews were held alongside many pro-Nazi Germans, who would sing fascist songs and rejoice when there was news of German victories.

Many of the guesthouse windows had been painted midnight blue by the army, and because the low-wattage lamps were red at night, a prisoner later recalled that "Camp Hutchinson looked like the red-light district of some sleazy harbor town." The Jewish internees included an array of important artists, intellectuals, writers, dancers, and actors, such as Arthur Koestler and Fred Uhlman. They were given free rein by the army to organize themselves, and soon they set up an internal administration to oversee all aspects of camp life. Each house in the camp was run according to its own rules, with inhabitants taking responsibility for cooking, cleaning, washing, and other chores.

Yet all the internees were locked behind barbed wire. These men who had been captains of industry, scientists, professors, and musicians in their home countries were treated as common prisoners. They kept up their spirits by turning to creative endeavors, and art and music in particular became a form of resistance. The internees began a series of lectures on culture and science, music concerts, art shows, and theater productions. Kurt Schwitters, a Dadaist, undertook one of the first performance art pieces ever — a forty-minute spoken poem titled *Ursonate*. The fashion designers somehow managed to get fabric to sew curtains for all the windows. A night school was opened, where internees could take courses on philosophy, science, and history. A camp newspaper was established that discussed daily events, commented on the news, and shared the prisoners' frustrations through caustic poems and stories.

Manfred thought it terribly unjust to be locked up, but he was pleased to find that he could pursue his passions: engineering and Jewish studies. He began exercising again, gained weight, and began classes in math, science, and the Talmud.

Study was not the only distraction available to the internees on the Isle of Man. For those who were sports-minded, soccer became an intense focus of life in the camp, and there was even an intra-camp league. It was on such a league that Peter Masters, also a recent internee of the camp, spent much of the day.

Peter had arrived in London with his sister and mother in August 1939. Nearly broke, stateless, and worried about their family in Vienna, the three had moved into a shabby boardinghouse in Warrington Crescent, Maida Vale.

Peter, who was only sixteen, was hungry and scared all the time. He rejoined the Boy Scouts and had his bicycle, but the events of the past eighteen months had traumatized him. When he heard a man whistling a fascist tune on the street, he thought the Nazis were coming for him and had a panic attack. The family became "curtain twitchers," alarmed by policemen strolling past the house and obsessively reading reports about Nazi agents in Britain. Peter avoided the backyard, where the local kids played, because he was too frightened to join them.

Soon Peter got a job at Frogmill Farm in Hurley, but as a sensitive artist he was utterly inept at agricultural work, and the farm's owner, a Mr. Long, jokingly called him "a no-good city kid." Peter escaped into something of a fantasy world, as he later remembered: "When I went to collect the chickens at night I pretended that I was stalking Nazis [with my stick]."

One afternoon in the summer of 1939 Peter was feeding hay onto a conveyer belt and thought he must be hallucinating when he saw a man

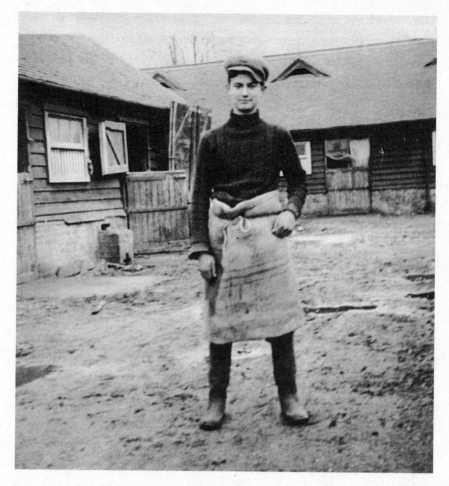

*Peter Masters at Frogmill Farm, Hurley, 1939*

walking toward him who looked just like his father, Rudolf, whom he had last seen when he left Vienna to escape the Gestapo. To his utter shock he realized that it was in fact his dad. "With the macho flamboyance of an ex-officer of the Austro-Hungarian Imperial Army, he threw off his jacket and rolled up his sleeves," he later recalled, and began to help Peter with his work. Seeing this improbable, heavily accented character, Mr. Long muttered that now he appeared to be stuck with two useless mouths to feed.

Rudolf had first tried to get into Britain by contacting George Bernard Shaw, who he assumed had real political leverage. He sent Shaw a homemade bust with a letter imploring the playwright to provide a statement in support of his visa application. Shaw wrote back, "Thank you for the very spirited bust. I have no influence on the Home Office but I have forwarded your letter thither. Good luck." When this avenue failed, Rudolf snuck into England by hiding in a coal pile on a steamer, then hitchhiked to Hurley. After having dinner with Peter on the farm, he turned himself in to the police.

When the war broke out, Peter and his father were classified as Group C aliens and Mr. Long's farm was declared a defense zone, so Peter had to return to London. Peter enrolled in art school and as in Vienna rode his bike everywhere. But, as with Manfred Gans's rude awakening in the summer of 1940, this period of uneasy calm in Peter's life did not last long. In June 1940 he was arrested. Being forcibly interned, he later wrote, was the third metamorphosis Jewish refugees like himself had to undergo during those terrible years: the first one "had been from a sheltered life of a more or less assimilated Central European middle-class high school student, to the harassed object of hatred, contempt, ridicule and ostracism in my home country." The second was the transformation from a citizen of a modern European country to "a penniless refugee." The third transformation was from a refugee to a prisoner "locked up behind barbed wire." There would be a fourth, more auspicious transformation for Peter and a select number of his fellow refugees, but in the summer of 1940 that was still only on the horizon.

While he tried to make the best of it, his circumstances at the Lingfield Camp in Surrey made optimism hard. For instance, during check-in he forgot to grab the toiletries given to new internees. When he attempted to go back to get them, he meekly suggested to the guards that he had a right to them. "Let me tell you something about rights!" a corporal screamed at him. "I have the right to bloody shoot you. You have no rights at all!" After a few months at Lingfield he was transferred to the Hutchinson Camp on the Isle of Man, where Manfred Gans was still being held.

Behind the scenes, however, the Boy Scouts were seeing what they could do for Peter. On August 11 a telegram arrived from Mrs. St. John Atkinson, the head of the Girl Guides in Britain, addressed to Peter's camp commandant. It requested that Peter be released to visit his mother, who was scheduled to undergo a major surgery. Mrs. St. John Atkinson told the commandant that if he didn't want to get on the bad side of "thousands of Girl Guides around Great Britain, the easiest thing was to let Peter go temporarily." The gambit worked: Peter was given a temporary leave from internment.

Within a few days he was back in London. After his mother's successful surgery, weeks of freedom became months, and it was obvious that the state had forgotten about him. Peter was free for now, but free did not necessarily mean safe as the Luftwaffe had begun the Blitz on London. As the bombs fell nightly and whole streets of London were turned into rubble, Peter, like George Orwell, marveled at the "highly civilized human beings flying overhead [who are] trying to kill me," with the additional question of whether he'd known any of them at school back in Vienna.

Being locked up in the UK was bad enough, but the camps in Canada and Australia were far worse than anything faced by the internees in the UK. The horrors of these colonial camps were experienced firsthand by another German-speaking Jewish refugee, Paul Hornig, who in a few years' time would assume the name Paul Streeten. He had been raised in Vienna by his mother and aunts after his father died and had come of age in a progressive circle that included Wilhelm Reich, the radical psychoanalyst who would create the phrase "the sexual revolution," and Karl Popper, the noted philosopher of liberal democracy. Paul was politically active from the age of ten, marching and demonstrating with like-minded Viennese socialists. As a teenager he began attending lectures in psychology given by Alfred Adler, and he decided he wanted to go to law school.

When the Nazis marched into Vienna, Paul's life changed overnight. There was no future in the Reich for a Jewish boy with big dreams, and to make matters worse Paul's name was on multiple lists as an agitator. He escaped arrest only because his family had recently moved to a new flat and the Gestapo gave up searching for him after checking his previous address.

Using his family's connections, Paul got a transit visa to England, where he began studying at Cambridge University. Eventually he was arrested and shipped to Canada when the British decided to extend their camp networks to Commonwealth countries in order to accommodate the thousands of "enemy aliens" they wanted to lock up. Paul was put on the hellish, overpacked HMS *Ettrick*. In addition to the 1,307 internees on board, there were 1,345 German prisoners-of-war, who were given the passenger cabins. The internees were put in the filthy hold, where they had to sleep in three layers: in hammocks, on tables, and on the ground. They felt that the Germans were protected because of the Geneva Conventions, but no one seemed to care about them. In Quebec all of the internees were strip-searched and had their possessions taken away. Eventually 700 of them, including Paul, were transported to the internment camp in Sherbrooke, east of Montreal. It was a grim and overcrowded block situated in two railway sheds with leaky ceilings and only a handful of toilets (which mostly did not work). Paul froze there for the next six months before being shipped back to the UK when the government decided to release all the Group C internees. He later recalled that "it was humiliating to have been rejected by the Austrians as a Jew, and imprisoned by the English as an Austrian."

Sent to Canada with Paul Streeten was a German Jewish refugee named Conrad Goldshmidt, who would come to be known as Brian Grant. Originally from a middle-class Jewish family in Berlin, Grant had arrived in England in 1936 and had settled in comfortably. He was a student at Cambridge University when he was arrested on May 12, 1940. A tall, fair-featured, delicate intellectual, Brian was unprepared for the horrors of internment. He would spend eight months imprisoned in Quebec, during which time his weight tumbled and he fell into a deep depression. Eventually he was shipped back to the Isle of Man along with hundreds of other internees who had been deported.

The internees read the newspapers whenever possible and eagerly waited for any good news from the continent. Unfortunately there was no good news to be found. France had collapsed, and although the British Expeditionary Force had successfully evacuated Dunkirk, they had left all their tanks and equipment on the beaches. On June 14, 1940, the Germans triumphantly entered Paris for a victory parade.

For reasons that are not completely clear, the British government decided in the summer of 1940 to ship thousands of German internees to the Australian outback aboard a converted passenger ship, the HMT *Dunera*. Among them was Hans Julius Guttmann, who would later be known as Ron Gilbert. He had suffered profoundly in Germany before escaping to England. During Kristallnacht in Singen, Germany, Gilbert had been forced at gunpoint to help tear down his own synagogue, and his fingers still had scars on them from ripping down the bimah. After that dreadful night a friend with contacts in the Gestapo told him that he had two weeks to leave Germany or he would be put in a concentration camp. On his escape, the SS boarded his train at the French border, found the Jewish passengers, and with customary cruelty threw their suitcases out the windows. Nearly everything Ron had was gone, but worse would follow. When he arrived in England, he learned that his father had had a fatal heart attack when the Gestapo ransacked his clothing factory in Singen. Soon thereafter Ron's mother was taken on a transport to Poland, where she would later be murdered in a extermination camp. And then Ron himself was forced to board the *Dunera*.

The *Dunera* set off from Liverpool on July 10. The ship had an official capacity of 1,600, but 2,732 internees were crammed on board. The majority, 1,450, were German and Austrian Jewish refugees who had been rounded up from a range of UK internment camps. Also on board were 244 German soldiers, most of whom were die-hard Nazi sympathizers, and 200 Italian survivors of the *Arandora Star*, a British passenger ship that had been sunk by the Germans en route to Canada (805 people had died).

Like Ron, most of the Jewish refugees had lost family members or had been in concentration camps themselves. From the moment of embarkation they were treated cruelly by the British seamen. Ron watched in amazement as their suitcases, passports, visas, letters, and even personal photographs were taken and later destroyed. Some of the refugees had managed to salvage Torah scrolls and Jewish ritual objects from synagogues the Nazis had torched. These were ripped from their hands and thrown overboard, and they were violently searched. One father who tried to keep his son's precious violin from being destroyed was viciously beaten, and the instrument was taken. No receipts were given for any of the confiscated property.

After this shocking treatment the refugees were stuffed belowdecks in the filthy hold for the journey from Liverpool to Australia, which would take fifty-four days. Once they were at sea it quickly became a voyage of the damned. On the first night the men were kept locked in the hold without food, water, or toilets. After that they were only allowed on deck for fifteen minutes of "exercise" per day. For the first few weeks the portholes were kept shut and it was nearly impossible to breathe. As the ship went farther and farther south, the heat was unimaginable. One man died from suffocation. Another, a man named Jakob Weiss, committed suicide after his visa to South America was confiscated. It turned out that Major William Patrick Scott, the officer in charge of the internees on the *Dunera,* was a rabid anti-Semite and sadist who enjoyed torturing the Jews in his care. Beatings were common, and bored guards made Jewish refugees run barefoot over broken bottles they had smashed, all while Nazi POWs howled with laughter.

The crew's anti-Semitism was rooted in the same type of anti-foreign sentiment that was common in the United States at the time, but the history was different in the UK. In 1290 the Jewish people in England, who had been there in small numbers since approximately 1066, were expelled following decades of massacres and hatred. By the seventeenth century small numbers of Jews were beginning to return, and the practice of Judaism was legalized soon after the passage of the Blasphemy Act of 1697. In 1753 the government introduced the Jewish Naturalisation Bill (aka the Jew Bill) to give foreign-born Jews extensive rights. It passed in the House of Lords but was opposed by the Tories in the House of Commons, and there was also so much public agitation against the bill that the government withdrew it from consideration. By the 1800s, however, Jews were allowed to serve in Parliament, and Nathaniel de Rothschild became the first Jewish lord. It seemed that Anglo-Jewry, which by then was mostly middle-class and highly assimilated, was becoming fully accepted into British society.

That changed after the exodus of Russian Jews to the UK following the pogroms and economic struggles of 1881. In the span of twenty-five years, the Jewish population in Britain increased from fewer than 65,000 to more than 300,000, and the majority of the new immigrants were poor, Yiddish-speaking, traditional, and lived in London's East End. During this time there was a violent backlash against them, reflected in the Aliens Act of 1905 and the Aliens Restriction Act of 1914, which radically curtailed the number of arrivals.

The Russian and eastern European immigrants faced intense pressure from the established, middle-class Anglo-Jewish community to assimilate and anglicize, which many did fairly rapidly. The reasons for the broad embrace of rapid assimilation were complicated and included the facts that many Jewish immigrants were deeply grateful to be in a country with a strong liberal ethos; the established Anglo-Jews served as role models of how assimilation could bring economic and social benefits; becoming anglicized could make them less susceptible to anti-Semitism; and they felt indebted to a country that gave them far more rights and freedom than they had had in Russia and eastern Europe. Nevertheless, anti-Jewish/anti-immigrant hatred continued in the 1920s and 1930s with the rise of Oswald Mosley's British Union of Fascists. The Rothschilds and other banking families, in particular, became easy targets of demagogues and rabble-rousers.

During World War Two, Britain would accept around 80,000 Jewish refugees (including around 10,000 children in the Kindertransport), but it would also refuse entry to perhaps hundreds of thousands of Jews trying to escape the Nazis. Most of these Jews, it should be remembered, ended up being murdered.

If the *Dunera* refugees had had to fear only their British tormentors, that would have been bad enough. But the ship also was under constant threat of U-boat attack and was often blacked out. Twenty-three hours a day the men lay on the iron floor, on wooden tables, or in hammocks. The filth was unimaginable, with one bar of soap for twenty men and vomit everywhere from seasickness. The refugees were given fresh water only a few times a week, and the food was infested with mold and weevils. The internees were regularly searched for anything they might have hidden — a wedding ring, a photo — and such items were confiscated or thrown overboard.

The smell belowdecks was rancid, and hundreds of men would crowd around each tiny porthole to get a breath of fresh air. Dysentery soon became a problem. The handful of filthy toilets that the thousands of refugees were allowed to use were on the other side of a gangway lined with barbed wire. One man sick with diarrhea was stabbed in the stomach by the guards when he tried to pass over the gangway. If refugees attempted to complain formally about their treatment, they were beaten, often to the point of unconsciousness. Some of the more sadistic seamen would attack vulnerable internees just for fun.

One of the *Dunera* passengers, Tony Firth (who at this point was known as Hans Fürth), wrote in his unpublished memoir that the guards "showed that you can be a subhuman brute without any special training." A fit, charismatic, dark-haired German Jew, Tony had moved to England from Halle in 1936 and was working as a film extra when he was arrested and placed on the ship. Tony had been raised in a happy, middle-class family. His father managed an oil refinery. His mother, Maria, had been raised Jewish but had converted to Catholicism to be able to attend university. Tony did not know he was Jewish until the Nazis came to power and his mother explained his true origins. After his father died of leukemia, Maria arranged for Tony to go to England to attend a school to learn how to be an auto mechanic. Maria would later be arrested by the Gestapo and murdered in an extermination camp.

After nearly two months of this hellish ordeal, the *Dunera* refugees arrived in Sydney on September 6. Told that more than a hundred passengers were severely ill, an Australian medical officer came aboard. He could not believe what he saw. He wrote a report detailing the horrors the refugees had experienced. The report was leaked to the press, and eventually Major Scott was investigated, resulting in his court-martial.

Once in Australia the Italians and Germans disembarked, while the emaciated and sick Jewish refugees were packed onto trains. As Tony later

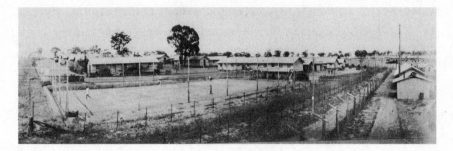

*Hay Internment Camp, c. 1940, Australia*

ironically wrote, "Since all our luggage had been stolen and/or thrown overboard by the British soldiers, loading it was not a problem." The train went 725 kilometers west into the flat, hot, kangaroo-infested bush, a trip lasting about thirty hours. They arrived at what Ron Gilbert dryly described as the "terrible camp in Hay."

Hay was a small town in the middle of New South Wales — dry, barren, and furnace hot. Some fifty years earlier, the great Bush poet Banjo Paterson had written about the special hell that was Hay in his famous poem "Hay and Hell and Booligal" (Booligal is the next town over):

> *No doubt it suits 'em very well*
> *To say it's worse than Hay or Hell,*
> *But don't you heed their talk at all;*
> *Of course, there's heat—no one denies—*
> *And sand and dust and stacks of flies,*
> *And rabbits, too, at Booligal . . .*

Among the Hay internees were prominent German Jewish scientists, artists, lawyers, and intellectuals. Sigmund Freud's grandson Walter Freud later wrote a private account of his internment at Hay. He said that the worst aspect was "the fact that nobody in the whole world seemed to like or want me or mine. We were thrown out of Germany under threat of death, and when we thought we had found a new home [in England] we were again thrown out unceremoniously. The earth did not seem to have a single spot where we could live undisturbed." From the moment they boarded the ship, the Jewish refugees received no information on what was occurring in the war, and while they were interned in Australia, they were not allowed to read newspapers. This news void was terrifying.

The internees lived in huts and were left to their own devices. They were still behind barbed wire, but there was nowhere to run to if they did escape. As at other internment camps, the men quickly organized themselves and started lecture series, cabarets, dance troupes, and art shows. They even created their own camp currency. The actors, including Tony Firth, put on productions of *Journey's End* and *The Importance of Being Earnest*. A number of the internees had been chefs back home, and they used the wealth of produce provided to them by local farmers to cook surprisingly sophisticated fare.

The internees quickly organized a letter-writing campaign to inundate the British and Australian Parliaments with accounts of their appalling conditions and to explain that they had been treated worse than German POWS. The British House of Commons debated their treatment as early as September 30, 1941, but the men remained imprisoned until Japan attacked Pearl Harbor in December of that year, whereupon they were told that they would soon be released. That was more than a year after their arrival.

Major Julian Layton arrived in Australia in early 1942 to determine which internees would be returned to the UK and to organize their transport. A mustached British Jew with a sympathetic demeanor, he was disgusted by what the refugees had been put through. As Tony Firth later recalled, Layton told the men that if they volunteered for the Pioneer Corps, they would get immediate transport back to England.

The Auxiliary Military Pioneer Corps had been created on October 17, 1939, as a labor force of sorts for the British Army. Based on the Labour Corps, which had been created in World War One to build bridges, dig ditches, clear roads, and perform other basic tasks to prepare for war, the Pioneer Corps was charged with noncombat work. That included all the manual labor that was necessary for the war effort: clearing roads, building bridges, packing trucks, cleaning up bomb damage. While most of the troops were based in Britain, occasionally units were sent into more active areas, such as Dunkirk and Normandy, to assist with the work there.

In part because it was mostly composed of recruits deemed unfit for active duty due to previous criminal behavior, poor fitness, or low intelligence, as well as many men (and later women) who had medical discharges from more active duty, the Pioneer Corps had a less-than-stellar reputation. Indeed, the Auxiliary Military Pioneer Corps was viewed so negatively by the public that in an inspired moment of rebranding in 1940, the name was officially changed to the Royal Pioneer Corps. Suddenly this group was "Royal" and no longer the "dumping ground of the British army." Most consequentially, at least for the refugees interned in Hay, the Pioneer Corps was the *sole* place in which the British Army would allow enemy aliens to serve.

Most of the internees chose to return to England and serve in the Pioneer Corps, but those who opted to stay — hundreds of cultured and educated Austrian and German Jews — would forever change the landscape of Australia. They would be known as the Dunera Boys and would become leaders in the arts, sciences, culinary arts, and industry during the twentieth century.

For the internees who opted to labor in Britain rather than remain in Australia, the trip back to the UK was just as dangerous as their initial voyage, albeit in new ways. On the return journey forty-seven of the refugees were killed when their ship was torpedoed.

It would have been understandable if the already brutalized refugees had their nerves shattered by their long ordeal. Yet when the survivors arrived back in Liverpool, they instead disembarked with a new sense of purpose.

Ron Gilbert, for one, had been a naïve, frightened young man before the *Dunera* voyage and Australian internment hardened him, as it did his fellow prisoners. But their letters and journals make it clear that they held surprisingly little animosity toward the British. The source of all the evil in the world was obvious to them, and many of them were now more determined than ever to find a way to fight the real enemy: Adolf Hitler and the Third Reich. If the best opportunity they could get for now was the Pioneer Corps, then so be it.

# THE PIONEER CORPS

THE MOURNFUL WAIL of the air raid siren meant that the bombs would soon be falling again. It was September 26, 1940, day nineteen of the Blitz, and the Luftwaffe had been pummeling London in the hope of crushing British morale. As Peter Masters turned out the lights and got ready for the blackout, there was a knock at the door. It was a detective from Scotland Yard. Peter and his mother invited him in.

The detective wanted to know why Peter had not returned to his internment camp on the Isle of Man when it was clear that his mother had recovered from her operation. As they drank tea and the police officer questioned them, suddenly there was a tremendous explosion. The whole house shook to its foundations. The three of them dived under the dining room table.

"By the way, I joined the Army last week," Peter told the detective, who was trying to regain his composure. Technically this was the truth; Peter *had* been accepted into the British Army. However, he did not think it worth mentioning that he was in the non-fighting, manual labor unit, the Royal Pioneer Corps.

"Oh really? Well, we can't intern one of His Majesty's soldiers, can we?" the detective replied, much to Peter's relief.

• • •

In the Pioneer Corps, German and Austrian Jewish recruits were segregated into "A for Alien" troops. Though they were generally highly educated, fit, and ready to fight, in stark contrast to many of the British corpsmen, they were not trusted to be armed. Instead, the "training" consisted of polishing uniforms, doing daily parades, and putting on gas masks.

Hugh Lewis, a Welshman who served in the Royal Engineers, felt that the alien troops "were given the thick end of the stick. All the worst jobs." He added, "In talking to them they weren't satisfied, they wanted something more active. They wanted to go at Hitler, they couldn't see that digging trenches would be any help at all. They were intelligent, educated men, dying to have a go at Hitler and his crowd."

Peter Masters was assigned to 246 Company Royal Pioneer Corps (RPC). Like him, most of the men were German and Austrian Jewish refugees, all victims of Nazi oppression. Some, like Peter, had volunteered for the Pioneer Corps in the hope that this could eventually lead them to an active service unit. Others, like Tony Firth and Ron Gilbert, had signed up to end their internments in Australia, while still others were sent to the Pioneer Corps from active fighting units after it was discovered that they were enemy aliens.

Masters's 246 Company RPC was assigned to a dreary existence that consisted of dull and unchallenging work. In his diary of January 1941 Peter described his daily life: doing morning parades, testing bridges, digging ditches, peeling potatoes. In his free time he smoked cigarettes (a new habit), had an occasional whiskey, sketched and painted, played tennis or soccer. Peter had grown into a handsome young man with jet-black hair and sparkling dark brown eyes. He had recently learned that his grandfather Arnold Metzger had been arrested by the Nazis in Belgium and his fate was unknown.

As Peter later recalled, "The war was going on before our very eyes. How were we supposed to satisfy our intense motivation to fight the Nazis by unloading freight cars?" He and those serving with him started writing letters to anyone they could think of to get the policy changed so that they could join combat units. The response was negative: the War Office was not budging.

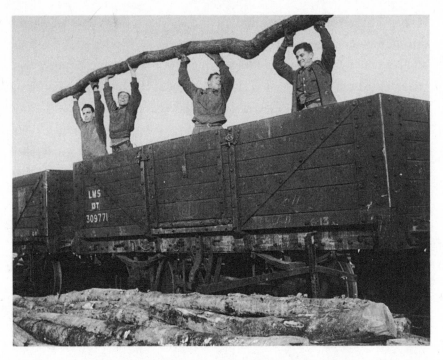

*Peter Masters, on the far right, in the Pioneer Corps*

Peter also continually applied directly to active units in the hopes that he could somehow slip through unnoticed. On July 22, 1941, however, Lord Croft, the joint parliamentary undersecretary of state for war, stated in a parliamentary debate that all applications from enemy aliens to transfer to combat units had been and would be refused.

A month after Peter began in the Pioneer Corps, Manfred Gans enlisted from his Isle of Man detention camp. By this point the British were finally having some military successes in the Battle of Britain, and by October Hitler's planned invasion of Britain, known as Operation Sea Lion, was postponed indefinitely. While the Führer's ambitions now focused on the east and North Africa, the Germans continued to bomb British cities nightly in an attempt to bring a weakened Churchill to the negotiating table.

Manfred began his training on December 5, 1940, and remained in the Pioneer Corps for nearly two years. Though grateful to no longer be behind barbed wire, he later recalled that he found his time in the Pioneer Corps "undoubtedly the most frustrating period of my life: I did not have the feeling that I was contributing much to the war effort."

Manfred spent his service in a range of locations: Yorkshire, Sedbergh (in the Lake District), and Scotland, where his unit first built a mess hall for American troops and then an ammunition depot. As he would later write, "Our intellectual powers, our education, the skills we had learned, our dedication to the cause of ridding Europe of the Nazi monstrosity were not being utilized."

Like Peter Masters, Manfred continually protested to his commanding officers that he was wasting his time doing this type of manual labor. He passed his pilot's examination with flying colors, but a few weeks later he received a letter stating that he could not join the Royal Air Force (RAF) because he was an enemy alien. Even so, it was a point of pride that he had been approved as a pilot, and for a long time afterward he carried around his acceptance letter.

In typical Manfred Gans fashion, he used his time in the Pioneer Corps to read and learn. He took correspondence courses and later in Glasgow studied advanced math at a local institute. He also read a "book a day" of the Penguin paperbacks that were then becoming commonplace. This introduced him to a range of subjects, and his fluency in English improved dramatically. His weekly diary transitioned from German to flawless English.

A strong, lean young man with the body of a runner and thick, dark blond hair parted on the side, Manfred attended lots of dances and had regular dates with Jewish girls who lived near where he was billeted. He also frequently attended concerts given by the Scottish National Orchestra. A few times a week he went to the movies, seeing anything that was showing: *Come on George!, Casablanca, The Great Dictator, I Stole a Million, Spare a Copper, Fantasia, Road to Zanzibar, Gone with the Wind.* Manfred had years of cinema to catch up on since the movie house in his hometown, Borken, had prohibited Jews.

Manfred continued to be a practicing Orthodox Jew, doing his best to keep kosher and pray three times a day. He won various middle-distance races and became a cross-country champion. By the summer, when live weapons training was allowed for some Pioneer Corps members, he was winning shooting competitions as well. Though he was frustrated by his inability to serve in a combat unit, his time in the corps made him stronger (due to all the manual labor), keener (due to the math courses and his voracious reading), and more focused than ever.

While other Jewish refugees were interned, Colin Anson had been put to good use training the younger orphans at the Wallingford Farm Training Colony. Although he had escaped internment, the impact of being classified as an enemy alien had a profound effect on him. It made him feel, as he later said, as if he had to "apologize for every breath of English air" he took. He now felt that he had to bend over backward to be more English than the English themselves, and for him "the primary driving force was to try and disassociate oneself from where one came from." This would be a central tenet of the way that Colin would live the rest of his life.

On October 28, 1940, eighteen-year-old Colin volunteered for the Pioneer Corps. He was accepted into 87 Company RPC, which was made up of German and Austrian refugees like himself. He was extremely pleased to pledge allegiance to the king, and by putting on the uniform he hoped to accelerate his transformation into being British.

Unlike Peter Masters and Manfred Gans, who were given boring, tedious work, Colin belonged to a unit that was assigned to London, where they cleared bomb damage. This also included fire watching and pulling people out of the ruins of buildings.

Interspersed with the hard manual labor were a lot of good times, and Colin finally loosened up a bit. With his sandy hair, cherubic features, dimples, and exotic looks, he was popular with the girls. He had his first kiss with a local girl when the unit was transferred to southern Wales during the summer of 1941. Having played the cello as a kid, he joined a dance band as a double bassist. The group even went on a small tour, which was not only great fun but also built up Colin's confidence.

• • •

While Peter, Manfred, and Colin were laboring on the home front, the German advance was continuing in the skies and across the Channel. All of western Europe had fallen to the Nazis. Britain was fighting a multifront war: still defending its homeland from Luftwaffe bombers while also using its navy to fend off U-boat attacks in the Atlantic; extending its air force to strike at targets on the continent; and mobilizing in the Middle East and North Africa to halt the expansion of the Axis powers. The British were determined to slow the growing might of the enemy and their seemingly unstoppable momentum.

On June 22, 1941, Hitler's long-planned invasion of the Soviet Union began with an attack on Soviet positions in occupied Poland. Stalin, who had somehow not foreseen (or simply ignored) the German military buildup, was caught unawares. Within weeks the Wehrmacht had pushed deep into Soviet territory.

As Hitler ran roughshod over Stalin's western domains, he also initiated a campaign of mass murder against European Jews. When Jews were rounded up, most of the local population merely stood by, while some actively assisted the Nazis, and only small numbers tried to help the Jews by hiding them and joining underground movements. The mass killings relied on an array of methods that the Germans developed over time to be more efficient. In eastern Europe, hundreds of thousands of Jews were murdered by carbon monoxide suffocation in mobile killing vans. Those who were not murdered outright were forced into ghettos in major cities and towns throughout German-occupied eastern Europe, including the largest one in Warsaw, established on November 15, 1940. Tens of thousands there died from starvation, disease, and executions. In September 1941 nearly 34,000 Jews were machine-gunned over open pits at Babi Yar in Ukraine.

There was nowhere to run and no one was helping. The United States was hamstrung by isolationism—a tendency reinforced by the pleas of prominent anti-Semites such as Father Coughlin, who urged the country not to get caught up in a war they claimed was driven by Jewish interests. America and most of the world were ignoring the cries of Jewish citizens to open their doors to more refugees. Even after the United States declared war on the Axis powers in December 1941, prodded into action by the Japanese attack on Pearl Harbor, the US government did precious little to help the Jews of Europe.

The pace of the exterminations quickened following the Wannsee Conference on January 20, 1942, to coordinate Germany's "final solution," or mass extermination of the Jews. Overseen by Reinhard Heydrich, senior members of the Nazi government planned the coordinated murder of Europe's remaining Jewish populations. Any Jews living in western European cities occupied by the Germans, including Athens, Paris, and Rome, along with those still alive in the ghettos of eastern Europe, were sent on overpacked trains to extermination camps such as Auschwitz-Birkenau and Treblinka, where they were murdered by the millions in gas chambers.

By the summer of 1942 Hitler's twin campaigns of industrialized genocide and warfare had reached their deadly apogee. German field marshal Erwin Rommel was driving the collapsing British Army back toward Alexandria in North Africa, and the Soviets were retreating east to Stalingrad. Even though America had finally entered the war on the side of the Allies, things were looking bleak.

Winston Churchill was desperate to fight back at the Germans any way he could — including guerrilla warfare. For the past two years commando units had been conducting raids in occupied Europe under the operational control of Combined Operations, which had been formed around the time of the fall of France in June 1940. Combined Operations was organized independently of the existing military structures and was a naval *and* army fighting force of men trained to undertake operations by land, sea, and air. By November 1940 the commando forces under Combined Operations became known as the Special Service Brigade, the name for commando formations at the brigade level or higher.

The British were making the best of what they had. Despite these extraordinary measures, however, Britain was losing, and losing badly.

Lord Mountbatten had commanded Combined Operations since October 27, 1941. An aristocratic eagle of a man, Mountbatten was a charmer and a scion of the British royal family, and he and Churchill chatted frequently. In one of those conversations, Mountbatten made a bold suggestion: they should create a new special unit of commandos, different from anything used before. Rather than coming from the ranks of the army or navy, No. 10 (Inter-Allied) Commando would be composed of soldiers made up of displaced nationals such as Poles, Norwegians, and Frenchmen. Each of the units would have their own distinct uniform (although they would all wear the famous green beret) and would be used for different missions depending on their native languages. They would be unified by the shared desire to drive the Nazis out of their home countries. These commandos, highly trained and highly motivated, would lead the way when the time came for the Allies' invasion of Europe.

This was exactly the kind of plan that excited Churchill. He told Mountbatten to pursue it and see if it was workable. Mountbatten got the ball rolling. The unit was formally created on July 2, 1942, under the command of Lieutenant Colonel Dudley Lister, a former amateur boxer, World War One veteran, and strict authoritarian whose imaginative swearing was legendary. No. 10 (Inter-Allied) Commando would include the following troops: French (No. 1), Dutch (No. 2), Belgian (No. 4), Norwegian (No. 5), Polish (No. 6), and Yugoslavian (No. 7). The "British troop" (No. 3), known as X Troop, would be composed of German-speaking refugees.

X Troop would be Britain's secret shock troop in the war against Germany. They would kill and capture Nazis on the battlefield. But that would not be all. They would also immediately interrogate captured Germans, be it in the heat of the battle or right afterward. The men's fluency in German would enable them to get essential intelligence that would guide the next moment's choices rather than having to wait to interview prisoners until they were back at headquarters.

Because these commandos would be used as fighters and as interrogators, they would have to be in peak form both physically and mentally. And because they were nearly all Jewish refugees from the Third Reich, they also would need to be diligently protected. The secrecy of this special unit was baked in from its very conception. As the intelligence officer of

No. 10 (Inter-Allied) Commando, Captain Johnny Coates, later described it, "It had to be [the most secret of all the troops] because if any of them were captured in battle and their true identity had been revealed, their fate would have been almost impossible to contemplate." This secrecy would endure throughout the unit's existence. Initially only six men, including Churchill and Mountbatten, knew of this top secret plan, and during the war only a few more were told that this "British troop" was really made up of German-speaking refugees from the Nazis.

The prime minister himself gave the group its distinct name. As Churchill explained, "Because they will be unknown warriors . . . they must perforce be considered an unknown quantity. Since the algebraic symbol for the unknown is X, let us call them X Troop."

An energetic, highly capable, and driven Welshman, Bryan Hilton-Jones, was chosen as the commanding officer (CO) of X Troop. Hilton-Jones was an accomplished and dedicated mountaineer with a first-class degree in modern languages from Cambridge; he was fluent in Welsh, English, French, German, Arabic, and Spanish. He had been raised in a wealthy family in Wales and had spent a lot of time in Egypt visiting his grandparents, who owned department stores in Cairo and Alexandria. He was willowy and dashing, with wavy brown hair and green eyes.

Hilton-Jones had joined the army on July 15, 1939, and had been commissioned as a second lieutenant in the Royal Artillery in June 1940. By May of 1941 he had been selected for the Intelligence Corps due to his keen mind and fluency in languages, especially German, which he had studied at the University of Bonn. In December, bored with a desk job, Hilton-Jones volunteered for the army's No. 4 Commando, where he took part in cross-Channel raids. In July of 1942 he was promoted to captain and assumed command of X Troop.

Now Hilton-Jones confronted his next big challenge: he had been given command of a unit that had no men. Somewhere, somehow, he would have to find the soldiers to fill it. As he later wrote in the X Troop war diary, he decided that he would use an unusually high standard to recruit

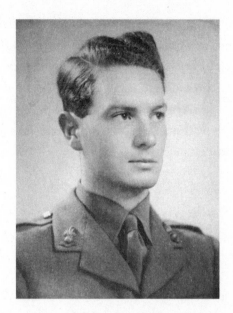

*Bryan Hilton-Jones*

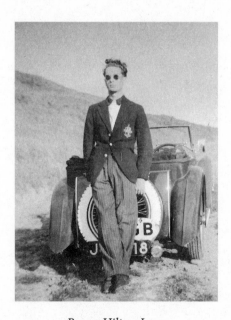

*Bryan Hilton-Jones*

only the very best and the brightest for this experimental unit. It was not hard to find volunteers for X Troop in the Pioneer Corps. Commanding officers were told to look out for German-speaking refugees who were smart, physically able, and eager to fight. Those in charge knew whom to go to first: men like Manfred Gans, Peter Masters, and Colin Anson, who were continually agitating to be transferred to fighting units and whose mailboxes were full of army rejection letters.

# JOINING THE FIGHT

COLIN ANSON HAD served with 87 Company Royal Pioneer Corps for just over a year when a mysterious new private named Hartmann showed up, seemingly out of nowhere, speaking German with a distinct Swiss intonation. Hartmann began grilling the men about their pasts and larger aims in life. Colin and the others were immediately suspicious, but, as he later recalled, "we were used to not asking too many questions. There was a war on."

One day Hartmann pulled Colin aside and asked him what motivated him, how he was with weapons, why he wanted to serve in the military. As Anson would later learn, Hartmann was not really a private in the Pioneer Corps but was in fact an officer in the Intelligence Corps, who was there to select men for Hilton-Jones's new unit.

Throughout the late fall of 1941 and on through the first half of 1942, this scene was repeated over and over in the far-flung "A for Alien" troops of the Pioneer Corps. Brian Grant, the wiry intellectual who had traded Berlin for Cambridge University before being arrested as an enemy alien in 1940, had returned from internment in Canada when he saw a notice calling for fluent German speakers who wanted to join a "Special Operations Unit." He immediately volunteered. Grant's fellow internee in Canada, Paul Streeten, the

Viennese native and aspiring lawyer, was recruited from 251 Company RPC to interview for X Troop after becoming a champion runner in his unit.

One by one, volunteers for X Troop were quietly assembled. It was a motley group of candidates for what Hilton-Jones hoped would be one of the country's most elite commando units. Before their training could begin, the pool would have to be narrowed.

In August 1942 Colin Anson and twenty-three other men from 87 Company RPC — among them Tony Firth, the *Dunera* survivor and former film extra — were given rail passes and a letter advising them to report immediately to the Hotel Great Central in Marylebone, London.

The Hotel Great Central was a massive redbrick building with a huge internal courtyard. It was one of London's many grand hotels, built during the Victorian era to coincide with the opening of the Great Central Railway's London extension. During the war a range of military offices from British intelligence agencies were housed there, including MI5, the internal security service that routed out spies, and MI9, which focused on supporting resistance cells in occupied Europe.

The potential X Troop recruits filed into the Hotel Great Central's cavernous, rather decrepit reception hall and checked in at the front desk. There they were given a shared room and were told to remain in the hotel until their names appeared on a notice board. As Colin Anson recalled, "We assembled in this great and mysterious place filled with corridors, and every time you walked along you saw someone disappearing around the corner in an exotic uniform or in tropical kit."

A number of the men at the hotel recognized each other from internment camp or the Pioneer Corps, including Colin and Tony Firth, who quickly renewed their friendship. No one had a clue what was happening, but it was all very exciting. As minutes became hours became days, some of the men would slip away to a nearby café to play cards or have a quick cup of tea. Each afternoon new men would arrive and others would disappear. First thing every morning Colin and Tony would rush to the notice board to see if their names had appeared on the list to be interviewed.

Finally, of course, their names did appear, and over the following days they went through a series of interviews and exams with medical, civilian, and intelligence officers. Colin was asked why he wished to join the unit and undertake especially dangerous operations. His answer was that his "father had been killed in a concentration camp." The interviewers saw the look in Colin's eyes and knew that he was the kind of man they wanted. Tony's charm and sense of humor also made a positive impression on the recruiters.

Both men made the cut for a final interview, which Tony would later describe in his memoir: "We were led into an office where we were met by a very young skinny officer who introduced himself as Captain Bryan Hilton-Jones and a six foot two unbelievably handsome enlisted man who was introduced as Sergeant George Lane, a Hungarian." The two men grilled Tony about his physical fitness, his languages, his education, and crucially his reason for wanting to join a special unit. As Lane himself would later say, "We were looking for people whose local knowledge and languages and hatred for Hitler was very much in evidence."

During the interview Tony was told that he would be given advanced explosives and weapons training. "I found it rather odd that one day I could not be trusted with anything more lethal than a broom stick and the next I was told that I was going to be a spy for the British," he noted in his memoir. "But who said that the English are logical?"

The Hungarian sergeant who had helped conduct the recruits' final interviews had, until recently, been in their shoes. George Lane was the first member of X Troop to be recruited (and the one who would later have the encounter with Field Marshal Rommel during the Normandy raid). Lane couldn't have been more perfect for the job. Originally from Hungary, he was raised Roman Catholic in Budapest by his Christian father, a banker, and his Jewish mother. An alternate on Hungary's 1936 Olympic water polo team, he was physically fit; fluent in Hungarian, German, and French; and very well-read. After his mother died of pneumonia in 1938, he was able to leave the country with the help of the archbishop of Budapest, who

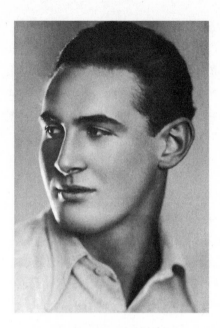

*George Lane*

was friends with his father. The archbishop arranged for him to live at the deanery of Windsor Castle with the dean of Windsor, Albert Baillie. Lane enrolled at Christ Church, Oxford, and then the University of London, where his charm and sophistication made him popular in influential circles. He also became close with Lady Baillie, who introduced him to many of the movers and shakers of Britain at the parties she held at Leeds Castle.

Lane later recalled that he had been "delighted with the declaration of war" in 1939 and decided that he would do whatever it took to join the fight. Using his contacts in high places, Lane was put in touch with Mark Maitland, a lieutenant colonel in the Grenadier Guards, an upper-crust regiment of the British Army. They met and at the end of the conversation Maitland asked him, "Do you play cricket, old boy?" Lane responded, "Yes, actually, I am the best Hungarian cricketer." Maitland then offered him a position in the Grenadiers.

Lane was one step closer to his goal of active combat, but then his commission was abruptly canceled when it was discovered that he was an enemy alien. Using his friendship with Lady Baillie and her connections with Anthony Eden (who would become prime minister in 1955) and several other influential men, he was able to get the order quickly rescinded. However, if Lane wished to serve in the military, his only option as an alien was in the dreary Pioneer Corps. He kicked his heels there for a full year until his luck turned yet again. He was selected for the Special Operations Executive (SOE), a top secret organization of the War Office formed in July 1940 to conduct espionage, sabotage, reconnaissance, and information-gathering operations in occupied Europe. Because the SOE was having difficulty recruiting Hungarian speakers, despite Lane's enemy alien status he was soon asked to volunteer for "special assignments." After some rudimentary parachute and weapons training, he was tasked with sabotage operations in Hungary. Unwilling to agree to the mission because it would mean the possible deaths of Hungarian civilians, Lane was released from the SOE and returned to the Pioneer Corps. Again he used his aristocratic connections and was soon transferred to No. 4 Commando, then under the command of the brilliant, dapper, eccentric, and phenomenally capable commando Lord Lovat.

When Bryan Hilton-Jones began to search for an enlisted man to help whip the new recruits into shape, he looked first among his previous unit, No. 4 Commando. The multilingual, highly intelligent, and very fit George Lane was an ideal choice. Lane had a deep independent streak, never shirked duty or danger, and was thrilled to be given the chance to be a commando. "I did not want to be a normal regimental soldier," he would later say. "I wanted to be an individual, standing on my own feet, making my own decisions." In this he would prove to be typical of the X Troopers whom he would help Hilton-Jones recruit and train.

During August of 1942, 22 men were interviewed at the Hotel Great Central and 10 were accepted to undergo training in advance of the final selection for X Troop. In September 120 more were interviewed; 50 were accepted. All 60 recruits were then posted to the Pioneer Corps Number

Six camp in Bradford to await the final MI5 vetting before being cleared to begin their training.

The interviews continued over a number of months, with an additional intake of 30 men in the spring of 1943 that included Peter Masters and Manfred Gans. Like the 60 recruits in the first round, all the second-round recruits were also sent to Bradford to await their MI5 clearances. There a number of the men recognized each other from the Pioneer Corps, the internment camps, or the *Dunera*. No one knew what the special duty was or what the unit was about. But they, like their predecessors, would soon find out.

Over the coming years, as some of the original men were killed, captured, or injured, there would be two additional rounds of recruiting. By the war's end a total of 350 men would be interviewed for X Troop, but only 87 would make it through selection and basic training and get to wear the distinctive green beret of a British commando. This low acceptance rate made X Troop one of the most selective units in the British Army at that time.

One afternoon soon after the first round of X Troop recruits had gathered at the Pioneer Corps Number Six base, Captain Bryan Hilton-Jones appeared and ordered all the men to line up. "You men are going to be trained as commandos," he said. "I am going to be your commanding officer."

The news could not have been better received. They were going to be part of an elite unit on the front lines taking the fight directly to the Nazis. Colin Anson later recalled, "It was such a leap from the ridiculous to the sublime, from the Pioneer Corps to commandos."

As the men tried to get their heads around this huge piece of news, Hilton-Jones singled out Tony Firth. "What is your name, soldier?" Hilton-Jones asked.

Though flustered to be addressed directly, Tony gave his original name, Hans Fürth.

"No, it's not," the captain replied. "After you leave here, Private Fürth will cease to exist. Every one of you will invent yourself a new British-sounding

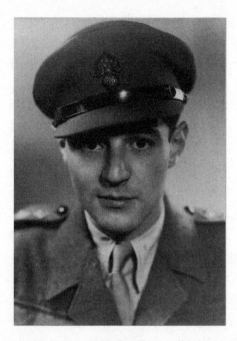

*Tony Firth*

name and a new cover story to go with it. You have fifteen minutes, and don't all call yourselves Montgomery." Along with new names, the men would have to invent backstories that would explain why, if they were British, they had German accents. Perhaps they had German-speaking nannies or fathers who were businessmen or diplomats who had worked in Germany or Austria. One way or another, they had to concoct their cover stories on the spot.

The men looked at each other in disbelief. A new name? A new identity? How could they do this in the span of a few minutes? This was a monumental decision for them, and yet Hilton-Jones was acting like it was no big deal—as if it was a choice between marmalade and jam on one's morning toast. Their names were one of the only ties they had left to their families in Germany and Austria. And now they had to shed them, possibly forever.

It might have seemed like a cruel and arbitrary command, but in fact it was essential for the task ahead. This was the first step of their transformation from stateless Jewish refugees into British commandos. And this adaptation, in particular, had been conceived with the men's best interests in mind.

Since the War Office refused to naturalize these men, Hilton-Jones knew that they would face a fourfold risk if captured: as Allied commandos, whom Hitler had ordered shot on sight; as refugees from Europe, who still had family who could be killed by the Gestapo; as Jews, who themselves were the targets of state-sanctioned murder; and as German or Austrian nationals, who would be considered traitors for taking up arms against their homeland. Assuming new names and identities would hopefully give the X Troopers a buffer of protection if they fell into enemy hands. This was not only to protect them individually, however; the British also did not want the Nazis to discover that there was an elite group of German-speaking commandos doing intelligence gathering both behind the lines and on the battlefield itself. This had to be a surprise shock troop that would hit the Germans without them even being aware of it. Hilton-Jones was so protective of the men's real identities that until the end of the war only one man, a secretary at MI5 who worked in the casualty division, a certain Mr. Dawkins, had access to the list of their real names and places of origin.

The men lined up outside the CO's office and were told to begin thinking about what names to choose. For a few of them the decision was not difficult. Tony Firth simply reverted to his stage name from when he was a film extra. However, many of the men struggled with this unexpected decision. Given so little time, they often chose names that echoed their previous ones: Gotthard Baumwollspinner became Gerald Barnes; Konstantin Goldstern became Kenneth Garvin. Many men kept their first names: Paul Streeten was originally Paul Hornig. Harry Nomburg chose to keep his first name but to adopt the last name Drew, because at his school there had been a teacher with that name he liked. He later recalled that he "found the name easy to spell and easy to sign on the paybook and it wasn't difficult to pronounce with a thick Teutonic accent."

Colin Anson, who at this time was still called Claus Ascher, found his mind completely blank as he was called into the office and saw Hilton-

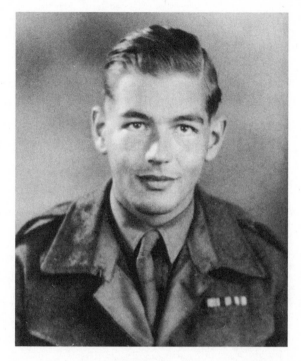

*Colin Anson*

Jones sitting behind a desk stacked with army paybooks. At that moment he heard an Avro Anson plane flying overhead. "Anson. I'll be Colin Anson," he announced. Hilton-Jones looked up and said, "Perfect. Right. There you go," and inscribed the name in his paybook. Along with their new names the men had army serial numbers and fake parent regiments. Claus was now officially Colin Anson, serial number 6436355, member of the Royal Sussex Regiment. Desperate to reinvent himself as British, Colin found this transition a positive first step on the road to a new identity.

For his part Peter Masters, originally named Peter Arany, at first decided that he was going to use the name Peter Arlen. He shared this surname with the man in front of him in line, Richard Abramowitz. When Abramowitz emerged from the CO's office, he declared to Peter, "I have taken the name Richard Arlen." Stunned, Peter exclaimed, "You bastard, you stole my name." Richard responded smugly that he had indeed taken

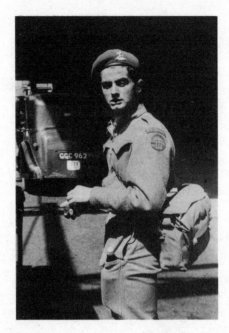

*Peter Masters in his commando uniform*

the name. Peter knew that Abramowitz had been a top-ranked boxer in his hometown of Brussels. When "he asked me if I wanted to make something of it," Peter later recalled, "I said, 'No, I'll think of another name.'"

As Peter stepped into the room, he recalled the surname of a commanding officer in the Pioneer Corps he admired: Masters. He told Hilton-Jones that Peter Masters would do. "Peter Masters it is," Hilton-Jones replied. "Army number 6837025, 'member' of the Royal West Kent Regiment."

For some recruits this identity transformation was particularly intense. Among them was the devoutly religious Manfred Gans. As a British commando he would be required to do battle during the sabbath, eat non-kosher foods, and miss the Jewish holidays. Under normal circumstances any of these requirements would have been anathema to Manfred; together, they represented a trial that might have stopped him in his tracks. As he stood in the line waiting to enter the CO's office, however, he remembered a heated dialogue he'd had with some fellow Orthodox Jews during their internment on the Isle of Man.

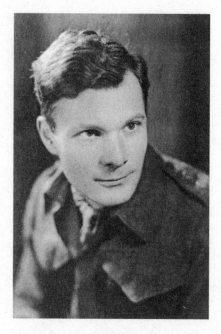

*Manfred Gans*

At the Hutchinson Camp, Manfred had shared his lodgings with the son of the prominent Hamburg rabbi Samuel Spitzer, as well as a yeshiva student named Yosele. When Manfred announced to the group one afternoon that he was intending to volunteer for the British Army when they were released, Yosele chimed in that this was the wrong choice because he would be "putting [his] secular consciousness far above [his] Jewish one." But Spitzer's son, an Orthodox Jew who was extremely well trained in Jewish law, responded that Yosele was incorrect since in fact it was a mitzvah (sanctified by Judaism) to fight Hitler.

This exchange exemplified what Manfred already believed: whatever it took would be worth it for the greater cause of fighting the Nazis. One might have thought it would have been difficult for him to assume a British identity and would have entailed some trauma, but Manfred was cut from a different cloth. When he set his mind to something, he just bloody well did it. If, to win this war, he had to pretend to be British, then by God he would, and not look back.

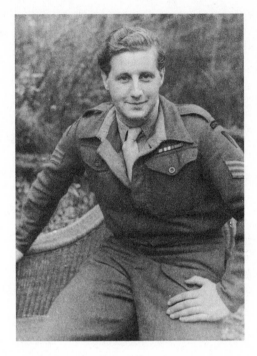

*Ron Gilbert*

When it was Manfred's turn to enter the office, he told Hilton-Jones he was going with his childhood nickname, Fred. Hilton-Jones then opened up a phone book that was in front of him and put his finger randomly down on the name Gray. Manfred agreed to the new last name, but he decided that once the war was won, he would return to being Manfred Gans.

Some of Manfred's fellow recruits found the moment destabilizing. Ron Gilbert, originally named Hans Julius Guttmann, already had lost every single remnant from home, first when the Gestapo threw his suitcase onto the train tracks in Holland, and later when the *Dunera* crew tossed his remaining belongings overboard into the Irish Sea. All he had left was his name. Now they were taking that from him as well. As he saw it, this name change represented a final stamping out of his old self. In this stale little office in a windswept Yorkshire army camp, he was officially being reduced to nothing.

He stood in the room, unable to speak or think of anything, until he finally came up with a random name: Ron Gilbert.

"Good show," Hilton-Jones said, and gave him his number and paybook. Gilbert saluted and stumbled outside. Well, he thought, this time last year I was a despised stateless Jewish refugee, and now I'm a British soldier. At least that was something.

The recruits weren't the only ones who endured this experience. Sergeant George Lane, originally named Lanyi György, had been the very first X Trooper to acquire a nom de guerre. "My dear chap," Hilton-Jones had explained, "after your commission you will be trying to impersonate a British officer, so you ought to have a very English name. What are you going to call yourself?"

"Smith," George replied, but coming out of his mouth it sounded like "Schmidt."

"Don't be a bloody fool, you don't even know how to pronounce it!" Hilton-Jones said.

George settled on something easier to pronounce: Lane.

The men were given the uniforms, caps, and badges of the different regiments they had supposedly volunteered for, and they were registered as members of the Church of England. Those killed in the war would be buried under a cross in an Allied war cemetery.

Once back in the barracks the X Troopers were told to gather up anything that connected them to their old identities: letters, photographs, mementos. All of these would be taken and stored away in a secure location.

"One other thing," Hilton-Jones said, "no diaries."

Peter Masters would later eloquently describe this metamorphosis from civilian to soldier, from Austrian to British, from refugee to elite military recruit, ready to begin his training and finally take the war back to the Führer: "First [you were] a hate object. Then if you were lucky and not killed you were a refugee. Then you were, in my case, a farmhand. These were all things I'd never dreamt about being. After that I became a soldier in the Pioneer Corps in the labor unit without weapons. And now comes the [ultimate] transformation like a butterfly out of a cocoon to the elite of the elite. Try and tell me that this isn't a thrilling thing to a young guy."

To some of the men the high level of security that accompanied this latest transition seemed ridiculous. But Sergeant Lane and Captain Hilton-Jones did not think it was absurd, for they were harboring a secret: it was not the first time they had conducted this ritual. A nascent unit had been formed a few months earlier from Sudeten German exiles — a tiny early version of X Troop.

As the men in Bradford were dismissed and began talking among themselves about how they couldn't wait to storm the beaches of France and get back at the Nazis, Hilton-Jones and Lane could only hope that when the X Troopers did attempt to liberate Europe, it would go better than it had for their predecessors.

# DISASTER AT DIEPPE

DAYBREAK, AUGUST 19, 1942. White Beach, Dieppe, was about to become the site of one of the worst Allied disasters of World War Two. The Germans were well dug in, fully supplied with ammunition, and had been waiting patiently for the last few hours. They now knew the Allies would land in daylight, which would make killing them all the easier.

White Beach, the code name of one of six designated landing zones along France's northern coast, was a stretch of waterfront near Dieppe, a small port and fishing town only seventy miles across the Channel. Although the time was not yet right for a full invasion of the continent, Winston Churchill felt a "butcher and bolt" amphibious raid could, perhaps, raise Allied morale against the seemingly unstoppable Germans. Operation Jubilee was to be the largest amphibious raid yet on mainland Europe and would include more than 300 ships, 700 aircraft, 6,000 mostly Canadian troops, 50 US Army Rangers, and 1,000 British commandos. The hope was that the operation would give Mountbatten the chance to field-test the men while sowing chaos among the enemy. If all went according to plan, Operation Jubilee would be over in a matter of hours.

When the landing craft set off from their parent ships before dawn, the Royal Navy ships bombarding the German positions ceased firing for fear of hitting their own men. This allowed the German defenders time to come out of their bunkers and assume their positions. As daylight came and the landing craft inched slowly toward the shore, the enemy opened fire with mortars, rockets, and their fearsome 88 mm guns, obliterating entire boats filled with soldiers.

The surviving landing craft pressed on, but when the bedraggled Allied invaders made it to shore, they were met with a hail of machine-gun fire from pillboxes positioned on the western headland just to the right of the beach, more mortars, howitzers, and sniper fire from the casino and town overlooking White Beach.

The brave, doomed advancing soldiers were, as one survivor later recounted, "mowed down like flies." Wounded and dying men littered the beach, screaming in English and French, begging for morphine or their mothers or death itself. One was trying to "stuff his disgorged entrails back into his sliced abdomen cavity," while others cowered on the sand in the fetal position, having lost their minds to the terror. Even those who managed to take cover behind the obstacles that had been laid out by the Germans did not find much respite. The defenders had set up machine guns in the buildings and towering cliffs that ran slightly perpendicular to the beach, and they were pouring enfilading fire on anyone courageous or foolish enough to raise his head.

Confusion reigned. As more and more landing craft clogged the water, some sergeants and junior officers ordered their men to press on toward the seawall. At the same time, other noncommissioned officers (NCOs) and junior officers began screaming at the men to get back to the ships any way they could. Small boats rammed into each other and capsized, and the vaunted Churchill tanks that were supposed to make their way easily across the steep shore stalled and were destroyed by the fixed artillery of the German 302nd Infantry Division.

Amid this shattered landing force was a small contingent of unusual soldiers, operating under the cover of the invasion to execute a special, highly secret raid of their own. This was the field test for a new, elite unit. Dieppe was the debut of X Troop — and it was not off to a good start.

· · ·

Two of these first X Troopers, Maurice Latimer (Moritz Levy) and Brian Platt (Brian Platschek), had left Newhaven, on the coast of England, the previous evening. In the anxious predawn hours, while squeezed into a landing craft with three Churchill tanks and their crews, as well as a jeep, a motorcycle, and a handful of sappers (engineers), they had been handed papers with their top secret orders. They memorized them and then destroyed the papers.

The crossing from Newhaven to Dieppe was calm, although the sky was dark with threatening clouds. While the main forces were engaging the Germans in a quick, full-frontal assault, Latimer, Platt, and the other commandos would hopefully have enough cover to advance into the town.

At 3:45 a.m. the quiet had been ominously broken by the sound of machine-gun fire. Something had gone wrong. The advancing convoys had been spotted by a German patrol boat. The Germans were now alerted to the enemy's presence, and although they did not yet realize the full scale of the raiding party headed toward them, the invaders had lost the most crucial aspect of their scheme: surprise.

The plan had been for the invasion to commence before dawn with landings at the two heavily defended beaches flanking central Dieppe, followed thirty minutes later by landings at the three other beaches, including the town's main waterfront, code named White Beach. The scale of the invasion became evident to the Germans when the Canadians landed at Blue Beach — the shorefront of Puys, less than two miles northeast along the French coast — sixteen minutes late, at 5:06. Crucially, they arrived after the sun had already started to rise, robbing them of the element of surprise.

The convoy to White Beach was supposed to be preceded by minesweepers and then at 5:15 a hammering of the seafront by four British destroyers and five Hurricane squadrons strafing the port town from the sky. But these advance attacks had been severely limited in order to protect French civilians, with the consequence that none of them would be enough to stop the Germans from returning fire.

As the soldiers on the incoming ships watched the half-hearted wave of air and sea attacks that were intended to clear their way, their alarm began to mount. A Canadian soldier later recalled, "We had been told that saturation bombing of the town front would [be so heavy that it would] perhaps obliterate landmarks. But one of the first things that had struck me was that everything was exactly as it had been described. Even the shop windows looked intact."

As light was breaking through, Latimer and Platt's flat-bottomed landing craft scraped up the single beach. The ramp was lowered and one of the Churchill tanks made it no more than a few yards before stalling. Latimer, crouched on the armored side of the landing craft, watched in horror as the pillboxes and artillery opened fire on them. An 88 mm shell hit a nearby landing craft and it exploded. Screams filled the air and the tank's ammunition began detonating. Men on fire plunged into the sea and sank.

Some landing craft did manage to disgorge their tanks, which drove slowly into the surf and stalled — more easy targets for the German 88s. In front of Latimer, sappers leaped from the landing ramp into the sea, which was already red with blood. Swimming clumsily with wire cutters in their hands, the engineers were intent on opening a path through the barbed wire for their comrades to stream through. But they didn't stand a chance. Some of the vanguard were killed immediately; others came back to the landing craft horribly wounded, still clutching their cutters. Of the 169 sappers who would try to land on White Beach, only 7 would make it back to England unscathed.

A frontal assault seemed like suicide now. Latimer had stared death in the face before, and he did not intend for it to take him here, on the shingle beach in front of Dieppe — not before he had gotten a chance to hit back at the Third Reich. A Jewish socialist from the Sudetenland, a region of predominantly German-speaking and German-identifying people along the Czech-German border, Latimer had been part of the International Brigades in the Spanish Civil War fighting the fascists around Barcelona. After the September 1938 Munich Agreement, when the Nazis had marched into the Sudetenland largely unopposed, he had sniped at an advancing Wehrmacht brigade from the forest. As a fellow commando would later note, Latimer was "the epitome of an X troop commando — intelligent, versatile, tough, stoic, burning with the cause."

"Retreat!" someone yelled back on the beach, but Latimer had been given his orders, and he was going to at least try to carry them out. Along with two Canadian sergeants, he went to the rear of the landing craft and jumped into the sea. The three men swam with weapons and full packs parallel to the beach. The raid had begun only minutes before, but the sea was already filled with corpses, upturned tanks, and wrecked landing craft. Somehow Latimer and the two Canadians made it to the shore uninjured and crawled behind a line of rocks.

The Germans were one hundred yards away, on Dieppe's seawall. With full daylight, the enemy had no problem machine-gunning the sappers who made it to the barbed wire. The screams of the wounded men could be heard by attackers and defenders alike. German officers were capitalizing on this fact by shouting to the Tommies to surrender or be slaughtered.

Soaked, pinned down, and without working weapons of any kind, Latimer realized that the game was up.

Behind him his landing craft began to pull away.

On it fellow X Trooper Brian Platt had been attempting to disembark by following a Churchill tank. Before he could get off, an officer had yelled at him to remain where he was; the attack was being aborted. The landing craft, tank, closed its metal ramp and reversed back into the waves. As he watched it go, Latimer told the Canadians that they had to somehow get back on board or they were dead.

Three other Sudeten Germans from the nascent X Troop were at White Beach that morning attempting to land: George Bate (Gustav Oppelt), Charles Rice (Karl Kutschaka), and Joseph Smith (Josef Kugler). They had all started off in the Pioneer Corps, had ended up in the SOE, and had been handpicked to undertake this raid. The group had already had SOE parachute, commando, and explosives training for sabotage missions in occupied Europe, and Latimer and Platt may have even been trained for Operation Anthropoid, the plan to assassinate SS chief Reinhard Heydrich.

Latimer had already done quite a few missions for the SOE, which viewed him as one of their finest recruits. In their assessment documents they described him as "intelligent, dedicated, popular and someone who would never let anyone down." In January 1942 he had been sent by ship to Freetown, Sierra Leone, using the fake name Max Lovrak. Once in Sierra Leone he seems to have conducted a raid (or raids) on the Vichy French port of Dakar under the command of the spymaster and well-known novelist Graham Greene. After four months in Africa, in April 1942, he returned to the UK, where he was soon transferred to X Troop for the Dieppe operation.

Latimer's fellow X Trooper Joseph Smith was originally from the German-speaking Czechoslovakian town of Nejdek, where his father was a miner. He was also a semiprofessional boxer and wrestler, and, like George Bate, knew jujitsu before being recruited from the Pioneer Corps. During the training and evaluation for the SOE, Smith received outstanding marks and was well liked. The officer evaluating him noted that he was "extremely keen on demolition work and sabotage and apparently made a study of sabotage and has studied several large works and factories and has already worked out his own plans as to how to get in and what to do." In other words, he was the perfect recruit for special operations behind enemy lines, particularly in Czechoslovakia.

Charles Rice, for his part, had come to England in 1939 as a political refugee from Brüx, in Czechoslovakia. A Roman Catholic, he had served for three months as a private in the Czech Army and then had been a member of an organization of Sudeten German Social Democrats actively opposed to the Nazi occupation.

As Latimer lay on the beach, he could not have known the fate of his fellow X Troopers — that Bate had just been killed, Rice and Smith were soon to be reported missing, and Platt would soon be injured.

The story of the Dieppe Raid is well-known and has been told in a number of history books, although the conventional account has been challenged in recent years by some scholars claiming that there was an additional reason for Operation Jubilee: to seize one of the Nazis' four-rotor Enigma encryption machines. The British were reasonably certain that there was an Enigma in the port of Dieppe, which saw heavy German naval traffic. They surmised that the machine and its codebooks were kept in the German headquarters there, assumed to be at the Hotel Moderne in the center of town. If they could get hold of a machine and its codebooks, they would take them to Bletchley Park.

Located sixty miles northwest of London, Bletchley Park was the headquarters of a top secret team of math geniuses, crossword puzzlers, and university professors who were attempting to decode the messages the Germans were sending through their supposedly unbreakable Enigmas. Mathematician Alan Turing was one of the leaders of this group of signal decoders collectively known as Ultra. The Ultra group had partially broken the three-rotor Enigma machine code in 1941, enabling the British to know where German U-boats were planning to attack British convoys. This had saved many ships and had helped prevent Britain from starving during the harsh winter of 1941–1942. But by February 1942 the Germans had switched to a four-rotor Enigma machine that created trillions of possible codes for each message. German U-boat wolf packs were again devastating British convoys. Britain needed one of the new machines, and fast. It was crucial, however, that the Germans never knew that this was one of the goals of the Dieppe Raid, because if they saw through the Allies' ruse, they would immediately change all the codebooks or create a new machine. Thus the attack on the Hotel Moderne had to look like a mere side element of a British amphibious invasion.

The mastermind of the "Enigma pinch," as it was called, was Commander Ian Fleming, personal assistant to the director of Naval Intelligence (and later author of the James Bond novels). Approximately half a mile offshore, beyond the reach of the German batteries but near enough to see what was happening on the beaches, Fleming watched in shock and horror from the Royal Navy destroyer HMS *Fernie,* one of the two headquarters ships, as reports of slaughter on the beaches came pouring in. Instead of this disaster, Fleming's commandos were supposed to have found the Enigma machine and its relevant codebooks and brought them to him, so that he could whisk the crucial goods back to England.

The evidence I've found on the X Troopers who took part in Operation Jubilee supports the theory that at the heart of the raid was the quest to get an Enigma machine, and the X Troopers appear to have been crucial to Fleming's plan. Their fluency in German meant that they could quickly evaluate the documents in the hotel and decide what they should bring to Fleming. It would also mean that they could do on-site interrogations of captured Germans.

The particular requirements of this operation explain not only how the men ended up in Operation Jubilee but perhaps also how X Troop came to be formed in the first place. Lord Mountbatten, who was overseeing the Enigma pinch as chief of Combined Operations, at that time was also administering the creation of the No. 10 (Inter-Allied) Commando. He likely suggested to Bryan Hilton-Jones that they pick a handful of fluent German speakers to join the Dieppe Raid.

The precise timing of X Troop's establishment lends further support to this theory. Hilton-Jones recorded in the X Troop war diary that on July 11, 1942, X Troop was officially formed and "the first raw material consisted of a Sergeant from the Pioneer Corps and six ex [Pioneer Corps] privates from Military Intelligence, War office." At first the handful of recruits who were chosen specifically for Dieppe were attached to No. 1 Commando, but on July 23 they were moved to Harlech, in northern Wales, where, according to Hilton-Jones, "10 Commando HQ was situated and itself was in the process of forming." It thus seems that two things happened simultaneously: German speakers were recruited for the Dieppe Raid, and when Mountbatten wanted a German-speaking unit for 10 (Inter-Allied) Commando, he used this group as his first recruits.

Segregating the men into their own unit of X Troop also would have solved a problem that the SOE was facing regarding how to use German speakers on its raids. According to a letter from an administrator of SOE files to the historian Ian Dear, "Many of the men were Sudeten Germans already in this country, and their inclusion in a raiding force presented many security difficulties; these were ultimately solved by the formation of a unit known as No. 10 Commando." The fact that X Troop came into existence at the same moment as the Dieppe Raid training period suggests that the formation of the troop was inextricably linked to the operation. (A group of men from the French troop of No. 10 [Inter-Allied] Commando would also participate in Operation Jubilee, but their goals were very different and not linked to the Enigma operation.)

At Kilwinning army base, Hilton-Jones continued training the five men as best he could in the limited time available, since he knew that Operation Jubilee was scheduled for mid-August. As he wrote in the X Troop war diary, "None of them really had the foggiest notion of where they were being sent nor why . . . Most had previous parachute jumps and special training but were woefully ignorant of elementary drill and weapons-training."

Due to a lack of equipment, the training was basic, but Hilton-Jones noted that "a start was made on field craft, map-reading, reconnaissance, swimming and above all on physical fitness." At one point he also had the recruits break into Harlech Castle, which was protected by the Home Guard, to retrieve documents (as they would need to do at the Hotel Moderne). Though Hilton-Jones only had a month to prepare this very first iteration of X Troop, no amount of training would have been enough for them to prevail in the circumstances of the botched operation at Dieppe.

Latimer and Platt, like all members of Fleming's assault unit, had been given their orders at the very last minute in order to ensure secrecy. Platt's classified after-action report notes that he and the others had "four tasks allotted to them" but does not specify what any of them were. Latimer's after-action report, also classified, says, "Our orders were to proceed immediately to German General H.Q. in Dieppe to pick up all documents, etc. of value, including, if possible, a new German respirator." The reference to "a new German respirator" is almost certainly code for the new Enigma machine, the real goal of the operation. The Ultra files on Enigma were not declassified until the 1970s, so it would not be surprising if Latimer had been told to use this term in his report.

To make the connection between X Troop and the Enigma pinch even more direct, George Lane, the Hungarian sergeant whom Hilton-Jones had selected to train the men, was married to Miriam Rothschild, a British-born member of the famous Jewish banking family (and a woman who would later become known as "the Lady of X Troop"). Rothschild at that time was working at Bletchley Park on Ultra, having been one of numerous brilliant scientists recruited to undertake code breaking. Indeed, she was working on naval codes in Hut 8, the section — initially overseen by Alan Turing — that was devoted to decrypting Enigma messages. According to the historian David O'Keefe, it was in Bletchley Park's Huts 4 and 8, which housed the naval section, where the Dieppe Raid was planned in cooperation with Fleming's men in Naval Intelligence. I believe that the fact that she was at Bletchley working in the hut where the raid was planned while her husband was selecting and training Sudeten Germans for Operation Jubilee strongly supports the thesis that the X Troopers were sent to Dieppe to help get an Enigma machine.

The planning for the raid was extensive, and the likelihood that X Troop was tapped for this purpose testifies to the operation's high stakes. But none of it went according to plan. The raid would go down in history as one of the worst disasters of the Allied war effort. As a member of the Royal Regiment of Canada later recalled, "The first three letters [of Dieppe] say Die. And when we got there that's exactly what we did."

Sheltering behind the rocks on White Beach, Latimer knew that he had to move or he would be killed. He and the terrified Canadian sergeants ran into the surf and began swimming toward the retreating landing craft, screaming at the boatswain to wait for them. Horrific stories of that morning tell of men wading through limbs and bobbing heads and more blood than sea. Latimer now was immersed in this carnage. Dumping his pack and gun, he swam on. Finally he reached the scramble netting on the landing craft's side and hauled himself aboard. He was gasping for air, pumped full of adrenaline, but miraculously unhurt. It is not known what became of the two Canadians who were with him.

The landing craft was badly damaged. It floated in the surf until it was spotted by a gunboat and towed back to Newhaven. As for Brian Platt, he had remained intent on making it ashore, but the minute the landing craft's ramp had been lowered for a second time, German mobile artillery fire had rained down upon them. Platt had crouched behind another Churchill tank as it had lumbered forward. He had barely gotten fifty feet before a mortar shell had landed behind him, sending shrapnel into his back and legs. An army medic had pulled Platt back into the landing craft and he lay there badly injured and losing blood as it floated unmoored in the surf. He would eventually be transferred to a rescue boat and brought to Newhaven for medical care. He survived, but his injuries would keep him out of combat, and he would serve out the rest of the war as the storekeeper for X Troop. The No. 10 (Inter-Allied) Commando war diary entry for August 29, 1942 (ten days after Dieppe), simply states that Bate, Rice, and Smith went "missing in action whilst taking part in ops. on enemy occupied territory." Bate, it turns out, was killed during the landing and was buried in the Dieppe Canadian War

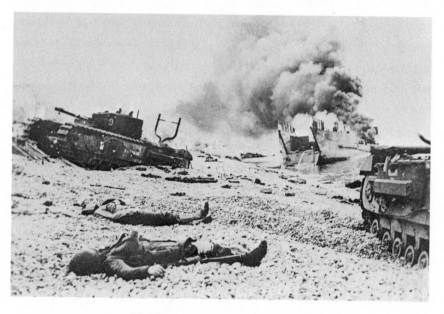

*The Dieppe Raid, August 19, 1942*

Cemetery at Hautot-sur-Mer under his original name, Gustav Oppelt. Rice and Smith were captured by the Germans and spent the war in a series of hard labor camps from which they continually attempted to escape. Maurice Latimer alone would return uninjured and would take part in many more operations for X Troop.

This first iteration of the troop is also interesting because it seems (based on the men's birth names and their brief bios from their SOE files) that only Latimer was Jewish. The other four had immigrated to the UK because of their political opposition to the Nazis. Moving forward, X Troop would be composed almost entirely of Jewish refugees except for a few notable exceptions, such as James Monahan, the troop's intelligence officer.

By eleven in the morning, just five hours after the initial assault, the withdrawal of the Allied forces began in earnest. As they pulled out, machine guns and mortars continued to mow down survivors. By two in the afternoon those men stuck onshore surrendered en masse. Lord Lovat's No. 4 Commando alone survived with the unit intact and their mission, to destroy one of the pillboxes on the flank, successful. For everyone else the day was an unmitigated disaster. Of the 6,086 men who took part in the Dieppe Raid, nearly 1,000 were killed, more than 2,400 were wounded, and nearly 2,000 were taken prisoner. The Canadians suffered the most, with an extraordinary rate of 63 percent dead, missing, or captured. The Germans reported only 591 casualties, and most of those were not deaths.

The day after Dieppe, August 20, 1942, Captain Bryan Hilton-Jones was in London at the Marylebone hotel interviewing volunteers from the Pioneer Corps to see if they had the mettle to join his unit. Having gone through the horror of losing most of his first group of men in a botched operation, Hilton-Jones vowed that this would never happen again. Not only would he select the best of the best, but he would train them harder than any other unit in the British Army. Once he was done with them, X Troop would be ready for anything.

# THE ELITE OF THE ELITE

ON OCTOBER 26, 1942, three X Troopers — Colin Anson, Paul Streeten, and Tony Firth — boarded a train at Bradford Exchange station in Yorkshire, heading southwest toward Wales. With them were fifty-three other recruits who had been selected for special training. Over the coming months other trainees would follow, including Manfred Gans and Peter Masters, who would arrive in mid-April 1943 with twelve other new recruits.

On the train that ran along the coast of Wales, Anson removed the peaked cap that had been set on the left side of his head, Pioneer Corps fashion, and took off the badge that was affixed to it: two crossed pickaxes below a crown. In its place he put the badge of the Royal Sussex Regiment, which featured the star of the chivalric Order of the Garter over the Roussillon Plume and was emblazoned with the motto "Honi soit qui mal y pense" (Shamed be the person who thinks evil of it).

Each of the men went through a similar ritual, changing their cap badges to correspond to their new identities. The X Troopers had just gotten to know each other and were still having trouble remembering their comrades' real names. Now they had to forget those names and memorize their aliases instead. Colin kept forgetting his own nom de guerre, and he had to be reminded by his fellow passengers that he was now Colin Anson, not Claus Ascher.

Such a metamorphosis did not come naturally, but by that evening, as the train puffed slowly along the Dyfi Valley, the men were mostly remembering who they were supposed to be. Ahead lay Aberdovey and with it the next stage of their transformation.

Aberdovey is a picturesque village of just under one thousand residents on the western coast of Wales, overlooking the Irish Sea. Perched on the northern shore of the estuary of the River Dyfi, the town sprawls up a steep hill from a small harbor and a long sandy beach. Aberdovey was made famous in the nineteenth century — when the town had a thriving shipbuilding industry—by a popular music hall song called "The Bells of Aberdovey." In 1936, six years before X Troop arrived, the tower of St. Peter's Church had been given a new set of bells that played this tune from a mechanical carillon, and many X Troopers would later remember with fondness how this lilting melody carried over the small town. But the song's lyrics are more ominous than its cheery notes suggest. They tell of a sunken Welsh kingdom destroyed in war, whose bells can still be heard peeling from beneath the waves of the Irish Sea:

> *Oft I listened to the chime, To the dulcet, ringing rhyme,*
> *Of the bells of Aberdovey. I first heard them years ago*
> *When, careless and light-hearted, I thought not of coming woe,*
> *Nor of bright days departed; Now those hours are past and gone,*
> *And when the strife of life is done, Peace is found in heaven alone,*
> *say the bells of Aberdovey.*

If the X troopers could have heard this message from the bells upon their arrival, it would have resonated with them that October evening. Already scarred by what lay behind them, they were full of nervous anticipation about what lay ahead.

In Aberdovey the men assembled at the station and then were marched up the hill. The townsfolk were used to commandos coming and going — members of the Norwegian troop of No. 10 (Inter-Allied) Commando had previously billeted there briefly — and this new batch likely looked little different from the others. But for the men of X Troop, their arrival in Aberdovey was exhilarating. Manfred Gans, now known by his cover identity of Fred Gray, looked around at the quaint Welsh village with mounting excitement: "I had dreamt that this would happen and now I was here in Aberdovey, the place where I would learn to become a commando. I finally would get an opportunity to fight back and bring an end to the Hitler regime in Germany."

A little over a month before the first set of recruits arrived, on September 21, 1942, Captain Bryan Hilton-Jones had officially established his billet and the headquarters of X Troop in an elegant house in the middle of the town. The place was inconspicuous, but that was the point: the very existence of X Troop was such a closely guarded secret that only an out-of-the-way proving ground such as this one would do. Conveniently, Aberdovey also was less than an hour's drive north from the headquarters of No. 10 (Inter-Allied) Commando in Harlech. Hilton-Jones had been raised in Wales and was pleased to be back in an area he knew intimately.

At X Troop headquarters each wave of the new trainees were ordered to fall in. Hilton-Jones briefly addressed the assembled men, after which they were told to remove their old peaked caps with their newly affixed but utterly spurious regimental badges. The men marched in turn forward, shook hands with the captain, and with much solemnity accepted their green berets. They also received the shoulder flashes of No. 10 (Inter-Allied) Commando and the Combined Operations insignia: an RAF eagle perched on an anchor with a tommy gun across its shank, set on a deep blue background. This, they must have thought, could not have been more different from the dreary pickaxe emblems of the Pioneer Corps.

Also that day the men were given rubber-soled boots to replace their army hobnail standards; they could be operating behind enemy lines and needed to be able to move extremely quietly. Not everyone wore them, however. Manfred Gans, for one, would insist on wearing blackened tennis shoes in combat because he found them to be even more stealthy.

With their new boots and headgear, the men were dispersed for the night. There was no central camp in Aberdovey. Unlike regular army soldiers, commandos were encouraged to be independent and self-reliant, and it had been decided that the men could be trusted to have their own billets. They were each given some cash (they earned 6 shillings and 8 pence per day, or roughly £2 per week, a good amount of money for the time), as well as extra ration cards, and were told to start knocking on doors until they found a room.

While some of the men headed to modest-looking houses in hopes that the inhabitants would want to take in well-paying lodgers with new ration books, Tony Firth decided that the best bet would be to find the largest house in town. He hoped that wealthy homeowners would feel guilty about living opulently during the war and would want to assuage that guilt by spoiling their guests. He was correct in his assumptions and ended up in one of the biggest houses in the village, that of Mr. and Mrs. Edwards on Church Street, up the hill overlooking the Irish Sea. The house was a radical change from what Firth had endured over the past few years.

After losing his father to cancer, learning of his mother's Jewish ancestry, and being forced to flee his comfortable life in Germany for a peripatetic existence in England, Firth had undergone the horrors of the *Dunera* voyage, followed by internment in the Australian outback and several monotonous years in the Pioneer Corps. Now as he looked around his new billet, he could not believe his luck: after countless nights spent in overcrowded rooms with bunks or hard cots, he had his own comfortable bed with cool cotton sheets and wool blankets. In Australia he'd had to share a terrifying "dunny" (outhouse) that stank and was often inhabited by snakes and spiders; now he had his own bathroom with a toilet. Colin Anson also had a room in the Edwardses' grand house, as did his friends from the Pioneer Corps: Ken Bartlett (Karl Billman), David Stewart (David Strauss), and Robbie Villiers (Egon Vogel).

When Peter Masters arrived with the later group of recruits in April 1943, he billeted with Dr. and Mrs. Wright and their two children in a house named Cartref, abutting the hill at the north end of the village. Over dinner the first night he told the Wrights that his accent was somewhat peculiar because his father had traveled a lot on business. After the meal he burned his possessions that bore his birth name, Peter Arany. He also practiced his new signature until it felt natural. Once this was done, he happily sewed his shoulder flashes and Combined Operations insignia badge onto his uniform, then put on his green beret and looked in the mirror. He was pleased with what he saw. "Out of the cocoon," he thought, "I am a butterfly at last."

Manfred Gans arrived in Aberdovey at the same time as Masters and found housing with an aged Welsh woman who was already boarding a young mother and daughter, evacuees from Birmingham. Over dinner he played the part of Fred Gray as best he could, but when the meal was over, he was relieved to get to the privacy of his room. He proceeded to make a package to send to the Wislickis, the couple he had boarded with in Manchester. It included his old clothes (which had his birth name stitched inside) and his diaries. His tallis and tefillin, Jewish prayer objects that he had been using daily since his Bar Mitzvah in Borken, were another matter. As an Orthodox Jew, he had been ordered by Hilton-Jones to get rid of everything that might connect him to Germany or his old life. He did as the captain ordered and put the objects in the package. "We were [now] in the uniform of the elite of the elites," Manfred would later write.

On their first morning in Aberdovey the new trainees paraded at dawn outside the headquarters in their khaki uniforms, with their caps perched comfortably on their heads. Captain Bryan Hilton-Jones and Sergeant George Lane inspected them, and then Hilton-Jones got down to business.

The captain told them that before they had breakfast, they were going to do an eight-mile run up and down the hills surrounding Aberdovey. Peter Masters, the art student, ever attuned to the colors around him, found that the "cold bluish" Welsh dawn and the "pale yellow-green slopes" added a bleakness to the setting. The men had mixed feelings about the run.

Manfred Gans, a keen long-distance runner who had always won Pioneer Corps races, looked forward to it. Colin Anson wondered if he would be able to do even one mile.

Wearing their new rubber-soled boots, they took off up the hills and were soon drenched with sweat. Encountering their first fence, which was an intimidating five feet high, the new recruits were baffled at what they were supposed to do. Masters watched with admiration as one man vaulted over it without missing a beat. "How on earth," Peter thought, "am I going to do that?" He gave it a go and was shocked to find that he actually made it over the first time.

Although most of them were reasonably fit from the Pioneer Corps, several keeled over or vomited after this first experience of the Welsh hills. Later, as the men devoured their breakfast of eggs, beans, toast, a double ration of sausage (standard for British commandos), and a cup of tea, Hilton-Jones explained that most days would begin with a long run that he and Sergeant Lane would do with them. This was just a taste of what he would be putting them through, he said. As he explained in the X Troop war diary: "The object was to produce a trained soldier thoroughly conversant with his own and his enemy's weapons and organization . . . Soldiers capable of moving unseen and unheard by day or by night without map or compass. This had to be accomplished from scratch since most of them had learnt little of use in their previous units [in the Pioneer Corps]. The problem was considerably simplified by their intelligence, enthusiasm, and discipline."

Since they would need to be highly skilled at both combat and intelligence gathering, their training would focus on developing their minds as well as their bodies. But they needed to be fit first. So on their second day in Aberdovey the commandos set out in full gear weighing forty pounds for an eleven-mile run that ended with a sprint. Soon this would be extended up to forty miles.

But these runs and speed marches would pale in comparison to later training exercises that took place on Mount Snowdon, some thirty miles to the north. Rising more than 3,500 feet above sea level, it was a perfect place to test the mettle of the recruits and hone their strength and endurance. Hilton-Jones had spent his childhood climbing Snowdon, and the X Troopers would also come to know the highest mountain in Wales like an old friend. They would spend a week there doing speed marches and runs in full kit. On the group's first fifty-three-mile run up and down the mountain, two of the X Troopers, George Lane and Maurice Latimer, raced each other to finish the course first. Sergeant Lane won despite carrying a fallen man's equipment for the final part of the route. Lane, with his dry wit and friendly manner, was well liked by the recruits, even when he pushed them to train harder and quicker. His movie star looks soon earned him the moniker "the Hungarian Hunk" from the other X Troopers. Lane would be the first member of X Troop to receive a commission when he was promoted to second lieutenant in August 1943.

Like his second-in-command, Hilton-Jones was phenomenally fit and expected everyone to be able to keep up with him. Unlike many British officers of the time, "the Skipper"—as the X Troopers now affectionately called him — always trained with the men and did everything he asked of them first. Manfred Gans, a superb runner, would sometimes outrun him during the final sprint, but most of the trainees, like Colin Anson, were simply grateful not to fall too far behind. To survive the relentless and intense physical regime, most of them gave up drinking and smoking within days of their arrival.

To a man, the X Troopers looked up to Hilton-Jones, admired him, and wanted to emulate him. Laconic and reserved, he seldom overpraised anyone, and his men lived for a curt "well done" or "good job." As Peter Terry (Peter Tischler) would recall, "He was a somewhat remote person but also a kind of superman." Fellow X Trooper Brian Grant later remembered that "the Skipper's leadership was by example. Whatever we were asked to do, he did as well, and better than any of us." Even in winter the exercises would often end with the men swimming across the harbor, sometimes in full kit. It was a miracle that none of them drowned.

Because the X Troopers admired the Skipper, they were desperate not to disappoint him. Peter Masters remembered one balmy day after a route march when several commandos sprinted home, leaving the rest of their fellow trainees collapsed by the road. The "usually unemotional Skipper was livid . . . 'Would you leave others if they couldn't carry on? From now on when I say there is no falling out, there is no falling out. If someone faints, you simply bring him along.'"

The men felt deeply such admonishments from the Skipper, but they were rare; most of the time Hilton-Jones's quiet, calm influence was enough to spur them on. Victor Davies described one time when the men were doing mountain training in the nearby town of Bethesda at the famous Idwal Slabs. He remembered "leading a team, my fingers grasping an overhang, my knees shaking like a drum and Hilton-Jones calmly talking me upward over the edge." Once the men mastered this, they moved on to one-hundred-foot crevice climbs. For Manfred Gans and the others, rock and mountain climbing were the toughest training they endured, and the extreme danger they faced came home to them one day when Ernest Lawrence (Ernst Richard) fell while climbing up one of the tallest slabs. Luckily, his partner, George Saunders (George Salochin), dug in his feet and pulled against the shared rope with all his strength so that once it was fully extended, Lawrence would not plummet to the ground. The rope jerked and Lawrence crashed against the cliff face, but Saunders kept his footing. Saunders and another commando together pulled their injured colleague back up the rock and saw to his injuries the best they could. Eventually Saunders, Gans, and the others carried Lawrence down the mountain to safety.

During their time in Bethesda, Manfred Gans was billeted in the same house as Colin Anson. One day their landlady quietly pulled Manfred aside and confessed that she had become aware that the men were not who they were pretending to be. She said to him, "I am not really British; my father is Jewish." For Manfred it was a nice reminder of who he really was.

The effect of the Skipper's leadership by example was profound. A Welsh local who had known some of the X Troopers in the Pioneer Corps could not believe the transformation: "I saw this group of men coming down the

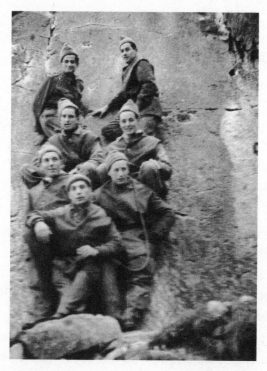

*X Troop training on Idwal Slabs, 1943. Clockwise from top left: Peter Masters, Gary Mason, Tony Firth, Ron Gilbert, Robbie Villiers, Leslie Wallen, Andrew Carson.*

trails jump into the river and swim across it without hesitation." As their strength and confidence grew, the men of X Troop began cohering into a tightly bound unit that would follow Hilton-Jones anywhere.

When the men had been in the "A for Alien" troops of the Pioneer Corps, they had not been trusted with weapons. But now, to their profound pleasure, they were given the newest and best firepower available. This included the commando weapon of choice, the Thompson submachine gun. The "tommy gun" was the ideal weapon for the commandos because it was shorter, lighter, and smaller than the Bren light machine gun or .303 rifle, and most important, the men could carry it while parachuting. Most of the X Troopers ended up bringing one into battle, but they were also taught how to use Lee-Enfield rifles, Sten and Bren guns, and the superior German MP40s and MG34s. Hilton-Jones also made them proficient in the use of pistols, Bangalore torpedoes, and a range of hand grenades, including ones containing liquid phosphorus.

The local sand dunes became the place where they would shoot and learn how to use explosives. They would also make their own handmade bombs and would practice using them in a house set up for just this purpose. As they moved stealthily and quickly through the building, they would practice blowing open the doors and windows and machine-gunning imaginary Germans.

The trainees found these sessions tremendous fun, although others living in the area felt the opposite. One afternoon an elderly lady who lived nearby had finally had enough and stuck her head out her window as they passed her house after one particularly loud session. She yelled down to the men, "This noise will simply have to stop!"

"There's a war on, madam," one of the commandos replied.

"I shall call Mr. Churchill and we'll see about that," she retorted, slamming the window closed with a loud bang.

Once the X Troopers had mastered the basics of these weapons, they had to use them while rock climbing, running, even parachuting. They also learned unarmed combat and silent assassination techniques; how to use a bayonet and knife; and lock-picking and burglary skills, in case the opportunity arose to sneak into German headquarters to steal documents. One of their comrades, Robbie Villiers, who, it turned out, was a master lock picker, taught them this skill. Some of the X Troopers even used what they learned from Villiers to break into their billets after a night out at the pubs whenever they forgot their keys.

The trainees also learned how to take apart and disarm a vast range of potential booby traps. For fun, some of them would fill a practice room with an array of traps — under tables, in bicycle wheels, below the floorboards — and the others would have to disarm them without triggering the mini explosives hidden inside.

These exercises did not always go smoothly. On one occasion, Colin Anson was undergoing training on the No. 69 grenade, a percussion explosive that had a small impact radius and could be thrown farther than the standard No. 36 grenade because it was made of Bakelite. The mild-mannered former cello player unscrewed the plastic cover, but instead of throwing the grenade, he watched in horror as the tape that triggered the device unwound before his eyes. Suddenly an arm reached over his shoulder and put a finger on the unwinding tape.

"You *are* a bloody fool, aren't you?" said the Skipper.

"Yes, sir," replied the terrified Anson.

This was not to be poor Colin's only near-fatal mishap. Another time he was taking over sentry duty from his good friend and fellow lodger Ken Bartlett when he accidentally pulled the trigger of his tommy gun. A bullet ricocheted off the ground and creased Bartlett's face, sending him to the hospital and leaving him with a permanent scar. (Bartlett, a musician from Munich, had made his way to England in 1937 to attend the London College of Music, after having been refused the chance to study at the University of Munich because he was half Jewish. His father, a judge, was later murdered in Sachsenhausen concentration camp.)

The men were also trained in map reading, code breaking, and interrogation techniques. They learned every detail of the Wehrmacht and its organization: all aspects of the Germans' weaponry, badges and insignia, military hierarchy, and colloquial military expressions. The goal, according to Peter Masters, was for the X Troopers to know "more about the German army than the Germans."

When not undergoing this arduous training, Masters, whose dream of attending art school had been interrupted by the war, pursued his passion for drawing and sketching. He kept detailed diaries on everything he was learning. There were annotated pages on every German unit, all the German weapons, and the hierarchy of the German high command, with Hitler sitting at the top. For the section of one diary that described how the X Troopers were to interrogate captured POWs in the field, he wrote down the strategies

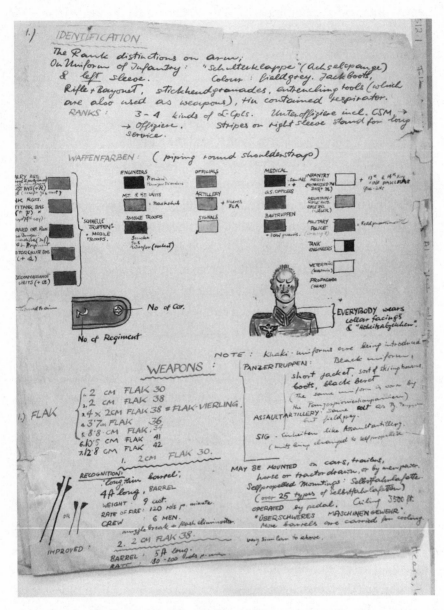

*Peter Masters's notebook page from training*

to gain information, such as setting the POW up by asking questions the interrogator already knew the answers to and using long, awkward pauses to encourage the prisoner to talk.

The first round of recruits, including Colin Anson and Tony Firth, also underwent a week of training in Harlech, the headquarters of No. 10 (Inter-Allied) Commando. This led to some interesting points of contrast with the foreign nationals in the other commando units. Officially, X Troop was known as the "British troop," so even around the other members of No. 10 (Inter-Allied) Commando they had to keep up the ruse that they were British, born and bred. While the Dutch, French, Polish, Norwegian, and Yugoslavian commandos were able to use their countries' prewar anthems as their troop marching songs, the X Troopers, severed from their diverse homelands, couldn't do that. Instead, they started using the battle hymn "Men of Harlech" as the X Troop anthem—an homage to the Welsh town that was home to their troop headquarters, and a way to keep up the pretense that they were British.

"Men of Harlech" may not have carried much personal meaning to the X Troopers, but it was a great improvement over the German songs they knew from their childhoods. One time, a commando recalled, the men were returning to their billets in Aberdovey when "one of us started singing a popular German song and everybody else joined in. All these Welsh ladies were looking out of their windows until Sergeant Lane said, 'Quiet, lads! If the Skipper hears about this we'll all be in big trouble.'" The men promptly stopped.

Over time the X Troopers loosened up a bit and learned how to swear and curse in the British manner — for instance, raising the first two fingers of the right hand and rocking them back and forth. This was often accompanied by the phrase "Up yours, mate."

Less than a month after the first recruits arrived in Wales, they were sent to Achnacarry, Scotland, for three weeks of intensive training, along with the other soldiers of No. 10 (Inter-Allied) Commando.

Lieutenant Colonel Charles Edward Vaughan oversaw the training camp at Achnacarry, and the men of X Troop quickly realized that he did not like their unit. They seemed to get worked a lot harder than the other troops, and they felt that Vaughan knew that they were not in fact British but a bunch of "ruddy foreigners." Vaughan's repeated attempts to break the X Troopers came to nothing, and they excelled in every exercise, drill, and race.

During their time at Achnacarry the troop learned "field craft," or how to operate behind enemy lines by making themselves almost invisible to the naked eye. This training was led by the men of No. 4 Commando, whose service at Dieppe had provided the only success story of the entire raid. That considerable feat had been attributable, in large part, to their commander, Lord Lovat. Lovat had extensive experience stalking deer in the Scottish Highlands, and at Achnacarry he and his men taught the trainees camouflage techniques. They were brought to a meadow and asked if they could see anything. As Colin Anson recalled, they said, "Yes, there is a little red flag stuck in the middle," but they could not see anything else. Suddenly the instructor blew a whistle and seemingly out of nowhere "a dozen or more men stood up in the middle of the field." Once they had learned the art of hiding in plain sight, the X Troopers would practice their own field craft on the villagers. They would ask them if they saw any men in their gardens. When they replied that they did not, they would be stunned to watch as several commandos stood up mere yards away.

The next exercise in field craft was learning to land, unnoticed, on the banks of the loch. As the men paddled to shore, the instructors would shoot live ammunition all around them. As Anson recalled, the men firing at them with Bren guns were "extremely good shots." This was meant to rid them of their natural fear and to force them to focus on the mission at hand. It seemed to work, for as Colin later noted, "We quickly got used to the sound of being shot at."

There were other exercises in field craft called night actions. To prepare the men for these exercises, the Skipper had required them to spend an entire month sleeping during the day so that they were as comfortable in the dark as they were in daylight. He told them that "the dark is your friend" and taught them how to navigate at night with a compass, as well as how to strip, load, and fire weapons in the dark.

Their stay at Achnacarry culminated in a two-day exercise that ended with the men rowing across the loch and stealthily making their way cross-country without being seen. The night crossing was so cold that by the time they landed, Colin noticed that his uniform had "frozen solid." The three-week Scottish training course was relentless, and Anson and the others sometimes were so tired that they would doze off while they marched. But those who survived Achnacarry could be confident that they had proved themselves worthy of the Skipper's trust. As X Trooper Brian Grant later recalled, a story circulated that Lieutenant Colonel Vaughan had made a bet with Hilton-Jones that his training program "would break the Krauts," but after watching the men's performance "he grudgingly conceded that 'these bastard foreigners were fucking fit.'"

Back in Aberdovey the men were delighted to discover that they now had a mascot: a white bulldog, appropriately named Bully, who would appear in group photos and was thenceforth always at the Skipper's side.

Hilton-Jones now had the X Troopers put all the training they had received so far into practice. They undertook numerous reconnaissance patrols, sneaking into restricted areas under cover of night and retrieving an object without being noticed. For one such mission they were ordered to break into an RAF airfield six miles away and return with detailed reports on what they had seen. Not only would they have to slip past the guards unnoticed, but there were also high fences around the base that they had to climb over. The commandos succeeded brilliantly, no one was hurt, and one of them even snuck into a barracks and stole an RAF cap. For Captain Bryan Hilton-Jones, this was "not quite cricket," and he made the X Trooper return the cap, unnoticed, the following night.

For Peter Masters, the Vienna schoolboy and artist, all this training called forth skills he had no idea he possessed. "I had been brought up to believe that I could not operate a machine more complex than a pair of scissors," he later recalled. "Suddenly, I found myself, while blindfolded,

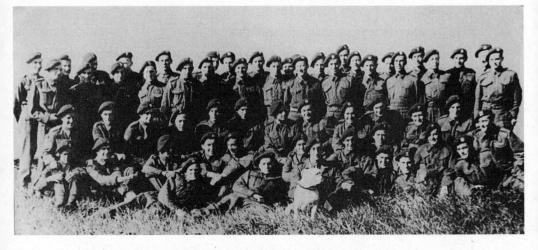

*X Troop at Aberdovey, 1943. Peter Masters is in the back row, second from the left; Colin Anson is in the second row from the back, twelfth from the left; Manfred Gans is in the third row from the back, third from the right; and Bryan Hilton-Jones is in the front row, just to the left of Bully.*

stripping and reassembling Bren guns, Tommy guns, and Colt .45 pistols." Nearly all of the X Troopers came from middle-class, cultured backgrounds and underwent a similarly momentous transformation. And although that was easier for some of them than for others, all of them persevered. Colin Anson, for instance, struggled mightily throughout training, but he did not want to fail the commando course, because he was desperate to get back at the Nazis, who had murdered his dear father.

Some of the men proved to be naturals in their new line of work. Hilton-Jones noticed Manfred Gans's keen intellect, and not long after his arrival in Aberdovey he was sent up to Cambridge University for secret intelligence training. Upon his return Manfred taught his troopmates what he had learned about interrogation techniques and new developments in field craft.

Around this time Manfred received news that his parents had been arrested by the Gestapo in Friesland, on the northern coast of the Netherlands, and transported to Bergen-Belsen concentration camp. Gans decided not only that he would help the British win the war but also that, if his parents were still alive, he personally would find them and save them.

Maurice Latimer also excelled during training. Latimer and Platt, who had been wounded during the Dieppe landing and now ran the troop's store, jokingly called each other "the Sudeten-Deutscher Volksverräter" (traitors of the Sudeten German populace). Latimer was so proficient in all the physical requirements of being a commando that Hilton-Jones promoted him to sergeant and used him to help train the others. Latimer took this role extremely seriously and worked the trainees as hard as he could. He never spoke about Dieppe, but he knew firsthand that surviving actual combat required luck, strength, determination, and a cool head. He couldn't teach his charges luck, but he could teach them the other skills.

Another X Trooper who distinguished himself was Geoff Broadman (Gottfried Conrad Sruh). While some of the other X Troopers would gripe privately about how hard the training was, Geoff loved every minute of it. He was from Vienna, where he had been obsessed with boxing, mountaineering, and skiing. After the Anschluss, the skis went into storage and Broadman, whose father was a trade unionist, also felt the call to battle and joined a nascent underground movement of revolutionary socialists fighting the Austrian fascists. They hatched their sabotage attacks and plans at the public baths. There, wearing bathing suits, the group would surreptitiously share information and plan their activities, all while swimming and doing gymnastics so no one would suspect them. When the group was betrayed, Geoff escaped and made his way to England. He picked the name "Broadman" because that had been his semiprofessional boxing moniker back in Austria. Once Hilton-Jones saw how capable he was, Broadman also received early promotion to sergeant.

Overall the men grew to love the hard work, the training, the skills they were learning, and the people they were pretending to be. Manfred Gans later described how they would even give each other tests, like sneaking onto trains without tickets and then jumping off and "rolling down the embankment before the train pulled into the station of our destination."

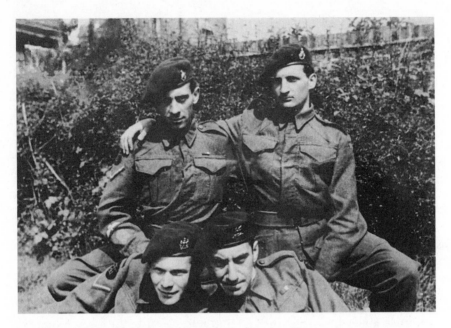

*Clockwise from top left: Maurice Latimer, Tommy Swinton,
Oscar O'Neill, and Manfred Gans, 1943*

As Gans wrote, "We were superbly fit, and consequently superbly self-confident." This self-confidence would be crucial in their new roles as commandos. Unlike enlisted men, whose job was to follow orders, commandos were expected to lead from the front, to make independent decisions, to think on their feet.

Outwardly the trainees were young British soldiers undergoing a toughening-up process and pushing themselves beyond their physical limits. But beneath the surface their experience in Wales was much more complicated. Many of them were still grappling with the trauma of being required to negate their identities at the same time the Nazis were wiping out their families. They were trying to master English and hide their German accents while also adjusting to new foods, ways of acting, and manners in the Welsh homes they suddenly found themselves inhabiting.

Despite all the precautions the X Troopers took to conceal their true identities, their cover stories were transparent to much of the community, who assumed that the men were being trained to do some type of subversive work against their own homelands. The police had been informed about what they were up to, and they and the citizens of Aberdovey were, according to Colin Anson, very "tactful" and kept quiet about it.

Hilton-Jones left it to the men to integrate into the community, and he was impressed that the residents chose to ignore their "Teutonic accents." As one Aberdovey woman recalled, it was "very funny because we knew that they were not British, and when we would ask them what nationality they were, they would say: 'Vee are English.'" Not only did their accents give them away, but some of the X Troopers also forgot or chose not to discard items such as books that still had their birth names in them. Some locals intuited that they were likely Jewish as well. As one recalled, "I think it must have meant a lot to them to be in an ordinary home with an ordinary family after what they'd been through in these camps. They'd had a rough time." While it must have been comforting to be housed with Welsh families, it also was a painful reminder of the parents, grandparents, wives, and children the X Troopers had left back home.

To hide their true identities, a complicated system was set up in which the X Troopers were told to let any surviving family members know that they could only write to them under their fake names and receive letters at fake addresses. Some of the letters got through and some did not. Manfred chose the Wislickis to receive his mail and serve as his cover. Both Leo and his wife, Luise, were doctors, who were used to being discreet, and they had no children who might accidentally spill the beans.

Manfred, now known as Fred Gray, used much of his free time to write letters, including long missives to the Wislickis. He also began to correspond with a Miss Joan Gerry in New York City, a young woman who in October 1943 sent a letter to him out of the blue at his cover address. Joan explained that she wanted to be pen pals with an Allied soldier and his name had been given to her. The two soon realized that they had a lot in common: a love of books, classical music, politics, history, and philosophy and an autodidact's desire for self-improvement. She was attending night school, while Manfred wanted to become an engineer after the war ended.

Several times he asked for more details about how she had come to find him, but she repeatedly and rather mysteriously avoided answering the question. Manfred also evaded Joan's questions about his past. He did not mention that he was Jewish, although he did discuss his mistrust of organized religion (which to him meant Christianity). Ever mindful of protecting his X Troop persona, he asked Leo Wislicki to cut out any information in his letters that might get Manfred or his correspondent in trouble with the censors.

The Aberdovey villagers found the personalities of their boarders intriguing. Not only did many of them occasionally slip into German accents, but they also did not seem to fit the stereotype of the hard-drinking, rough soldier. As Bryan Hilton-Jones commented in the X Troop war diary, "The prosperous and rather snotty seaside watering place, Aberdovey, was not at first keen to take into its bosom a crowd of rude and licentious commandos, but on the arrival of the Troop, distaste turned to justifiable curiosity, and later, largely due to the exceptional behavior of the men, to real affection." Or, as Mrs. Margaret Evans, one of the X Troopers' hosts, recalled, "I had two commandos and I had them for nine months. And they were the nicest boys. They didn't drink or smoke. They were lovely. Such good manners." One villager whose mother billeted X Troopers later wrote in a letter to the historian Ian Dear that in many cases the commandos became "a part of the family."

Relations between the X Troopers and the community were so good that the town council held weekly dances at the village hall, where the local women were only too pleased to dance with this "handsome bunch of young men." Two of the X Troopers, Max Laddy (Max Lewinsky) and Dicky Tennant (Richard Trojan), even ended up marrying Aberdovey women. When Dorothy Paine started dating Dicky, her father was deeply suspicious of his origins. "You don't know what he is," he grumbled. "He could be an Italian fishmonger." Their brief courtship was followed by a long marriage, however.

While there were numerous romances between X Troopers and Welsh women, there were also homosexual relationships among the men that elicited surprisingly little comment from their comrades. Jewish exiles from Nazi Europe knew, of course, of the brutal treatment of homosexuals under the Third Reich, and perhaps they thought it would be hypocritical to discriminate against the gay men in their midst. Such relationships were allowed to develop in peace.

As they and their fellow refugees had done in the internment camps, the highly educated X Troopers organized cultural events in Aberdovey. Discussions and debates were set up at the town hall, including a memorable one between Paul Streeten and the Welsh novelist Berta Ruck about the pros and cons of the welfare state. Ruck, the author of ninety romance novels during her lifetime (and married to the equally prolific horror writer George Oliver Onions), was likely unprepared for what hit her. Streeten was a devoted socialist, who had been raised in cultured circles in Vienna and had briefly studied at Cambridge. He argued forcefully to the audience that the welfare state was required to meet every citizen's basic survival needs.

In addition to the X Troopers, the people of Aberdovey had an unusual but thoroughly English guest in their midst, in the person of Miriam Rothschild, Sergeant George Lane's wife. The famous Rothschild family, of course, possessed one of the largest private fortunes in the world, along with a huge array of castles and estates in England and France. The fact that they were so fabulously wealthy while also being Jewish had made them the target of anti-Semitic attacks and conspiracy theories. The Austrian branch of the family was forced to surrender their estates to the Reich before they were able to flee the country.

Miriam Rothschild was born into the English branch of the family, which in addition to being a powerful banking dynasty was filled with committed philanthropists, naturalists, and conservationists. Her father, Nathaniel Charles Rothschild, was a banker who spent every free minute collecting and analyzing fleas. He amassed thirty thousand of them in his own museum and discovered more than five hundred unknown types. When Miriam was fifteen, he committed suicide after learning that he had a terminal illness. Miriam went to live with her uncle Lionel Walter Rothschild, who had built an extensive natural history museum on his estate in Tring, in the southern English county of Hertfordshire. According to Miriam, he had "two and a quarter million butterflies and moths, three hundred thousand bird skins, two hundred thousand birds' eggs and a hundred and forty-four giant tortoises." Uncle Lionel was also a world expert on zebras, had two species named after him, and used the supposedly untrainable animals to pull his carriage through the streets of London on his visits to Buckingham Palace.

Miriam never attended any formal school; instead her teachers were the outdoors and her father's and uncle's extensive libraries and natural history collections. She also collected insects, and by the time the war broke out, she was on her way to becoming a noted entomologist and botanist. In the lead-up to the war Miriam personally petitioned the British government to accept more Jewish refugees and housed forty-nine Jewish children at her own estate, Ashton Wold. This property also became a transit camp for more than six thousand American servicemen, including the film star Clark Gable — "a very pleasant companion for shooting at rooks but a rather conceited man," according to Miriam. This was far from her only contribution to the war effort. Miriam's intelligence drew the attention of the War Office, which sent her to Bletchley Park to become a code breaker in the top secret Enigma decryption program. She worked there from "four in the afternoon until eight in the morning, with two days off every fortnight." Like Miriam, her brother, Victor, did his part in the war effort. At MI5 he headed the explosives and sabotage section and also oversaw the "fifth column operation" to find Nazi sympathizers in England.

Miriam met George Lane in 1941 when he was recovering from an injury on her estate. George fell hard for this funny and intelligent woman with wavy dark hair and piercing brown eyes, and she for this suave, fit, smart gentleman. It couldn't have hurt that Miriam's mother, Rózsika Edle von Wertheimstein, like George, came from Hungary and was extremely gifted at tennis and half a dozen other sports. Miriam and George married in August 1943 in a secret registry office ceremony — secret because marrying an unnaturalized Hungarian could have immediately cost Miriam her British citizenship, as well as sparked a scandal that would have been impossible to keep out of the newspapers.

Miriam, who found being one of the Bletchley "girl code breakers" tedious and unrewarding, decided she would use her marriage to George as an excuse to quit Bletchley and billet with the rest of the X Troopers in Wales while doing her own scientific work to help the war effort. Surprisingly, Bryan Hilton-Jones had no objection to this; she even initially ended up sharing his headquarters house and moved with the men when they went to Scotland and England for additional training. The X Troopers joked among themselves that Miriam and George were a couple because with Lane's good looks and Miriam's brains, they were going to create perfect children.

Miriam's charisma was infectious, and she made a big splash in Aberdovey. Within a few weeks of her arrival with the first recruits in October 1942, the wife of "the Hungarian Hunk" had earned her own name, "the Lady of X Troop." She was always there to provide encouragement, tea, and sympathy, as well as witty, hilarious, and often deeply irreverent conversation. She later remembered the recruits as being nothing like typical soldiers: "You don't expect groups of soldiers to spend their time talking about Schopenhauer, about philosophy, but that's the sort of stuff we discussed the whole time. They were very intellectual." Miriam was fiercely loyal to the Jewish refugees turned commando trainees. She lent them books, sought to get them the best equipment and rations available, and nursed them when they got injured during climbing expeditions or strenuous route marches.

Rothschild did all of this while continuing to perform her own scientific research. She became obsessed with wood pigeons and began to wonder how they could be used to help with pest control. She kept a couple of the pigeons in a cage under her bed, along with a suitcase "full of codes" (which were really math puzzles). When her landlady discovered the pigeons and "code books," she called the police, and Miriam was immediately arrested as a spy. When the report eventually made its way to MI5, it was read by her brother, Victor. He found out where Miriam was being held, got her released, and afterward called her to ask what on earth she had been doing in Wales with a pair of pigeons in a cage under her bed. As she later recalled, "I said, 'What a lot of people are doing these days — following in the footsteps of true love.'"

During this extended period of training in Wales, the men of X Troop began renewing old friendships and making new ones. Their interactions were all now in English. They avoided talking about their previous lives because the less they knew about each other the better; if they were captured and tortured, they did not want to be able to betray their fellow commandos. Also, for many of them talking about their old lives was extremely painful. By the end of their time in Aberdovey the men had bonded with each other and deep friendships had formed. Some, like Manfred Gans and Peter Masters, remained close for the rest of their lives. But for many the friendships forged in training ended abruptly when one of them was killed in battle.

On May 23, 1943, the Skipper plucked four men out of training — Hugh Miles (Hubertus Levin), George Franklyn (Günter Max Frank), Colin Anson, and Paul Streeten—to take part in Operation Husky, the first large-scale operation on the European continent that would include British, Canadian, and American forces. The Germans had invaded the Soviet Union in the summer of 1941, and they had suffered their first major defeat, at Stalingrad, in the winter of 1942. Hitler had declared war on the United States following the Japanese attack on Pearl Harbor on December 7, 1941. The following November the Allies had attacked Axis forces in North Africa, embarking from El Alamein in the east and Algeria in the west. What should have been a straightforward pincer campaign had been complicated by the brilliant tactics of one of Germany's best generals, Field Marshal Erwin Rommel. By May 1943, however, the Allies were able to force the surrender of the Axis forces in Tunisia, and that region was now under their control. Mainland Italy and Sicily were their next targets.

The other X Troopers, desperate to see action, looked on with envy as the four commandos packed their kit for an unknown destination. To Colin

Anson it made sense that Paul Streeten had been selected: he was smart as a whip, and like Manfred Gans he had been given special intelligence training; he had also been recently promoted to corporal. But Colin was confused as to why he had been chosen over top performers like Manfred Gans and Maurice Latimer. Perhaps it was because the Skipper saw something in him that he did not yet see in himself. One way or another, he would soon find out.

# ITALY

IT WAS MIDNIGHT plus thirty, July 10, 1943, somewhere off the coast of Sicily, and Corporal Paul Streeten thought he was going to die.

There were waves. Big waves. Big, black, freezing waves, pounding the sides of the flat-bottomed landing craft and rocking it from side to side like a toy boat in a bathtub. Streeten had been a long-distance runner before joining X Troop, but he was not as capable a swimmer. Not that swimming ability was going to make any difference in his current predicament. Like the men of No. 41 (Royal Marine) Commando with whom he was now attached, he was loaded down with fifty pounds of kit: grenades, wire cutters, shovels, rations, smoke bombs, spare ammo, maps. When the inevitable happened and the landing craft capsized, Streeten and his new comrades were going to plummet to the bottom of the Mediterranean—if this really was the Mediterranean. Who could tell in the pitch-black?

Some of the men in the landing craft were praying, but Streeten was an atheistic Jewish socialist from Vienna with no god to pray to. He kept his mouth shut.

Buffeted by the waves, the landing craft flipped at a 45-degree angle to port, then to starboard, then back to port. Anyone who hadn't already thrown up their breakfast of tea and toast now did so.

Despite his best efforts to keep his weapon dry, Streeten's tommy gun was soaked, and he wondered if it would work if they ever made it to dry land.

"Let's give the bastards hell!" someone said over a loudspeaker.

They were near the shore at last.

Streeten found that he was not afraid. He was, as he later recalled, "too cold and wet and sick and cramped and sleepy and weary to feel fear."

He and the others did not know that the heavy winds and rain had wreaked havoc on the American paratroopers who had attempted to land, before the amphibious assault, in order to seize crucial bridges. They were now scattered all over southeastern Sicily, and most of the British gliders tasked with capturing inland sites beyond the beaches had ditched in the sea, with hundreds drowning in the black night. The advance support that was supposed to facilitate the full invasion was in total disarray.

When Paul Streeten, Colin Anson, and the two other X Troopers were hand-picked by the Skipper for this secret mission, none of them had any idea where they were going. The only clue was their tropical kit, which they joked was a decoy — they were really heading to Norway. After a month of amphibious assault training with Nos. 40 and 41 (RM) Cdo., the commandos boarded the HMS *Derbyshire*, a passenger ship that had been converted to a troopship, in Greenock, Scotland. On the ship the men were packed be-lowdecks, sleeping either on the iron floor or in hammocks slung side by side.

A few days out of Greenock, Major General Robert Laycock, who had succeeded Mountbatten as chief of Combined Operations, told the men that they were going to Sicily, off the toe of Italy's boot, which they were tasked with taking from the Axis.

There were many reasons for the invasion. Now that the Allies had re-taken North Africa, getting control of Sicily would secure the Suez Canal for the transport of oil and other supplies coming from the Middle East and India. It was also considered important to open up a second front against the Axis in order to relieve the pressure on the Russians on the eastern front. At the Trident Conference in May 1943 Churchill convinced the Americans to support the upcoming Allied invasion of Sicily, and it was determined that the invasion of France would be put off until May 1944 at the earliest. In the best-case scenario, taking Sicily would knock Italy out of the war. The Germans, of course, knew this too. (Miriam Rothschild's cousin Ewen Montagu had helped run Operation Mincemeat, which in April 1943 used the staged death of a British officer — complete with false identification and intelligence documents—to convince the Germans that the Allies were planning to invade Greece.)

The invasion of Sicily was to be led by Field Marshal Bernard Montgomery's Eighth Army and US General George Patton's Seventh Army. Canadian and Highland divisions and Nos. 40 and 41 (RM) Cdo. were to land first. In one of the ironies of history, Paul Streeten, an Austrian Jew, was going to be at the very front: he was on the first boat, in the first wave, as the Allies began their liberation of Europe.

The landing craft plunged through the surf and ground violently onto the beach. A sergeant began screaming for the men of No. 41 (RM) Cdo. to "move, move, bloody move!"

No one was quite sure where they were or what to do next.

The water was cold.

The sky was black.

No one was shooting at them. Yet.

Streeten and the other commandos hit the surf and came to a line of barbed wire strung out along the sand. They immediately began cutting it. They had to do this fast and then find the shore defenses and wipe them out quickly, because behind the commandos in an hour or so there was going to be a full landing of the First Canadian Division. The Marines wanted to do a good job — they owed the Canadians, who had lost so many men in the Dieppe disaster. No one could afford another fiasco. This wasn't just another raid. This was the overthrow of the Third Reich.

Streeten cut through the barbed wire and stacked it the way he had been trained to do. Holding his tommy gun in two hands, he made his way toward the dunes. To his left two commando officers were arguing with each other as they realized that in the storm they had landed on the wrong beach.

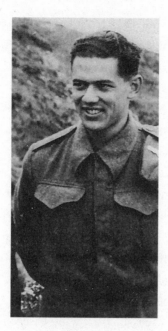

*Paul Streeten*

Chaos was beginning to assert itself.

The more senior of the two officers found a beach path and ordered a small contingent of Marines to follow him, but he was immediately cut down by machine-gun fire. Mortars and flares lit up the sky. As the Marine commandos lay in the sand and waited for the shooting to stop, Streeten became aware not of imminent danger, but of a "sharp, strange, sweet, spicy smell . . . as of vines and southern leaves and fruits."

Eventually he was ordered up, and No. 41 (RM) Cdo. launched a counter-attack on the shore batteries and trenches. Streeten managed to fire his tommy gun in the direction of the enemy, but he didn't know if he had hit anything.

It didn't much matter: after a brief gunfight the Italian defenders gave up. The prisoners were put under guard, and a party went back to clear out the rest of the barbed wire.

Streeten was exhilarated. Their very first mission had been a success. He hadn't let down No. 41 (RM) Cdo. or X Troop or the Skipper. This was the

moment of military success he'd been itching for since he had been forced
to flee Vienna with the Gestapo on his tail.

Twenty minutes after Paul Streeten's landing craft left the *Derbyshire*, Private Colin Anson with No. 40 (RM) Cdo. climbed aboard his own landing
craft. As it chugged through the nine-foot swells, Anson, sitting at the stern,
was sure—as Streeten had been—that the boat was going to flip over and
they were all going to drown. Shaking with nerves, he looked with awe at
the other Marines staring stoically ahead. He had not been able to believe
his luck when Captain Bryan Hilton-Jones had selected him to undertake
this secret mission. But now he, again like Streeten, wondered how they
could possibly make it to land. Perhaps his first instinct had been correct:
he was a lousy X Trooper and the Skipper wanted to get rid of him.

As the landing craft moved into the sheltered bay near the landing site in
the southeast corner of the island, the wind eased. The navy coxswain cut
the diesel engines and suddenly all became still. From his perch at the stern
Anson could even hear the song of the cicadas. The landing craft ground
to a stop, and the front ramp went down. Anson helped a comrade with a
bulky radio set, lifted the extra gear above his head, and rushed forward with
the rest of the men, successfully keeping the electronics from getting wet.

Years later Anson would recall the uncanny sensation of his new sur-
roundings washing over him: "I can still remember the smell of warm
tropical vegetation coming over the shore." The wind had died down, the
night was comparatively gentle, and for a moment it seemed that they were
invading paradise. In an instant the serenity was broken as the Italians,
hidden in pillboxes along the beach, started firing wildly at them with machine guns using tracer bullets.

The Sicilian beach might have turned into another Dieppe were it not
for the fast thinking of the commandos and the poor preparation of the defending troops. Noticing that the Italian pillboxes were, quite unbelievably,
covered with hay to camouflage them, Anson and the other Marines hurled
phosphorus grenades, which burn with a ferocious white heat. One by one

the pillboxes erupted into flames as their surviving occupants — some of them on fire — ran for their lives.

Anson's unit proceeded inland through the blackness, dodging random machine-gun bursts and friendly fire. Halted by a report of snipers hidden in an olive grove, they fired mortars into the trees until the snipers were killed or retreated.

Beyond the olive grove a man on point spotted a large machine-gun post. The commandos fixed bayonets and Anson reloaded his tommy gun. He found himself yelling with the others as they charged the post. The Italians seemed to be taken completely by surprise, and after a violent melee they surrendered. There were no British casualties; one Italian was killed and fifteen taken prisoner.

Anson felt strangely exhilarated after his first taste of combat, although, as he later recalled, he "would always remember the screams of the men frying inside those awful pillboxes." As an intelligence specialist, he was tasked with interrogating the prisoners. Speaking little Italian, he did his best, then passed the information back to headquarters.

After a long, nerve-racking day the sun began to set and the order was given to make camp. The men opened their sodden ration packs and settled in for the night. Anson found a spot to sleep on the rough ground below an olive tree. Mules brayed all around him. As he waited for sleep to come, Colin replayed the day's events in his head.

Ever since his father's murder at Dachau, Anson had dreamed of taking the battle to the enemy. As a refugee in Britain he had felt intense pressure to show that he fit in and that he was worthy of the country that had given him a new life. Here in Sicily he had finally had the chance to prove to everyone that he had the goods to be a real British commando. He had shot at the enemy. He didn't think he had actually hit anyone, but he hadn't hesitated and he had kept his nerve. He had charged when he had been ordered to charge. He had debriefed the prisoners. And in the process he had done his fellow X Troopers proud. Now he just had to keep it up for as long as the mission lasted.

Anson knew how important it was to make a good impression. Reports on his performance would be sent back to the Skipper. If he screwed up or showed how scared he was, it might jeopardize the entire unit. As part of the first group of X Troopers to land on the continent, they needed to show the other commando units preparing for the large invasion of France that they were trustworthy and efficient warriors.

In the next few days Colin Anson and No. 40 (RM) Cdo. received orders to move up the east coast of Sicily toward Syracuse, which they wanted to capture to prevent the Germans from landing more men and supplies.

Anson was part of a reconnaissance mission that was soon hit by mortar fire, and the officer in charge was badly wounded. Much to his amazement Colin found himself taking charge. He seized a ladder from a nearby farm and organized an ambulance party to carry the stricken officer back to the field hospital, then regrouped the men and got them out of the range of the mortars. Once the wounded lieutenant was safely at the aid station, Anson, who was determined to maintain good relations with the community, returned the ladder and thanked the farmers for its use. "I said thank you," he later recalled, "but could not remember the [Italian] word for ladder. I made a stair-climbing motion with my fingers. And the father of the family piped up, 'Ah! La scala!' he said. 'Si, la scala,' I replied and began singing a scale: 'Do-re-mi-fa-so!' and everyone laughed." The other soldiers assumed that Anson, who was known to be fluent in German, was fluent in Italian as well, so they started to use him for their interactions with the locals. He had to try to learn the language as quickly as he could.

No. 40 (RM) Cdo. continued northward along the coast highway through intense heat. At night they slept in tents along the road, and by day — parched with thirst, drenched with sweat — they went into the fields along the road and gorged on pears and ripening melons. Sometimes Anson shared his rations with the local children who tagged along with the men.

Italian resistance was crumbling and within days they had advanced to Syracuse. They pushed on toward Augusta, a little more than twenty miles farther up the coast. There the Germans were tenaciously defending the Primosole Bridge. The bridge was crucial because if it was taken, the British Eighth Army could drive the Italians and Germans into a narrow pocket on Sicily's right shoulder.

On July 16 Anson was chosen with some other men from No. 40 (RM) Cdo. to take an assault boat up the coast to outflank the bridge's defenders. His boat was being carried by the HMS *Queen Emma,* originally a Dutch passenger ship that had been converted into a troopship. (For those who believed in bad luck, it was a bad omen that the ship had been used in the ill-starred Dieppe Raid.) Anson boarded the *Queen Emma* the night before the operation. It was oppressively hot and humid, so he decided to sling his hammock on the quarter deck to get some air. He fell asleep and awoke to the *Queen Emma* being attacked by German Stuka dive-bombers, which had spotted the vessel when its smoke screen blew away. As Colin rolled off his hammock to lie flat on the deck, the force of one of the bombs knocked him unconscious.

Below on the mess deck a bomb hit a store of explosives, which ignited. Many men were killed instantly and others had limbs blown off. As Anson came to, the ship was listing badly. He went belowdecks to see what he could do to help. He spotted a fellow Marine, Nobby Wood, from No. 40 (RM) Cdo., whose abdomen had been ripped open by shrapnel. Anson pulled him into a gangway and attempted first aid. The Stukas came in for another pass, sirens screaming, their bombs exploding in the harbor. Anson gave Wood a sip from his canteen and put his helmet on his injured comrade's head. As he did so, he noticed some blood dripping down from his own skull. Anson got Wood to an aid station and spent the rest of the night seeing to the injured and helping to evacuate them. In all, fifteen commandos were killed and fifty-eight were badly wounded.

The next morning Colin finally sought out a medical officer. The X Trooper who wanted to be more British than the British said in an offhand, stiff-upper-lip way, "Look, if you have any bandages left I think I've scratched my head somewhat." When he removed his helmet, the officer gasped and told Anson to sit in the corner and not move.

Colin thought, "What is he making a fuss for? I'll bet he's seen a bit worse tonight." He did not yet realize that he had been hit by a piece of shrapnel during the first assault when he was knocked unconscious, and it had made a hole in his skull. Later, when the doctors got him into surgery, they found that his brain was visible under the operating lights.

Anson's fellow X Trooper Paul Streeten was having better luck than his comrade in No. 40 (RM) Cdo. Over the two weeks following the initial invasion of Sicily, including the fateful day when Anson was wounded, Streeten and his fellow fighters in No. 41 (RM) Cdo. marched their way up the rugged coast of Sicily toward Messina, the crucial northeast tip of the island, which was being used to evacuate retreating Axis forces. If the Allies could take Messina, they could capture prisoners and major supplies.

Tall and skinny, with jet-black hair and olive skin, Streeten looked like one of the locals, and as his Italian improved he became a kind of morale officer, organizing games and theatrical performances among the children in the area. Streeten was promoted to sergeant within days of the landings, although he never discussed what he had done to earn this promotion.

Sergeant Streeten was soon seconded to the Long Range Desert Group (LRDG), a reconnaissance and raiding unit of the British Army, newly arrived in Sicily after a successful campaign in North Africa. Paul, who had been trained in deep penetration tactics, did well with the famed LRDG, and his knowledge of German and some Italian enabled him to interrogate prisoners during their operations.

With Axis forces in full retreat to Messina, a plan was hatched for the LRDG to land behind enemy lines on the coast, in the shadow of Mount Etna. As was usual with LRDG incursions, the aim was to reconnoiter the area, capture prisoners, get intelligence, and, if possible, open a bridgehead for an Allied assault. On July 9 the group worked their way behind the lines and made their way to a small bridgehead, intending to enlarge it for the upcoming attack. Almost immediately things began to go wrong.

Mortars and 88 mm shells started landing all around them. The order was given to evacuate. Then a shell exploded close to Streeten, and the last thing he remembered was the sky filled with a brilliant white light.

Somehow the LRDG got Streeten back to Allied lines, where it was found he had devastating injuries down the left side of his body. For days he was delirious, slipping in and out of consciousness, though morphine helped keep the pain at bay. He was evacuated first to Alexandria and then to the Fifteenth Scottish General Hospital in Cairo. The doctors did the best they could to save him, but no one expected him to survive.

Streeten was not the only X Trooper fighting for his life in the Egyptian capital. After a brain operation at a Canadian field hospital in a Sicilian olive grove, during which his heart stopped, Colin Anson was transported to North Africa for multiple operations in late July 1943, first in Tripoli and then in Cairo. There he was also admitted to the Fifteenth Scottish General Hospital, considered the best military hospital in the Middle East.

Anson, who was in good shape despite the surgeries, soon discovered that Streeten was only a few wards away, and he spent days reading to Paul as he lay in a near-comatose state. Soon, however, Streeten was airlifted back to Britain to continue his recovery, leaving Anson behind in Cairo. With Streeten out of commission the honor of X Troop fell even more disproportionately on Anson. Contrary to his expectations Colin had managed to suppress his fears on the battlefield. Now, reflecting on his time in combat, he knew not only that he *could* do this but also that he *wanted* to do this. But first he had to endure months of brain operations, including a bone graft to close the hole in his skull. For Anson these "soul destroying months" in Egypt were the worst period of the war. He later recalled that there was "nothing but tents and sand, bugles and bullshit, from morning till night." Anson did everything he possibly could to get permission to go back to his unit, including writing to his comrades in X Troop imploring them to persuade Bryan Hilton-Jones to get him released. Finally, after eight months, he was deemed well enough to return to Italy, by which time the Allies had landed in several places on the mainland and were fighting their way up the peninsula.

In March 1944 Colin Anson boarded a ship in Alexandria and after a rough trip landed at Bari, a port on the eastern shore of the heel of Italy's boot. From there he took a train to Naples. While he had been recovering in North Africa, No. 40 (RM) Cdo. had become part of No. 2 Special Service Brigade, Central Mediterranean Force, which consisted of a combination of British Army and Royal Marine units. This move was in keeping with a broader reorganization of Britain's commando forces around this time. To adjust to the expanding ranks of and demands on these elite fighters, the War Office divided the Special Service Brigade — which had been operating as a single group since its inception in 1940 — into four distinct subgroups, each of which contained an amalgam of commando units from the army and navy.

As Anson's train rumbled past Mount Vesuvius, he marveled at the thick, gray billows of smoke pouring from the first active volcano he had ever seen. From Naples Anson was sent to rejoin No. 40 (RM) Cdo. on Vis, an island off Croatia that had become a vast armed camp, filled with more than ten thousand Yugoslavian partisans led by Joseph Tito. Tito was the communist leader of the Yugoslavian partisan movement, which had been responsible for numerous armed guerrilla attacks against the Nazis since their invasion of Yugoslavia in April 1941. Tito and his men had taken the island back from Italy, and it was now a perfect base from which to raid German positions on nearby islands. Because of this the Vis airfield was under continual attack from the Luftwaffe, and life on the island was precarious.

In addition to the thousands of partisans on Vis, there were seven hundred British commandos, several auxiliaries, and on one memorable occasion the novelist Evelyn Waugh, who had trained earlier in the war as a commando and was flown in to meet with Tito. Along with two other X Troopers, Hugh Miles and George Kendell, Anson was assigned to the intelligence section of No. 2 Special Service Brigade, which was commanded by Brigadier Tom Churchill (no relation to the prime minister). Anson's task was to take part in amphibious raids against nearby German positions around Vis, to assist in the capture of prisoners, and to interrogate prisoners for actionable intelligence. When not on missions he wrote articles for the Vis newspaper put out by the intelligence section of No. 2 Special Service Brigade. Around this time Anson was promoted to sergeant. This must have been both a surprise and a relief for Colin, who was perhaps suffering from impostor syndrome.

Over in Yugoslavia the Wehrmacht was slogging it out with Tito's partisans. Tito had become a thorn in the Nazis' side, and on May 25, 1944, the Germans undertook Operation Rösselsprung on Drvar, Yugoslavia, where Tito was said to be hiding in a network of caves.

In response to this German operation, the British hastily organized Operation Flounced. The aim, according to the war diary for this operation, was to use men from Nos. 40 and 43 (RM) Cdo. and the Twenty-Sixth Dalmatian Division of partisans to make it seem as if a full-scale attack on Yugoslavia was underway. The operation would begin on the German-held Dalmatian island of Brač, which had two heavily reinforced battalions of the 118th Jäger Division, totaling about two thousand men.

The hope was that the Germans would get word that the partisans, working with the British, were planning a huge invasion of the island, and they would respond by diverting their troops from Drvar to Brač. If they did this, it would give Tito and his partisans a chance to escape. Anson and the other commandos would land and noisily make their way across the island in an attempt to convince the Germans that they were a large invasion force. It was a bold, risky scheme, but if it would help throw sand in the gears of the German war machine, Colin Anson was all in.

Before midnight on June 2, 1944, Anson boarded a landing craft packed with commandos and partisans. As it came to a stop on the southwest coast of Brač at 3:45 in the morning on June 3, the partisans went ashore first. Anson and the others were shocked to see them light cigarettes as they moved up the beach. They wanted the Germans to know they were there, but not yet, not while they could be machine-gunned in the water. The commandos politely and not so politely yelled at the partisans to put out their cigarettes. The four hundred or so partisans and Nos. 40 and 43 (RM) Cdo. headed inland, up the rough, scraggly, steep hills, to await further orders.

Lieutenant Colonel "Mad Jack" Churchill, who was in charge of the operation, soon called a meeting of his officers and intelligence men, including

Sergeant Anson. Churchill was an extraordinary figure — a former competitive archer, male model, and actor (he had appeared in *The Thief of Baghdad*
and *A Yank at Oxford*) — who always went into battle carrying bagpipes, a
Scottish broadsword, and a longbow. By this stage of the war he had already
killed a German officer with the longbow and won a Distinguished Service
Order.

Anson had previously had two memorable encounters with the eccentric
colonel. He had run into him during a brief leave in Italy, where Mad Jack
had given him a lift in his open jeep. Anson later remembered "skidding
around the hairpins of the gravel road up from the coast and Churchill
scaring the daylights out of me." Another time he had spent the night drinking at a bar and singing partisan songs with Jack and his younger brother,
Brigadier Tom Churchill, in whose brigade intelligence section Anson was
serving in Brač.

Lieutenant Colonel Churchill told the British soldiers they were to attack the German command post perched atop the mountain at Nerežišća,
a tiny village in the center of the island. The command post was a concrete bunker surrounded by two rows of barbed wire and mines, and it was
heavily defended by an ad hoc band of soldiers from various Waffen-SS
units. In the proposed attack, Anson's unit was given one of the riskiest assignments: to advance straight up the hill toward the German stronghold
while other forces attacked the flanks.

On the signal from Churchill they began running up the hill in the
predawn light. The ground was rocky and the hill was steep, with shrubs,
stunted almond trees, and small, thorny bushes. The only sound was the
heavy breathing of the men and the rocks crunching under their feet, until
the silence was abruptly broken by the rumble of aircraft. Anson heard two
German Messerschmitt fighters heading toward the beach where the Allies
had come ashore, evidently intent on destroying their landing craft.

Just as suddenly, two British Hurricanes dropped out of the sky behind
the Messerschmitts. A spectacular dogfight ensued, ending with the Hurricanes chasing the Luftwaffe away.

Watching from the slope below Nerežišća, Anson and the other commandos cheered and saw this as a good omen. But then the Germans began firing at them from their heavily fortified positions at the top of the hill. Men were falling left and right, and what was left of the night was lit up on all sides by flares and tracer and mortar fire.

Any hope of surprise, Anson knew, was gone. They wouldn't be able to capture the enemy position, but it didn't really matter. Their purpose on the island was always supposed to be diversionary; taking down the garrison would be considered a positive side effect, but the main aim was to convince the Axis forces that a huge Allied force had landed. In other words, they just had to sit there and take it. They had to find cover and return fire as best they could until they got the order to withdraw. "Ours not to reason why, ours but to do and die," the poetry-loving Mad Jack Churchill may well have reminded his men as he waved his broadsword at the enemy.

Anson found cover behind a boulder wall. It was with some alarm that the lightly armed commandos discovered that the German defenders seemed to have armored cars, or possibly tanks, to defend their position. These vehicles were now heading straight for them. As Anson dryly noted, "We sat there on the mountain with SS panzers heading for us; [it was] a particularly hazardous time and rather uncomfortable to find the masked-headlights of an SS Division coming closer and closer." The Marines fired their mortars and rockets at the Germans until they retreated, possibly believing that they were in fact dealing with a much larger force. The Germans also sent probing attacks down the hill, during which the commandos sustained multiple casualties, including the death of Anson's CO, Lieutenant Ian Laidlaw of No. 40 (RM) Cdo.

As the battle wore on, Churchill attempted to rally his men by playing his bagpipes. The Scottish tradition of having pipers with their regiments during battle had been banned since World War One (German snipers had often killed the pipers to sow confusion), but Churchill had refused to relinquish his own pipes. That day on the island of Brač, German snipers tried multiple times to kill the "mad bagpiper," but no one was able to hit him.

The order was again given to attempt to take the top of the hill, and Churchill — carrying his pipes, broadsword, and longbow — led the men straight toward the German lines. Anson remembered the colonel playing "Will Ye No Come Back Again?" (an ode to Bonnie Prince Charlie, who fled Scotland after the disastrous Battle of Culloden) as they attempted to take the ridge. The fighting was bloody, visceral, and intense. At times Anson's troop found themselves in vicious hand-to-hand combat with German soldiers using bayonets, knives, and even trenching tools to attack them at close quarters.

After a day and night of sustained fighting, at 8:30 in the morning on June 5 the surviving men from Nos. 40 and 43 (RM) Cdo., along with the partisans who had undertaken the raid with them, were ordered to withdraw back to the beach. There they were picked up by landing craft and exfiltrated back to Croatia. According to the war diary for Operation Flounced, it had been a success: "The Germans were deceived into thinking that a full scale invasion of Yugoslavia was about to take place." Three thousand Axis troops were diverted from Drvar, allowing Tito and his partisans to escape and delivering a blow to the Nazis' efforts on the Adriatic front. What's more, the Allied soldiers and partisans killed 350 Germans and captured 160.

But this success had come at a cost. No. 40 (RM) Cdo. suffered six confirmed dead, forty-one wounded, and thirteen missing. No. 43 (RM) Cdo. had also taken losses — including Lieutenant Colonel Churchill, who had been captured by the Germans after being knocked unconscious by a mortar shell. An unknown number of partisans had been killed.

As Colin Anson's landing craft, infantry, slipped into the Adriatic after unimaginable carnage and horror, he could not believe that he had again survived. The Yugoslavian partisan women began singing folk songs, and some of the soldiers found themselves in tears.

# THE FIELD MARSHAL, THE WATER POLO STAR, AND THE CODE BREAKER

ON MAY 22, 1943, the night before the Skipper ordered Colin Anson and Paul Streeten to pack their kit for an unknown assignment, a dance was held at the Aberdovey Town Hall in honor of X Troop. The trainees and the villagers tried to enjoy themselves, but the mood was somber. They had recently found out that the X Troopers were being moved to Eastbourne, a seaside resort town in the south of England, to continue their training. The men were sad to leave their adopted village and its inhabitants; the locals, for their part, knew that things would not be the same in Aberdovey without this pack of intelligent, polite, interesting men in their midst.

The X Troopers, who were now very physically fit according to Bryan Hilton-Jones, were being transferred to Eastbourne to undergo extensive group training with the other units of No. 10 (Inter-Allied) Commando, under the leadership of Colonel Dudley Lister. Lister, the salty former prizefighter who the previous summer had been assigned by Mountbatten to command them, wanted to turn all the units into one cohesive force, but the reality would be very different: the eight commando troops would continue socializing and training among themselves, often in their own

languages. For X Troop this meant that Bryan Hilton-Jones continued to
oversee everything, although he would now adapt his lessons to the countryside around Eastbourne, including the Seven Sisters chalk cliffs, which
could be used for rappelling.

The X Troopers soon began attending dances at a local town hall, enjoy-
ing showing off their newly muscular bodies and flirting with the attendees.
They also took advantage of the town's relative closeness to London by train
to travel there on weekends and go to shows, concerts, and restaurants.

Peter Masters, who was billeted with two other X Troopers in the home
of married Salvation Army officers, had a memorable afternoon when a
Salvation Army general was invited to lunch with them. The three X Troopers
put on their best English accents for the meal and laughed inwardly when
afterward the officer proclaimed them "the flower of Britain's manhood." At
the conclusion of the meal, the officer asked the commandos to kneel and
pray with him to Jesus Christ for their safe return from battle. Peter and the
other Jewish commandos knelt with him in prayer (a position never taken
by Jews), as they had "no intention of blowing the cover."

Colonel Lister must have quickly realized that his plan to make a homo-
geneous unit out of these disparate troops would not work, so he switched
the focus to building cohesion within the troops themselves. As part of this
plan, a number of competitions were introduced, including an intercom-
mando cross-country race. An X Trooper, George Saunders, won; another,
Manfred Gans, came in third. In fact X Troopers took most of the top fifteen
spots. Manfred was over the moon when he received a rare compliment
from the Skipper: "I hear you lads did very well in the races."

By September 1943 X Troop was recognized as a highly trained, cohesive
unit, and they were moved again, this time to Littlehampton, a coastal town
west of Eastbourne. Bryan Hilton-Jones noted in the X Troop war diary
that the men were delighted to leave Eastbourne, and it "cheered everyone
immensely" that they were "regaining their full identity as a separate troop."
In Littlehampton Manfred Gans, Peter Masters, and Tony Firth all bunked
together while they trained for parachute raids on the French coast. D-Day

was coming up, as everyone knew, and the men were extremely happy to be at the point at last where they could prepare for real operations.

They were also sent for a few weeks to the Parachute Training School in Ringway, near Manchester. For the initial jump off a twenty-foot-high platform Hilton-Jones, as always, went first. His harness, however, malfunctioned and he plummeted to the ground. Though bruised all over and suffering a badly sprained ankle, the Skipper calmly got up and did the jump again.

Amid the intensity of their training, there were also occasional opportunities for respite and reflection. The parachute training, for instance, was conducted during the Jewish High Holidays, Rosh Hashanah and Yom Kippur, and one evening Manfred Gans caught a bus to Manchester to celebrate with the Wislickis. It must have felt good to drop his alias temporarily, but the visit may also have reminded him of his childhood sweetheart, Anita Lamm, who was now safely in New York and who had broken off her correspondence with him around the time he had been boarding with them.

Once the X Troopers had finished all their practice jumps — including one from a horrifying balloon contraption at night, an exercise they called "jumping from nothing into sweet fuck-all" — they moved on to eight airplane jumps. Now used to jumping into "sweet fuck-all," they were expected to leap from Halifax bombers with full packs, weapons, and even climbing ropes and rappelling spikes. Though none of them died, the jumps were not without severe injuries, including concussions, broken limbs, and twisted ankles. Victor Davies ended up damaging his leg so severely that he had to wear a plaster cast for months.

In March 1944—as Colin Anson was traveling from Egypt back to Italy after his recovery in Cairo, and Paul Streeten was still recovering in a hospital in the UK — Captain Hilton-Jones had his recruits undertake their last training exercise: a feat of survival mimicking that of the ancient Spartans in the *agoge*. They were dropped into a remote area in Scotland with nothing to eat, according to Bill Watson (Otto Wassermann), except "grass and snails." After a week the men had to make their way back to Littlehampton within twenty-four hours. Watson did this by stealing a motorcycle and riding it until it ran out of gas, sneaking onto a train, and then, for the final leg, stealing a jeep. Everyone made it back, except for one X Trooper who was arrested as a spy because he was wearing a British uniform but speaking with a German accent. The Skipper quickly got him released.

The men of X Troop had spent months training and preparing for operations in Europe. Everybody knew the invasion of the continent was coming — including, of course, the Germans — and it was clear that it would take place somewhere along the northern coast of France. The question was not *if* the Allies were going to invade; the question was *where*.

The answers were known only to the top Allied planners. Due in part to Hitler's lack of naval experience, he assumed the Allies would take the shortest route to France and this would mean they would land on the Pas-de-Calais. Field Marshal Rommel, however, made no such assumption, and when he was put in charge of the Atlantic Wall, the series of German defensive fortifications along the coast of continental Europe, he reinforced all the possible landing sites from Belgium to Spain. The Allies ended up choosing Normandy because of its wide, long beaches and because the German defenses were slightly weaker there; the panzer divisions, being held in reserve, were located closer to the Pas-de-Calais. The buildup to D-Day would involve preparing an invasion force of more than 150,000 men, including two US Army airborne divisions, commandos, US Army Rangers, Free French Forces, and American, British, and Canadian soldiers who would land on the five designated beaches on D-Day itself.

Apart from a handful of men, most of the X Troopers still had not seen combat. For those who had not been deployed in other units before being selected for X Troop (like George Lane, who had been in the SOE) or who had not been picked to join other commandos in the Mediterranean theater (such as Colin Anson and Paul Streeten), their best hope of seeing action during this period was being chosen for small-scale raids into France — forays that were intended to harass the enemy while also laying the intelligence groundwork for the coming invasion. With their advanced commando and intelligence training, fluency in German, and parachute instruction, the men began to be selected for a number of these missions. One of them was Operation Crossbow. X Troopers, including

Manfred Gans and Peter Masters, were to parachute near the Pas-de-Calais and make their way to German V-1 flying bomb sites to gather information about the new terror weapons. The intelligence would be sent back by radio and by carrier pigeons that they had strapped to their chests. (One wonders if Miriam Rothschild had a hand in the pigeon part of this plan.) Operation Crossbow was canceled at the last minute, however, due to bad weather, which was deeply disappointing for the men.

They did participate in a number of successful small-scale secret operations, the full details of which remain undisclosed. In his unpublished memoir Tony Firth discusses going on such raids across the Channel into France for "intelligence gathering" or "sometimes for capturing a prisoner." George Lane also mentioned in interviews that he had successfully completed parachute missions into France, and he had even been trained in the art of safecracking for one operation that never took place. (Lane received instruction from a convict who had been released from prison for two days to teach him the ropes.) He never shared any details of these operations, however, which remained tantalizingly classified throughout his life.

Operation Tarbrush, however, did take place. It was this series of raids conducted in the weeks before D-Day that brought George Lane to the shores of France and face-to-face with none other than German field marshal Erwin Rommel.

Operation Tarbrush comprised eight raids led by Captain Bryan Hilton-Jones and executed by men from a range of units in No. 10 (Inter-Allied) Commando. The plan was both extremely dangerous and extremely audacious: after landing at night on the heavily defended French coast, the commandos would attempt to snatch one of the mines that had been laid in the waters off the Normandy beaches and return it to England for analysis, all while avoiding German patrols.

This would be a highly risky operation to be sure, but a grim necessity. In April 1944, intelligence had surfaced suggesting that the Germans had a new and more deadly type of antipersonnel mine in their coastal defense network around Normandy. With the D-Day landings scheduled for early

June, the Allies had precious little time to figure out what they were up against and, if possible, how they could protect their invasion force against this new threat. If they couldn't, they might have to delay the entire D-Day attack.

In April, when RAF bombers attacked a German pillbox at Houlgate, on the Normandy coast, a camera on one of the planes recorded a massive underwater chain reaction that seemed to occur when one of the bombs landed in the sea short of its target. When the aerial film was examined, it sent panicked ripples up the command chain. Was this yet another new German terror weapon?

Hilton-Jones selected Lane, his second-in-command, for Operation Tarbrush because of his intelligence, fitness, and SOE and commando training — as well as the champion swimmer's brilliance in the water, an important quality for anyone mounting this sort of clandestine amphibious raid. Many years later Lane told an interviewer, "I knew the [D-Day soldiers'] lives would be very much in danger, and the more they knew about the beach, the safer they were. Knowing it was up to me, I had to forget all about myself, which is what I did, and just concentrate on the job in order to help the eventual people who came to land." Hilton-Jones also understood the extreme danger of the operation, writing later, "We didn't know if the mine would go off if we [simply] looked at it."

The Skipper knew that Lane would be up for the job, and he was right. Upon returning from gathering intelligence on the mines, Lane reported to command and control that it was not a new terror weapon but instead a standard anti-tank Teller mine. There was no new explosive or new device; rather, because the Germans had been putting Tellers on stakes in the sea, the impact of the RAF bomb, along with the seawater having corroded the safety pins, had made them go off in the chain reaction the aircraft had filmed. The upshot of all this was that the Nazis did not have some new advanced technology and the invasion did not need to be postponed.

If not for Lane's information, D-Day might well have been put off until July or even August of 1944, with untold consequences for those living under Nazi occupation. Still, the planners were skeptical of Lane's explanation, and he was sent back two more times to obtain further information about the beach defenses.

It was on this last mission, Tarbrush 10, on May 18, 1944, that Germans scouting the French coast in an E-boat (an inshore Kriegsmarine patrol craft) spotted Lane and his comrade, Captain Roy Wooldridge, a mine expert with the Royal Engineers, as they made their way back to the motor torpedo boat from which they had deployed. After narrowly avoiding death on the beach, Lane and Wooldridge now faced death on the water.

The two soldiers watched in horror as the German E-boat came closer and closer. At first they planned to pretend that they were French fishermen lost at sea, but under the full spotlight they knew that wouldn't work. As the Germans aimed their weapons at them, Lane and Wooldridge threw their equipment into the sea and raised their hands in surrender.

Unbeknownst to Lane and Wooldridge, as they had been paddling frantically north toward England, Captain Bryan Hilton-Jones, who had been waiting on the motor torpedo boat to pick up the dinghy and take them back to England, had gone back to the beach to try to find them. He stayed as long as he possibly could and only withdrew when, according to the report in the war diary on the operation, "a longer stay would have jeopardized the whole expedition." Alas, the men could not be found because they had already been captured by the Germans.

The two men were taken ashore and locked in separate cells in the basement of a German command post. Their initial interrogators frequently used the dreaded words "Gestapo" and "SS." Lane thought about Miriam, now pregnant with their first child, and his responsibility to the X Troopers back in England. The next day he and Wooldridge were driven into the French countryside without being told where they were being taken. But rather than ending up in a clearing in the woods where they would be summarily executed, they found themselves in Field Marshal Rommel's headquarters at Château de La Roche-Guyon.

During his training in the SOE and No. 10 (Inter-Allied) Commando, Lane had been taught to give only his (fake) name, rank, and serial number if he was captured. But instead he found himself having an extended conversation

with the field marshal over tea. Lane fortunately recovered his composure
and didn't say anything that would give him and his comrade away.

After their interview with Rommel, Lane and Wooldridge were taken
briefly to Fresnes Prison, outside Paris, which was run by the SS. Lane was
terrified that his good luck had run out. He spent two sleepless nights listening to the sounds of men screaming in agony as they were tortured. On
the third day, likely due to Rommel's personal intervention, the men were
transferred by train to Spangenberg Castle in the wooded hills of central
Germany. Lane and Wooldridge's new prison, Oflag IX AH, was a medieval
fortified castle with a moat, which had been turned into a prison for three
hundred British officers.

Lane knew that his Welsh cover would be useless because the prisoners
would recognize his fake accent. He found the camp's Allied commanding

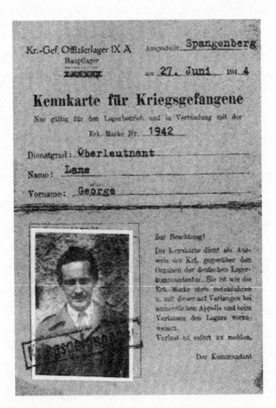

*George Lane's POW identity card issued after the Tarbrush 10 raid of May 1944*

officer, Colonel Euan Miller of the King's Royal Rifle Corps, and explained to him that he was really a commando of Hungarian origin and a member of X Troop.

"You will need to lie low until we can verify this," Miller responded cautiously.

Once his story checked out, Lane told Miller and the senior officers the bizarre tale of having tea with Field Marshal Rommel. Lane also described the environs of Rommel's château: how the building was surrounded by trees that seemed to grow out of ramparts.

"Oh, I know exactly where that is," one of the officers exclaimed, and he went off to the prison library. A short while later he returned with a copy of *The Voyage* by Charles Morgan. The book described exactly the location of the castle and gave its name as Château de La Roche-Guyon.

Using a hidden homemade wireless set, the prisoners transmitted Lane's information to London. A few months later, on July 17, during the Normandy campaign, Rommel's staff car was strafed by RAF Spitfires as he drove from Château de La Roche-Guyon to the front near St.-Lô. The attack left Rommel, one of Germany's best and most creative generals, with serious injuries, and from that moment on his participation in the war was effectively over. (He was later forced to commit suicide after being implicated in the plot to kill Hitler.) It is perhaps not too big an exaggeration to suggest that George Lane's ill-fitting blindfold affected the course of World War Two.

Having made himself known to the camp's senior officers, Lane settled into prison life and composed a letter to Miriam telling her that he was still alive. According to Miriam, however, she already knew. Soon after apprehending him, the Germans had announced over a secret radio transmission that they had captured two British soldiers. This message was intercepted by the Dutch Underground and then relayed to No. 10 (Inter-Allied) Commando's Dutch troop, who passed it on to Miriam in person. She took this information to General Robert Laycock, who told her that this was good evidence that her husband had not been killed immediately. Miriam, ever hopeful, soon received the news that George was indeed alive and was being held in a POW camp.

There was little food in the prisoner of war camp and it was freezing cold, but there were plenty of books to read, and Lane bided his time while plotting to escape the fortress.

For their success in Operation Tarbrush, Bryan Hilton-Jones and George Lane were awarded the Military Cross in August 1944. The Skipper's commendation note read that "the whole of the Tarbrush operations were only made possible by the outstanding leadership and organizing ability of Captain Hilton-Jones. In spite of lack of sleep on seven consecutive nights, it was largely due to his untiring efforts that these urgent operations were brought to such a successful conclusion."

In Lane's citation it was noted that the intelligence about the mines had "a direct bearing on the final plans for *Overlord*. The operation was of the highest importance," and due to Lane's "tenacity and purpose [he] assisted in obtaining the vital intelligence," which meant that D-Day could go on as planned. Locked away in Spangenberg Castle, Lane surely would have been heartened to know that he had contributed to keeping the invasion on track.

Medals and praise were all very well, but what mattered most to Captain Hilton-Jones and Lieutenant Lane were the men they had spent the past two years molding into shape and the mission upon which they were about to embark. D-Day would be the ultimate crucible and testing ground for the secret Jewish commandos of X Troop.

# SOUTHAMPTON, JUNE 4–5, 1944

PETER MASTERS WAS doing his best to seem relaxed among the rest of the Special Service Brigade gathered together on Southampton Common on a brisk morning. Everyone knew that the invasion of Europe was imminent, it was just a matter of when and where. The brigade had been in a sealed transit camp on the outskirts of Southampton for weeks; only one hundred miles of English Channel separated them from France. Even if the officers knew when the attack was scheduled to occur, they would not tell the enlisted men. The location and timing of the invasion were the most jealously guarded military secrets of the war.

It was rumored that Brigadier Lovat was about to come to address the men. Lieutenant Colonel Simon Fraser, fifteenth Lord Lovat, was a popular commander. Lovat had been promoted to lead No. 1 Special Service Brigade, which was composed of four commando units: Nos. 3, 4, and 6 Army Commando and No. 45 (Royal Marine) Cdo.

Peter Masters knew that if the invasion was being postponed, there would be no formal announcement. A visit by Lovat, the commandos' commando, could only mean one thing: they were about to embark for France.

Lovat was already a near-mythic figure. His ancestors had battled with the Scottish revolutionary William Wallace against the English; fought for Mary,

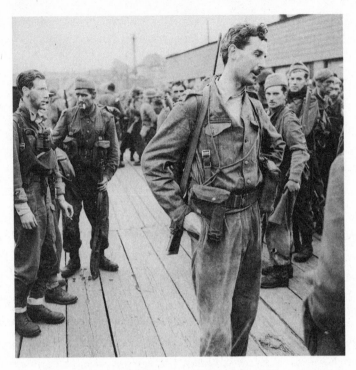

*Lord Lovat, Dieppe Raid, August 1942*

Queen of Scots, against her foes; and taken up arms with Bonnie Prince Charlie at the devastating Battle of Culloden. Fraser's father, fourteenth Lord Lovat, had won a Distinguished Service Order (Britain's second-highest medal for gallantry) in the Boer War and a knighthood in World War One. Lovat himself had already received a Military Cross in July 1942 for a reconnaissance raid on the French coast. After that he had become the CO of No. 4 Commando, which was the sole unit that was successful during the Dieppe Raid.

A tea station had been set up. The tension was mounting. The smell of body odor, strong English tea, and cheap British Army Woodbine cigarettes was overpowering.

Finally, a hush fell over the men as Lovat appeared with his walking stick, wearing his green beret, waistcoat, and trademark wool sweater, as if he was just popping out for a stroll on another rainy day on his Highland estate. Cigarettes were put out and the men came to attention. Lovat ordered them to stand at ease.

Lovat cleared his throat and announced simply that "the big show" was on. A cheer went through the crowd and then, nervously, they quieted to listen. "You will shortly be embarking on ships for the invasion of France," Lovat said. "You are the tip of the spear, the fine cutting edge of the British Expeditionary Force. You men should expect a physical encounter in which you have had no equal. You know your job and I know that you will not fail. Remember the bigger the challenge, the better we play. History will tell that in our age there were giants who walked the Earth and by God we are going to prove that tomorrow!" Masters found himself cheering with the rest of the commandos.

In total forty-three X Troopers would be deployed with eight commando units for D-Day—the largest amphibious assault in history, intended to turn the tide for the Allies. Since the peak of German power in 1942, the Nazis had been increasingly weakened with losses in North Africa, Stalingrad, Leningrad, and Kursk. In Italy Mussolini had been overthrown, and the Allied armies were close to liberating Rome. But so far the Germans had not been seriously challenged on the western front—in France and the Low Countries, which was precisely the area that the Allies were now poised to strike. By attacking the French coast, they could force Hitler to devote huge quantities of men and materiel to yet another front—a commitment the beleaguered Germans could not afford.

The brigade was, according to Lovat, being given the formidable task of holding the left flank of the Allied bridgehead. The plan was for its four commando units to land at Ouistreham, a small port on the Normandy coast about ten miles north of Caen and on a stretch of beach code-named Sword, the easternmost of the Allies' five designated amphibious landing zones. Once ashore at Sword Beach, they would pass through the assault troops of the British Third Infantry Division, which would have arrived earlier, and then head inland to meet up with two brigades of the British Sixth Airborne Division, which would have already landed by parachute and glider.

Once assembled, the four commando units would support the Sixth Airborne Division, now fighting to take two vital bridges, one over the

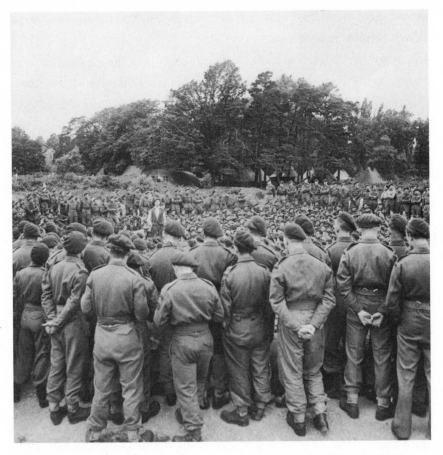

*Brigadier Lovat addressing the commandos in Southampton before embarking on the D-Day operation, June 5, 1944*

Caen Canal outside Bénouville — soon to go down in history as Pegasus Bridge — and the other over the Orne River at nearby Ranville. Another of their tasks was to help capture the Merville Battery, which was firing on the troops landing at Sword Beach. Once they had met these objectives, they were to advance and take a series of villages in the area east of the city of Caen.

The X Troopers attached to the brigade included Lance Corporal Peter Masters, Corporal Gerald Nichols (Heinz Herman), and Private Harry Nomburg, all of whom were attached to No. 6 Commando, a unit that had returned from a string of successes in North Africa, where they had gained skills in desert warfare. Nichols, with headquarters, would be in charge of the X Troopers in No. 6 Commando, while Masters would be his second-in-command.

A group of X Troopers was also attached to No. 45 (RM) Cdo., commanded by Lieutenant Colonel N. C. Reis. A brand-new unit, it was seeing its first action on D-Day, which meant that the handful of X Troopers who were seconded with it — Corporal George Saunders, Private Richard Arlen, Corporal Percy Shelley (Alfred Samson), and Sergeant David Stewart — did not have as much trouble sharing in the group's esprit de corps as some of their comrades in the battle-hardened units.

By this time Bryan Hilton-Jones had been promoted to major and was now officially the second-in-command of No. 10 (Inter-Allied) Commando under Lieutenant Colonel Peter Laycock. The younger brother of the chief of Combined Operations, Robert Laycock, Peter had taken over as head of No. 10 (Inter-Allied) Commando from Dudley Lister in May 1944. For D-Day the Skipper was attached to the brigade's headquarters, while also overseeing the detached X Troopers in the commando units.

Peter Masters listened, transfixed, to Lovat's rousing words. For him and the other members of X Troop, the invasion was deeply personal. As he explained later, "You were praying for war. Not because you were bloodthirsty, but because if you didn't fight, then you and all those you loved would be killed." Peter's mother, father, and sister were in England, but many members of his extended family remained in Austria. He could only hope that the invasion was not coming too late to save them.

When Lovat's speech ended, the commandos broke into another rousing cheer and began shaking hands and clapping each other on the back. Rum was passed around, and some groups started singing old army or traditional English songs. While the others celebrated, Masters made his way to the intelligence section of No. 1 Special Service Brigade and discovered there a full-scale model of Sword Beach with tiny houses, anti-tank obstacles, and minefields. Peter memorized the route off the beach, then returned to his billet and cleaned and recleaned his Thompson submachine gun. There was nothing else to be done. After all those months of hard training, he was as ready as he would ever be. Yet that night, as the men prepared to leave, they were told, much to their disappointment, that the invasion was being delayed twenty-four hours due to bad weather. They would leave on the afternoon of June 5 instead. There followed a sleepless night of drinking and smoking and playing cards as they awaited whatever fate lay ahead.

The following afternoon buses arrived to take them to the nearby town of Warsash to board the ships for Normandy. Most of the trip across the Channel would take place on frigates and other small warships. As they neared France, the men would switch to a range of landing craft for the final approach. The X Troopers felt relief, as well as a bit of apprehension. The long-awaited moment had finally arrived.

As they were on their way to the boats, X Trooper Corporal Gerald Nichols took Masters aside. "You ride a bike, don't you?" Nichols asked.

"I do," Masters replied.

Nichols was a rather dashing blond charmer from a factory-owning family in Berlin. Due to his Aryan looks, he had been selected to participate as a flag carrier in the 1936 Olympics by organizers who had been unaware that he was Jewish. (This grim irony was immortalized with a brief appearance by Nichols in Leni Riefenstahl's propaganda film *Olympia*.) Nichols had been transported on the brutal HMT *Dunera* and spent a year in the Hay Internment Camp in Australia. Like Masters he was eager to get back to Europe to strike a blow against the Nazis.

Nichols explained to Masters that he had been assigned to the headquarters unit and they needed an X Trooper with a stripe on his arm for Bicycle Troop (officially No. 1 Troop of No. 6 Commando). This, according to Nichols, would be the "most interesting" of all the units. He wondered if Masters would be willing to switch his assignment at the last minute. Bicycle Troop would have one of the potentially most dangerous missions on the morning of D-Day. Their bikes would enable them to bolt ahead of the rest of the commandos, leading the way across the fields and roads of Normandy to Pegasus Bridge. As part of this assignment, they would likely be among the first to encounter the enemy who had amassed inland.

Although he hadn't trained with the Bicycle Troop at all, Masters readily accepted Nichols's invitation.

The bicycle that Nichols gave to Masters was nothing like the heavy German bike Peter had ridden around the streets of Vienna when he was evading anti-Semitic thugs or going to soccer matches. It was also nothing like the bike he had ridden to his London art school before he was interned as an enemy alien. In fact it was unlike any he had ever seen before. It folded in half, and in place of proper pedals there were metal stems for his feet.

Masters mounted the strange contraption and rode it the rest of the way to his designated ship. In that brief run down the dock, he could see that he would need more time to get the hang of it. Yet as an X Trooper he was accustomed to mastering skills that others had spent much longer acquiring. After a bit more pedaling up and down the dock, he reckoned he would be able to keep up with the rest of the troop.

Masters knew that as a newcomer to a unit that had already spent months serving and fighting together in Africa, he would have to work hard to gain his new comrades' respect and get special assignments such as going on advance patrols. The Skipper was also aware of this unique challenge the X Troopers would face in their new units, and he had told his men, "Your [new] commanding officers will be busy and have a lot on their minds, so don't come back telling me they didn't use you. Pester them until they do. Make nuisances of yourselves; I know you can be pretty damn good at that." It was advice that Peter Masters did not forget.

X Troop had never fought as a distinct unit because on May 15, 1944, all the men had been distributed to various frontline commando detachments in anticipation of D-Day. As Bryan Hilton-Jones noted, the men had been very much sought after by other companies — not just No. 1 Special Service Brigade but also its sister group, No. 4 Special Service Brigade — due to the "high and repeated praise for [their] work, both as individuals and as a Troop." No. 4 Special Service Brigade was a new brigade created for D-Day, which meant that the X Troopers were the "most seasoned" of the men and the others looked up to them. With their extensive commando training, language skills, high intelligence, and personal drive to beat the Nazis, the men of X Troop were too valuable to risk being wiped out in one unlucky shell burst. Instead, they would be sent in groups of two to six to other units. In the course of the war no other British fighting unit would be so carefully husbanded.

Before the Normandy landings, the Skipper also promoted as many of them as he could. This was crucial because it would give them the authority to make command decisions and take on leadership roles in their new units. Interestingly, as he noted in the X Troop war diary, those who he had not managed to promote ended up getting promoted anyway in disproportionately large numbers due to their outstanding work in the field.

By the end of April 1944 the Skipper had also arranged for eleven X Troopers to be sent to the Officer Cadet Training Unit (OCTU), or officer training school. After meeting this group of men, the president of one War Office Selection Board (WOSB) told Hilton-Jones that the men of the X Troop were the "finest lot of OCTU applicants he had ever come across." Seven of these eleven were ultimately selected for officer training, including Manfred Gans, Tony Firth, and Victor Davies. Manfred, however, refused the offer: D-Day was imminent and he did not want to miss the action by undergoing weeks of additional training. He was, he felt, sufficiently prepared to take on the Nazis, and nothing was going to stop him from being part of the invasion of occupied France. As he saw it, "We were reborn in Aberdovey. As far as I was concerned, five years living as a pariah and four years of being an enemy alien were behind us, and we were somebody new now."

Manfred didn't want to waste time becoming an officer; all he wanted to do was to fight. His parents were in danger in occupied Europe, and he was determined to somehow get the Nazis before they got them. He did not know it, but the clock was ticking, as the extermination of the Jews was continuing at a frenzied pace. The deportation of hundreds of thousands of Hungarian Jews to Auschwitz-Birkenau had begun just the previous month, and over the following three months the gas chambers and crematoria there would work nonstop: up to nine thousand Jewish children, women, and men were being murdered at the camp every day. This included many of the parents, siblings, friends, cousins, wives, and children of the X Troopers.

No. 4 Special Service Brigade was tasked with securing the flanks of the invasion beaches. The brigade included Manfred Gans and Maurice Latimer, with No. 41 (RM) Cdo., which would land at Hermanville-sur-Mer, by Sword Beach, and then destroy the German coastal defenses westward to Luc-sur-Mer.

The Southampton camp where the X Troopers awaited D-Day was surrounded by barbed wire in order to sequester the men from the outside world and ensure that any invasion details would remain secret. Or at least that was the plan; in fact many of the soldiers would sneak away to meet women or go to a pub.

The boredom of camp life was also relieved by regular visits from prominent military men. Field Marshal Bernard Montgomery showed up to give speeches based on the tactics he had learned leading the British Eighth Army for the North Africa and Sicily campaigns. An intelligent, professional soldier, he was admired equally by the enlisted men and his fellow officers. But his success in North Africa had perhaps gone somewhat to his head, and as the war went on his worst characteristics became exacerbated. Although Monty was always something of a martinet, his colleagues now feared that his vanity had impaired his judgment on several occasions. By the time of D-Day, fortunately and unfortunately, he was Britain's obvious choice to lead its contingent of invasion forces. The British public would have demanded no less, but there were serious doubts in the high command that the ever-cautious Montgomery could achieve all his objectives on time. Still, he was no fool, and when he was cautious, he was cautious for a good reason: he didn't want to see his men slaughtered the way they had been in World War One. Monty was popular with the rank and file, no matter what his superiors thought of him.

In one of Monty's speeches at Southampton he reminded the soldiers that it was crucial that they not be "beach happy" and freeze on landing; otherwise they would be mowed down by German machine guns. Manfred Gans, who was determined to kill and capture as many Nazis as possible, later wrote that he told himself "this was not a trap that I was going to fall into."

· · ·

Once they were loaded onto the landing craft for the initial leg of their passage across the Channel, the commandos settled in as best they could. As the convoy with No. 1 Special Service Brigade left Warsash at 5 p.m. on June 5 with Lord Lovat's ship in the lead, his personal bagpiper, Bill Millin, played "The Road to the Isles," a rousing marching song written originally for those going off to World War One. Although Lovat had been told that he could not take a piper with him, he told Millin that "since they were both Scots, what the English War Office said did not apply to them."

The convoy went past the Isle of Wight in darkness and then out into the English Channel. As the ships pitched about, many soldiers began vomiting up rum and their dinner of self-heating soups and cocoa. Masters had avoided the rum because he wanted to keep his full focus, and now he found that abstinence had another benefit: he wasn't sick like the others.

The boats in this convoy were headed to Sword Beach, the easternmost of the five invasion beaches, which extended about five miles from Lion-sur-Mer to Ouistreham at the mouth of the Caen Canal. The plan was to eventually have 29,000 men land at Sword.

During the night the US 82nd and 101st Airborne Divisions and British airborne and glider troops had landed in Normandy in an attempt to capture key roads, towns, and bridges. The RAF had bombed the coastline. Then came the minesweepers and air and naval bombardments. Sword, like the other beaches, was protected by German beach obstacles and 75 mm and 155 mm guns from shore batteries and by 88 mm guns inland. There were also snipers, mortars, and machine guns trained on the beach from the summer houses along the shore, as well as pillboxes in the dunes. The British Third Infantry Division would land at 7:25 a.m. and secure the beach while the Royal Engineers would clear the mines and the obstacles. They would be followed shortly thereafter by the commandos.

Huddled belowdecks in his landing craft, infantry (small), in the early morning hours of June 6, Peter Masters knew they were in the vicinity of Sword Beach when suddenly all the naval guns in the world seemed to let loose at once. The Royal Navy was softening up the coast in advance of the main invasion.

While some of the men on the landing craft began singing to calm their nerves, Masters remained silent and focused. He thought about the fact that finally he was getting his chance to strike back. He was confident that if he could get off the landing craft in one piece, he could bring the fight to the enemy. "I felt well-trained," he would later recall, "and definitely a better-than-even match for what I was likely to encounter." As the surf got rougher, Masters battled his seasickness by reading the comic novel *Cold Comfort Farm*. Finally, after hours of being tossed about in the midst of the naval shelling and rocket fire, the beach was in sight. As sirens began to sound, Masters optimistically dog-eared his paperback and put it in his pocket.

"Attention on deck! Attention on deck!" a naval rating yelled.

The shelling continued and Masters thought he could hear return fire coming from the shore.

"Get your bicycles and prepare to land!" someone shouted.

Peter went up to the chaotic, heaving deck and desperately tried to find his bicycle among the tangle of bikes that had been stacked in a messy pile.

"Attention on deck!" the naval rating kept yelling. On the horizon behind him, Peter could see an enormous flotilla of ships that seemed to go on forever. Ahead, the beach was obscured with black smoke.

More men were throwing up now.

Spray was coming over the sides of the landing craft.

Peter could see the muzzle flashes from machine-gun fire up beyond the dunes.

The landing craft hit the shallows. Masters looked at the shore and noticed that the houses he had seen in the model back at Southampton were no longer there; they had all been blown to smithereens.

"Attention on deck! Attention on deck!"

Heavy gears began turning and the ramp in front of him began to creak downward. Peter was hit with a startling realization: "This may be the last thing I ever do."

It was 8:41 a.m.

# SWORD BEACH, JUNE 6, 1944

THE RAMP WAS steeper than Peter Masters had been expecting, and it was already slick with diesel, vomit, and greasy sea spray. The landing craft was pitching up and down in the surf like an angry sea monster. France was burning, the sky was gray, men were yelling, sometimes screaming. This was not a good day or a good place to die. At the very least, Masters decided, he was going to get off this bloody boat.

Wheeling his bike with one hand, he held his tommy gun and the guide rope with the other and jumped into the cold, waist-high surf, which to his horror was turning red from the blood of the dead and dying of the Eighth Infantry Brigade, which had struggled ashore before them.

Staggering through the waves, Masters labored to stay upright with his bike; his tommy gun with its thirty-round magazine; his heavy backpack containing extra ammunition, four grenades, a pickaxe, and a two-hundred-foot hemp rope that would be used to cross the canal if the Germans had managed to blow up Pegasus Bridge. All over the Normandy beaches that morning Allied soldiers were drowning under similarly heavy loads.

Peter made it through the breakers and stumbled onto the sand. Field Marshal Montgomery, Brigadier Lovat, and Major Hilton-Jones had told

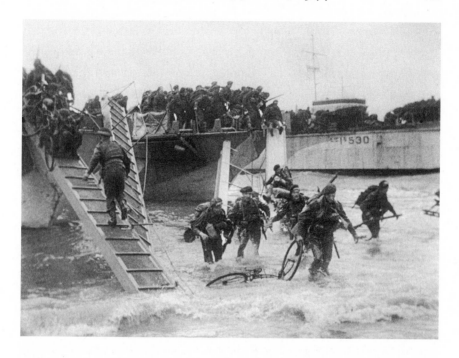

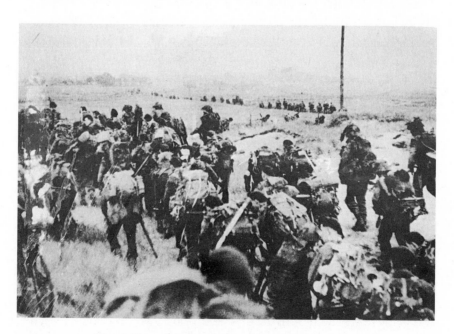

*Bicycle Troop landing at Sword Beach, June 6, 1944*

the men over and over, "Don't stop on the beach! Advance! Advance!" These words were ringing through his head as he stood there gasping. The very worst thing would be to get stuck between the sea and the German defenses, an easy target for the enemy. Although Masters did not know it, this very situation was happening on Omaha Beach, a few miles to the west, where American soldiers were being slaughtered by the hundreds as they struggled to get off the heavily defended beach exits.

But Masters found it hard not to stop and gape at the horrific scene in front of him. The air smelled of diesel and brine, gunpowder and death. Behind him dead men and parts of men were being pitched about by the surf. In front of Masters a dying soldier kept trying to stand up in slow motion, but he had lost too much blood. Nearby Masters saw two men digging frantically into the sand, trying to hide from the bullets and mortars. It was a Sisyphean task as the waves kept filling in their useless trench.

A few brave men charged the enemy defenses and were mowed down. Others were frozen in fear, just sitting on the sand, a look of emptiness in their eyes. Everything seemed to be going wrong. The beach should have been cleared already. The commandos were supposed to be doing their fighting inland. Peter stood with the other members of Bicycle Troop, unsure what to do next.

Then Peter saw the towering figure of Brigadier Lovat, still wearing his white turtleneck sweater under his battle dress uniform, emerging from the very next landing craft and wading through the surf. The next man out of Lovat's landing craft was shot in the face and fell into the sea. The man after him was Lovat's personal piper, Bill Millin, wearing his full kilt and carrying his bagpipes. As his kilt floated away from his body into the surf, he began playing the jaunty "Hieland Laddie," one of Lovat's favorites.

As Masters watched in amazement, next down the ramp was the Skipper. Lance Corporal Peter Masters stood at attention and absurdly found himself saluting his CO, Major Bryan Hilton-Jones. Lovat, Millin, and Hilton-Jones all began moving forward, and Peter would be damned if he was going to stay there with the dead and dying, so he moved forward too.

• • •

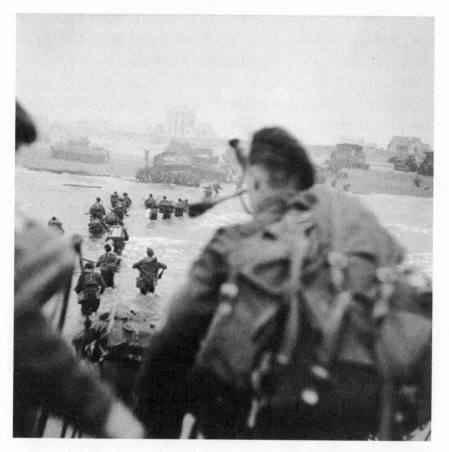

*Piper Bill Millin disembarking after Lord Lovat at Sword Beach, June 6, 1944*

A few minutes after Peter Masters landed, X Trooper Private Harry Nomburg also arrived at Sword Beach with 3 Troop, No. 6 Commando. Few knew that behind Harry's easy smile and effervescent personality lay the scars of intense tragedy. On May 21, 1939, at the age of fifteen, he had been sent to Britain on a Kindertransport train. The last time he saw his parents was on the excruciating day when they waved goodbye to him at the train station in Berlin. It was a Sunday, which also happened to be Mother's Day, as well as Harry's mother's birthday. He had not heard from either of his parents since then, and he would later learn that both had been murdered by the Nazis.

As Nomburg descended the ramp of his landing craft, his first thought was gratitude to be off the stinking, vomit-filled ship. Raising his tommy gun over his head to keep it dry, he charged forward—and then watched in horror as the magazine clip from his submachine gun fell into the white surf. Years later he would recall that he had "hit the beaches of France and stormed the fortress of Europe without a single bullet in my gun."

Harry was looking for cover when he heard the sound of Lovat's bagpiper up ahead. Millin was now playing "The Road to the Isles," marching back and forth along the blood-soaked beach to rouse the troops as mortar shells landed all around them. Harry could hardly believe what he was seeing.

At the same time, Lovat was gathering his men for a concerted push inland. Nomburg went up to Lovat and shyly touched his belt from behind for luck. As he did so he thought, "Should anything happen to me now, let it be said that Private Nomburg fell by Lord Lovat's side!" Nomburg wasn't the only who thought Lovat had a protective aura about him. Lovat and his commandos had been the only ones who had been successful at Dieppe and had not suffered major casualties there. Some people thought that Lovat was unkillable. The coming days would test those beliefs.

As Harry moved off the beach, the first two Germans he saw put their hands in the air in surrender and Nomburg conducted his first battlefield interrogation, asking them in German, "Where are your gun emplacements? Your minefields?" The prisoners told him and he shared this intelligence with his commanding officer, Captain Alan Pyeman. Pyeman led the men through the minefields into the lush, damp June countryside beyond. They were going to the brigade assembly area, a large clump of tall, bushy trees near the village of Lion-sur-Mer that was clearly visible at the end of a plowed field, about a quarter mile inland. All the commando units of No. 1 Special Service Brigade were to meet up there before heading farther inland toward their various objectives in support of the airborne troops.

At 8: 45 a.m. X Troopers Manfred Gans, Maurice Latimer, and Peter Moody (Kurt Meyer) were landing with No. 41 (RM) Cdo. at the westernmost point of Sword Beach. They were part of a convoy of five landing craft, infantry, each of which held about two hundred men. The X Troopers were the new-comers to a unit that had already fought (along with Paul Streeten) in the Sicily invasion and the Italian campaign. The commandos' goal that day was to capture the small coastal villages between their landing point and Luc-sur-Mer. This would require an advance of nearly three miles through German-held territory.

None of this seemed even remotely possible to Manfred as he stepped off the ramp into a scene of carnage. It turned out that No. 41 (RM) Cdo. had landed a few hundred yards from the intended site and were now in an area that hadn't been softened up and was taking heavy, sustained bombard-ment. The air was thick with smoke, and the din of artillery fire and naval guns gave off a "cacophony of the devil." The unit's war diary recounts the scene in this part of Sword Beach with atypical emotion: "[The beach] was littered with the dead and the wounded and burnt out tanks . . . The beach was quite obviously still under fire with mortar bombs and shells crashing down fairly plentifully."

As Manfred Gans ran through the surf, he kept reminding himself to keep moving even though there were bodies everywhere. His first thought, he would later recall, was "At last I've come back!" Ahead of him were Ger-man machine guns, some of which, he thought, might even be manned by his classmates from Borken. Now they were *literally* gunning for him, and Manfred was happy to reciprocate.

British sappers blew a gap in the steel barricades that the Germans had laid all along the beach. Manfred ran through the opening and found a platoon of about twenty-five Germans putting their hands up. He accepted their surrender. Although he'd been told to interrogate prisoners, he was not interested in any lengthy interrogations this morning; he just wanted a safe way off the beach. He briskly addressed the Germans in their mother tongue: "Good morning, gentlemen. Where is the path through the mine-fields?" The POWs must have been shocked to be addressed so politely by a Brit in flawless German, and they pointed out the path through the mines.

"Come on, boys, follow me!" Gans yelled to a dozen or so Marines, who followed him along the path the POWs had indicated. They made it to the rendezvous outside Lion-sur-Mer with no injuries or deaths. They were the first ones there. They waited on the outskirts of the village, not realizing that nearly half of No. 41 (RM) Cdo., including many officers, had been killed or wounded back on the beach.

The final group of X Troopers to arrive at Sword Beach, at 9:10 a.m., were with No. 45 (RM) Cdo. The commandos' task was to assist the Sixth Airborne Division in capturing the Merville Battery, a heavily fortified structure with six-foot-thick, steel-reinforced gun casements surrounded by layers of barbed wire. The battery's firepower of 100 mm guns, 20 mm antiaircraft guns, and machine guns was mainly directed at Sword Beach.

One of the X Troopers was George Saunders, a near legend among the men. He was extremely handsome and charismatic, had a knack for picking up women, and was completely fearless. Before Hitler came to power, George's family had been minor nobility in Munich, where they owned and operated a liberal newspaper. In 1937, after their paper published an anti-Hitler article, a sympathetic member of the SS warned George's mother that they should leave Germany immediately. George, his brother, and their parents made it to the UK. After being interned in Canada, Saunders volunteered for the Pioneer Corps and was then selected for X Troop.

Following a botched initial landing when the craft was too far from shore, Saunders alighted on a beach, as a fellow commando later noted, that was filled with "dead bodies, living bodies and all the blood in the water, giving the appearance they were drowning in their own blood for the want of moving." George ran for cover under the dunes to await further instructions.

Sergeant Manfred Gans was waiting for backup at the assembly area near Lion-sur-Mer. He was relieved at last to see a fellow commando running toward him along the beach path. A whole troop would have been useful, but one more man was better than nothing. And this wasn't just any commando but another X Trooper, Corporal Maurice Latimer. The Sudeten

German had made it through the Spanish Civil War, Germany's annexa-tion of Czechoslovakia, and the Dieppe Raid, and thus far his luck was holding out on D-Day too. Latimer and Gans congratulated each other on having survived the landing and then conferred about what to do next.

Latimer suggested that they stop waiting and head into the village. Man-fred agreed with this assessment and explained to the others that it was up to them to take Lion-sur-Mer. They would begin the liberation of Europe by themselves, right here, now.

# PEGASUS BRIDGE, JUNE 6, 1944

AFTER SALUTING THE Skipper at Sword Beach, Peter Masters wheeled his bike over the sand and found the other members of Bicycle Troop. Their troop commander, Captain Douglas Robinson, ordered them to mount their bicycles and pedal down a road leading inland, ignoring the pleas from the sappers to wait until all the mines had been cleared. They couldn't wait. If all had gone according to plan, a party of 181 parachutists and infantry, led by Major John Howard, should have landed by glider and taken Pegasus Bridge over the Caen Canal near Bénouville, as well as the nearby bridge over the Orne River at Ranville. At first light the Germans would have almost certainly counterattacked, and this small coup de main force would need support and reinforcements as quickly as Bicycle Troop could get there.

Behind the beaches was bocage, or hedge, country and a winding creek that forced Masters and the others to wade chest-deep in slimy, muddy water, clutching their bikes and clinging to their packs and ammunition. They had scarcely made any progress crossing the field when they came under sniper fire, forcing them to scatter to find cover. They were trying to figure out what to do next when they heard the distinctive grumbling engine of a lone Sherman tank chugging up behind them. Peter noticed with surprise that the hatch was open and a soldier was standing with his head exposed. Masters caught his attention and warned him about the snipers in the trees.

"OK," the soldier said, and then he "closed his hatch and blazed away into the woods with his cannon and machine guns."

Bicycle Troop had no problem crossing the field after that.

With relief they rode into the brigade congregating area, where those not encumbered with heavy bicycles had arrived before them. There Masters again spotted Lord Lovat. Carrying his walking stick and hunting rifle, he looked, Peter thought, "perfectly at ease in spite of the shooting." With him was piper Bill Millin, who had made it from the beach entirely unarmed except for his ceremonial dirk.

Spotting a couple of captured prisoners, Masters remembered Hilton-Jones's order to always take the initiative, and he headed over to them. As he did so Lovat called out, "Oh, you're the chap with the languages, aren't you? Ask them where the Howitzers are." Peter began to grill the POWs in German, but they said nothing back. Looking at their paybooks, he saw the men were Russian and Polish, so he tried French, guessing they might have learned it in school. Lovat, fluent in French, joined in, but they quickly realized the POWs knew precious little of the language.

Soon George Saunders and the surviving men of No. 45 (RM) Cdo. also arrived at the rendezvous. As they filed past, Lord Lovat said "Good morning, gentlemen" and "Good show, chaps" to each of them. Like everyone else, Saunders was deeply impressed by Lovat: "Every time there was a burst of machine-gun fire he ignored it, nonchalantly unscuffing the sand from his highly polished shoes."

Around this time Manfred Gans and some of the Marines of No. 41 (RM) Cdo. arrived at the outskirts of Lion-sur-Mer. As they made their way cautiously through the village, they began to encounter jubilant French civilians. With his schoolboy French, Gans was able to learn that the Germans had retreated to a strongpoint at the far end of the village, where they had camouflaged machine guns and heavy artillery.

The commandos would need to take that position before the road could be cleared for Allied vehicles. Manfred knew that he was going to have to come up with a plan of attack. He was the senior sergeant and, frankly, was far better trained than most of the Marines present. Gans reminded the others to avoid the road and go slowly from house to house to avoid being shot at. They did so and took no casualties. Eventually the commandos reached a large house overlooking the strongpoint, and as Gans entered it to view the German positions, a bullet from the house next door almost hit him. He cautiously went into the neighboring house to investigate, creeping upstairs in his tennis shoes. On the second floor he discovered an Algerian man happily shooting at the Germans with an "1871 rifle from the Franco-Prussian War." Gans, using his broken French, persuaded him to stop shooting and to join them in their attack.

Meanwhile at the brigade congregating area, Lovat ordered Bicycle Troop to head toward Pegasus Bridge. Peter Masters and the bicyclists rode silently through a nightmare landscape shelled to near oblivion by the naval guns. There were dead Germans everywhere, dead horses and cows, and dead Allied parachutists hanging from trees. For Peter it was a heartbreaking sight.

It was hard going on the poorly designed bikes. To ride them required each man to strap his tommy gun across his chest or back, then place his backpack in a holder in front of the handlebars. The weight of the pack would push down on the bike's front wheel, causing it to constantly stop. This, as Peter recalled, inevitably seemed to happen when someone was shooting at them and they were in a hurry to pedal out of the way. Bryan Samain, the intelligence officer for No. 45 (RM) Cdo., noted of Masters's unit that "of all the things to go to war with, perhaps a bicycle was the worst."

Masters kept thinking of the Skipper's advice to make a nuisance of himself. Yet every time he volunteered to scout ahead, Captain Robinson chose one of the men from the North Africa campaign whom he already knew and trusted. Peter felt that his new commanding officer saw him "as a preposterous character with an accent whom he had only met that morning." This made Masters even more determined to show that he was capable of using his initiative.

As Bicycle Troop rode through the small villages, people opened their doors and yelled, "Vive La France, vive les Tommies!" In one small hamlet the bicyclists pedaled hard to avoid a sniper in the church steeple. They continued east toward Bénouville.

On a hill before the village their lead cyclist was killed by machine-gun fire. He fell to the ground with, as Masters vividly recalled, "one wheel of his bike . . . spinning in the air as if it, too, had been mortally struck." Captain Robinson ordered the men to ditch the bikes and deploy behind the hill. They could not proceed until the enemy was dealt with.

"Ah, Corporal Masters," Robinson said. "Now there is something you can do. Go down to that village and see what's going on."

Masters, happy to finally be chosen, asked how many men to take with him.

"No men, Masters, just you."

Fine, thought Peter, I can do that. He explained to Robinson that he would sweep around the village and approach from the side to get the needed intelligence.

"You still don't seem to understand what I want you to do. Go down this road and see what's going on in this village," Robinson said.

Masters understood. They were going to send the funny-talking stranger to draw the Germans' machine-gun fire. Miriam Rothschild had warned the X Troopers when they were training in Aberdovey that the Brits might see them as an expendable suicide squad, and now it seemed her warnings were coming true.

To Masters it "felt rather like mounting the scaffold leading to the guillotine." But he didn't take it too personally; drawing the enemy's fire might truly be the most effective and quickest means of getting through Bénouville and reaching their objective, even if he was killed in the process. Peter walked alone down the middle of the road, like a hero in one of the Westerns he had watched in the Welsh cinemas. He was terrified but reminded himself that this was for the greater good. It was just a pity, he thought, that all his years of training in Aberdovey were going to go to waste.

Then he remembered a different movie, one he had seen in 1939 called *Gunga Din,* starring Cary Grant as Sergeant Archibald Cutter, a British Army warrant officer in colonial India. To disarm an angry mob in one scene, Cutter had yelled that they were all under arrest.

Perhaps that could work here.

Where the lead bicyclist had fallen, Masters cleared his throat and bellowed in German: "All right! Surrender, all of you! Come out! You are completely surrounded and don't have a chance! Throw away your weapons and come out with your hands up if you want to go on living. The war is over for all of you."

There was an eerie and unnerving silence, but no one fired at him.

Masters looked back at Captain Robinson, who motioned at him to keep moving forward. So Peter continued down the road until the inevitable happened.

A German popped up from behind a small wall. He looked at Masters, considered him for a moment, and then shot at him. In response Masters went down on one knee, aimed his tommy gun, and fired back. Both of them missed.

Peter pulled the trigger a second time. The tommy gun jammed. He dived for cover to give himself time to clear the gun. The German fired another burst. Masters tried to shoot back, but his gun jammed again. He ripped out the magazine, cleared the breech, cocked it, and just as he was about to fire he heard a noise from behind him. The men of Bicycle Troop were charging with fixed bayonets. He got up and joined them, and they roared into the village as most of the Germans hightailed it across the fields, perhaps persuaded by Masters's *Gunga Din* speech and certainly encouraged in their flight by the glint of the fixed bayonets.

As the commandos cleared the area, Corporal George Thompson found two of the enemy hiding in a ditch and shot both of them. Masters interro-

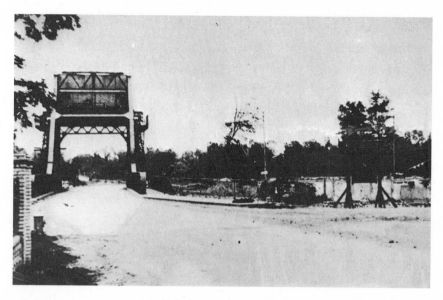

*Pegasus Bridge, D-Day*

gated the less seriously hurt one and learned that they were mere teenagers from Austria. Hearing this, Thompson was quite shaken, and he asked Masters to apologize to them in German.

The troop retrieved their bikes and rode on toward the center of the village. As they did, some of Major Howard's men emerged from their positions and shouted encouragement. When they finally reached Pegasus Bridge, they were relieved to find that it was still in the hands of British paratroopers, who waved their red berets in the air and cheered.

As they dashed across the bridge, sniper bullets clanged against the iron girders, and the airborne soldiers yelled, "Give 'em hell." They rode on toward the second bridge at Ranville, which was about a third of a mile away. One man was hit by sniper fire as they crossed.

Popular lore stemming from later accounts of D-Day, such as the book and movie *The Longest Day* and later fictions, has it that Lovat and his bagpiper were the first ones from the beaches to reach Pegasus Bridge, thus relieving Major Howard and thereby completing the commandos' first mission of the day. But in fact it was No. 6 Commando's Bicycle Troop that reached the bridge first, with Peter Masters, a Jewish lad from Vienna, among the improbable little vanguard.

After Bicycle Troop came the rest of No. 6 Commando, including Harry Nomburg, followed about thirty minutes later by Lord Lovat, with his piper by his side. As they began to cross Pegasus Bridge, Lovat told Millin, "No matter what the situation, just continue. Don't stop." Playing "Blue Bonnets over the Border" while sniper bullets flew all around, Millin encouraged Lovat's substantial relief force to push back the German counterattack. It was, as Millin recalled, by far "the longest bridge I ever piped across." Both he and Lovat lived to fight another day.

Back in Lion-sur-Mer, the rest of No. 41 (RM) Cdo. had caught up with Manfred Gans's commandos and their Algerian accomplice. After a few skirmishes Gans and the men pinned the Germans down to a position on the outskirts of the village. Gans informed the unit's commanding officer, Colonel Tim Gray, about the enemy positions, and the two of them toured the Allied portion of the town.

When Gray and Gans came across a South African unit that had just arrived from the beach road with three armored cars, Gray told them to launch a frontal attack on the German stronghold, which would be followed by the commandos. The Skipper had taught Manfred never to attack frontally when there were other options available, although perhaps using the main road was the only choice in the bocage. The French Resistance also had warned them that there would likely be a German anti-tank gun aimed at the road. But what could a humble sergeant say to a colonel?

To his horror Manfred watched the three armored cars trundle slowly down the road in a direct assault, accompanied by the infantry. A 50 mm Pak 38 anti-tank gun opened fire at very close range, blowing up all three vehicles. It was a complete slaughter, and Y Troop of No. 41 (RM) Cdo. suffered nearly 50 percent casualties.

After this catastrophe Colonel Gray decided that they would wait until the following day for another go at the German position. In the meantime Gans was ordered to report to the temporary headquarters at a farm just outside the village, where Manfred told the intelligence officer what he had seen and heard.

That done, Manfred found a spot in a barn and made himself a meal from his dehydrated food pack. A few years earlier he would have likely found a minyan of ten Jews — the minimum necessary for the thrice-daily prayers — with whom to say his evening prayers. But those days were in the past. In order to seem truly English he could not perform even the basic rites of Judaism, such as reciting daily prayers or mourning the dead.

As he settled in for some sorely needed rest, Gans reviewed the day. He had been focused on his mission and felt that he had performed well in battle. He did not yet know that 140 men of No. 41 (RM) Cdo. had been killed or wounded that day on the beaches and roads of Normandy. The X Troopers also had suffered a heavy toll. The wounded included Didi Fuller (Eugen Kagerer-Stein) and Eric Howarth (Erich Nathan); among the dead were several of his mates, including George Franklyn, Ernest Webster (E. G. Weinberger), and Max Laddy, who had recently married an Aberdovey woman.

Manfred told himself that if he survived, he would make sure to find the graves of fallen X Troopers. He would put a Magen David (Star of David) over them and say Kaddish, the Jewish prayer for the dead.

As the first day of the invasion drew to a close, Harry Nomburg with 3 Troop was continuing to Bréville-les-Monts, a village just east of Bénouville. There they were to connect with the Ninth Parachute Battalion to try to take Bréville, which was crucial for the Allies' strategy because it lay in the watershed of the Orne and Dives Rivers. Also aware of its importance, the Germans were regrouping and moving back along the west side of the Orne.

On the outskirts of Bréville the commandos came under sniper fire from a large house overlooking the main street. Captain Alan Pyeman led the attempt to storm the house but was shot dead through the neck. Though only twenty-three years old, he was already a seasoned and distinguished veteran of the North Africa campaign, and Harry Nomburg had found him to be a brave and competent commander. His death was a huge blow to the unit, but with German mortar fire intensifying there was no time for mourning. The most senior surviving officer, Lieutenant Donald Cahoon, took control of the troop and ordered the men to retreat, carrying the wounded with them. Leaving the village temporarily in the hands of the Germans, 3 Troop was ordered to rejoin No. 1 Special Service Brigade in Amfreville and would attempt to take Bréville once they had artillery support. By the end of the day Nomburg's unit had suffered twenty-one casualties, yet they had taken sixteen prisoners and killed at least twenty-four Germans.

Meanwhile George Saunders and the Marines of No. 45 (RM) Cdo. had crossed Pegasus Bridge on their mission to help take the Merville Battery and the nearby town of Franceville-Plage.

Somewhere in the vicinity of Sallenelles, on the road to Merville, they came under artillery fire and Saunders became separated from the others. He took cover in the basement of a large farm and helped himself to the red wine and Camembert stored there. Once the German guns had quieted, he left the cellar and found a bicycle. He mounted it and headed back toward the advance units of the brigade, which by then had reached Merville. The sun was setting, and he saw a group of men standing at a crossroads. He assumed they were Allied soldiers and waved to them.

"Das ist ein Englander," one of the soldiers exclaimed, and began shooting at him. Saunders leaped off his bike and scrambled into a nearby ditch.

For the next two hours in the darkness, they hunted the "Englander." Every time the Germans seemed to be getting close, he would toss a hand grenade or fire at them and move to a different position. Saunders was thankful that he was overloaded with kit and armed to the teeth. He knew that when the grenades ran out, he still had his tommy gun, knife, and Colt .45.

Yet Saunders was aware that he could not elude the soldiers forever, and more and more Germans were arriving to help with the search. Desperate, he finally resorted to hiding in a cold, stagnant pond with a camouflage net draped over him. The Germans finally gave up the search, and using the field craft the Skipper had taught him, Saunders was eventually able to make his way back to British lines.

Out of 450 commandos from No. 45 (RM) Cdo. who had landed at Sword Beach that day, 20 had been confirmed killed, including 3 officers; 28 were missing; and many others were wounded.

Peter Masters with Bicycle Troop was now on the outskirts of the village of Varaville, just east of Pegasus Bridge. The First Canadian Parachute Battalion had landed there during the night and was in a fight for this strategically important village that would have to be captured if a German counterattack from the east was to be thwarted. Captain Robinson asked the Canadians if they wanted assistance, but he was told they were close to taking the village and did not need help at this time. While resting there Masters was asked by the Canadians to come and interrogate a captured German officer.

"How come you speak such perfect German?" the officer asked after Masters's initial questions.

"I'm the one who asks the questions here!" Masters responded. The officer confirmed the existence of large German formations to the south. After the interrogation Bicycle Troop received orders to hold the German positions that the Canadians had captured until additional men arrived.

Masters and the bicyclists made tea and assessed the situation. Peter saw that only thirty or so of the original Bicycle Troop were left. Yet he could feel pleased with what they had done. They had accomplished their goal of making it to Pegasus Bridge before the rest of the brigade and then on to Varaville, farther than most of the other units had gone.

In fact all the X Troopers had been central players in the Allied successes of the day. Manfred Gans and Harry Nomburg had both gotten crucial intelligence about the location of minefields that had saved commando lives; Gans had effectively led his men through a village under heavy fire by showing them the safest way to proceed; Saunders had killed several Germans and occupied many others looking for him; and Masters had helped take a German machine-gun nest by drawing out their fire. None had flinched from danger, and all had assumed leadership roles in crucial moments in a way that would have made the Skipper proud and that directly saved Allied lives.

Masters sipped his tea and made sketches of the scene at Sword Beach.

As the evening wore on, Bicycle Troop's radio operator lost contact with No. 1 Special Service Brigade headquarters and then all the nearby units. Peter wondered "if perhaps the whole invasion had been repulsed and we were the only Allied troops still left alive in Normandy." In case this was true, and to prepare for a counterattack, they blew up two small bridges over a nearby river and fortified the abandoned German trenches.

Eventually Bicycle Troop's radio operator managed to find a broadcast coming from the BBC's German Service. The newsreader gave details of the invasion and claimed that it had been a success at all five beaches. Peter relayed the news to the others, who received it with great relief. Soon afterward they began to hear vehicles somewhere down the road, and they knew the enemy was mustering in the darkness.

Peter put away his sketch pad and pencils. He cleaned and dried his tommy gun to make sure it wouldn't jam again.

Just after midnight the German counterattack on Varaville began.

# VARAVILLE AND BEYOND, JUNE 7–15, 1944

FLARES AND STAR shells lit up the sky.

"Ready, lads. Ready! Here they come."

It was D-Day plus 1, 3 a.m.

The men were dug into the abandoned German trenches on the westernmost edge of Varaville. Peter Masters heard the *BUDDA BUDDA BUDDA* of a heavy machine gun spraying the field ahead of them, and to their rear a château that had been an ammunition dump took a direct hit and exploded.

Masters and the other Bicycle Troopers began shooting into the darkness with their captured Maxim machine guns, weapons from World War One that had been abandoned by the German infantry units when the Canadians had forced them to retreat. Some of the commandos also had figured out how to fire the formidable 7.5 cm Pak 40 anti-tank gun that the Germans had left fully loaded in their abandoned trenches.

Knowing where the anti-tank gun was located, the Germans lobbed mortars at it. A man next to Peter was killed, and several others were badly wounded. Assuming they had lost their sole big weapon, Peter thought,

"Well, that's the end of us." But after an ominous silence someone started firing the anti-tank gun again. Although the situation was desperate, Captain Robinson refused to withdraw to a better position without orders from headquarters. The radio operator kept trying to make contact but to no avail, and the radio was now nearly dead. Peter realized that once dawn broke, it would be a simple matter for the Germans to wipe out the surviving members of Bicycle Troop.

Finally, just before first light on June 7, the radio operator managed to contact headquarters and a response crackled back: "If you receive this, return to HQ immediately. Avoid Bréville on your way back. It has been retaken by the enemy. Repeat, return immediately."

"Grab your bikes and kit and retreat," Captain Robinson ordered.

The bedraggled group cycled through the fog of a gray dawn as the sound of gunfire faded behind them. They found a deserted farm where they had a breakfast of raw eggs and dried rations, and then they set out across an open field outside Bréville, intending to skirt the town on the way back to headquarters, as instructed.

The field was littered with crashed gliders, shell craters, and dead men. As they pushed their bikes in single file diagonally across the open field, they came under direct fire from a German artillery pack. Three of the men were wounded and later picked up by Red Cross field ambulances. The others pedaled furiously across the field, trying to get back to Amfreville without any more casualties.

On the outskirts of Amfreville, Masters spotted an Allied soldier waving at them. It was another X Trooper, none other than Peter's good friend Corporal Gerald Nichols, who had arranged for Peter to join Bicycle Troop back in Southampton. Nichols had gone out on his own to try to find the bicyclists, and he was deeply relieved to find Masters alive and unwounded. "Thank God, Peter!" he exclaimed. "You were all posted as missing! Now let's get the hell out of here: they say some Tiger tanks are on the way."

Bicycle Troop continued on to their next assignment: to assist No. 45 (RM) Cdo. in taking Franceville-Plage, the town on the outskirts of the crucial Merville Battery, which the Germans apparently were still holding. The men headed north toward the coast on a tree-lined country road.

At the Sallenelles crossroads en route to Franceville-Plage, a few miles from where they had seen Nichols, Masters was sent to do some advance intelligence gathering. He was surprised to find a bar open and packed with patrons who were excited to share everything they knew about German positions in the area. They all told Peter the same thing: the Germans were still massed at the Merville Battery, which they had been reinforcing all night.

As he was speaking with the villagers, Masters heard the sound of a jeep screeching to a halt outside. The bar door swung open and he was stunned to see another X Trooper, Corporal George Saunders, who was attached to No. 45 (RM) Cdo., the unit that Bicycle Troop was being sent to assist. Delighted to find each other still alive twenty-four hours after the invasion, they drank to their health and the Allied successes.

After George left, an elderly French woman invited Peter to have a quick wash. She gave him a china pitcher filled with luxuriously hot water and led him to a sunny bedroom with a washstand. He scrubbed himself clean. When he looked in the mirror, he barely recognized himself: his face was gray, drawn, and thin. The first day and a half of nonstop fighting and terror had marked him. How deeply, he could only guess.

Although D-Day had been more successful than the Allies could have hoped, there were still significant failures that were now becoming serious causes for concern. After the shock of the first landings, the Germans had begun to recover and start their counterattacks. The British had not taken Caen on the first day as Montgomery had planned, and the city was now a major focal point drawing Allied soldiers from other fronts. More crucially there was still the huge problem of getting supplies and men ashore. Until the two temporary Mulberry harbors were completed — one in the British and Canadian sector, the other in the American — all supplies and reinforcements had to be landed on the beaches.

The stalemate would only worsen as they faced the difficulties of fighting in the bocage, where high, strong, thick hedges impeded the advance of tanks and men. Over the coming weeks the Allies would keep trying to break out, but their efforts would be largely unsuccessful as the Germans tenaciously held on.

Lord Lovat was surely not the only one who was surprised to find that the commandos were still fighting in the bogs and fields and hedges of Normandy as the weeks ground by. "We thought we'd be ashore for about three days," he later wrote, "and be treated as shock troops who would bust and knock out the opposition and then be withdrawn." Instead, after their early operational successes, his brigade was kept in the field, where it was steadily worn down by attrition.

This was a depressingly common phenomenon among the British armed forces. The military planners had created many such specialist units filled with highly motivated, highly intelligent soldiers who in the days after D-Day were simply turned into cannon fodder. Major Howard's extraordinary coup de main force on Pegasus Bridge, Lord Lovat's commandos, and even the X Troopers themselves were often shoved into the front line with the regular infantry to fill gaps in the line. The X Troopers, however, were no doubt glad to still be in the field rather than having been withdrawn as Lovat had assumed would happen. The last thing they wanted was to be taken out of the fight.

After leaving Peter Masters at the bar at Sallenelles, George Saunders had not proceeded more than a mile or two northeast when he joined No. 45 (RM) Cdo., massing for the attack on the small seaside town of Franceville-Plage. A cluster of little villas separated by narrow cobblestone streets, the village provided plenty of attics where snipers could hide.

Saunders and fellow X Trooper Corporal Percy Shelley were scouting the town ahead of the other commandos. Shelley came from a Hamburg banking family and was an intelligent, somewhat eccentric individualist who had simply borrowed the name of his favorite English poet for his nom de guerre. To top off his artistic persona, he wore a "non-regulation silk scarf," Peter later remembered, "cut from a parachute silk" to look like a cravat. Like their equally eccentric commander, Lord Lovat, Shelley was proving to be a born leader on the battlefield.

As the two entered a cobblestone courtyard, they came under attack. Bullets from enemy snipers pinged all around them. Saunders dove behind a pillar but was hit in the leg by shrapnel from a grenade. Shelley dragged his friend to safety.

"German ambush," Shelley yelled as a warning to the commandos coming up behind them. They heard a tank heading toward them. Spotting a coal bin grid, Shelley removed the grid and both men squeezed inside. Shelley pulled the grid over them just as a tank rumbled overhead.

"That's a Panzer III; we can take that," Shelley said.

Saunders watched in amazement as Shelley climbed out of the bin, ran up to the tank, unclipped one of his phosphorus grenades, and tossed it into the tank's air-intake valve. Panicked, the German crew opened the hatch and tried to get out. Shelley tossed a grenade into the open hatch and took cover as it exploded. The X Troopers had learned about this method of attack during the Skipper's blackboard lessons on German panzers. Once again the Skipper's training was proving its use on the battlefield.

As Shelley sought help for his injured comrade, Saunders started to limp back toward the Allied lines. He discovered that two German ambulances had driven into their staging area by mistake. Pointing his tommy gun at one of the drivers, Saunders yelled at them in German, "If you do exactly what I tell you to do you will survive this."

"Yes sir," the German corporal replied.

Saunders helped fill the German ambulances with eight severely wounded Brits who needed immediate attention. He sat in front with one of the drivers and ordered him to drive south as he was intent on getting his comrades medical help.

The X Trooper and his precious cargo didn't get far before the ambulances were stopped by a German patrol. Saunders whispered to the driver that if he kept the X Trooper's cover, he would make sure the driver was taken care of by the British. The driver, who was "shit scared," as Saunders later recalled, did as he was told. He explained to the German patrol that he was simply carrying the wounded to safety. The ruse didn't work and the Germans commandeered the ambulances. The wounded men were taken to a dressing station for treatment and then on to the German hospital at Pont l'Évêque. Saunders was held in a temporary pen for POWs. After an interrogation in which his cover stayed intact and then imprisonment for a few hours, he managed to climb over a barbed wire fence and make it back through the lines to No. 45 (RM) Cdo., which was still outside Merville.

He did not enjoy his freedom for long. Sent on a patrol the very next night, Saunders got caught again when his lame leg prevented him from running away. He was brought to the same German officer from whom he had escaped the previous day. The officer labeled him a troublemaker and threatened to shoot him, but Saunders argued that if the German shot him, he would have to live with it for the rest of his life.

Saunders was put on a train to a POW camp, but even then he didn't give up. As the train moved slowly across the French countryside, he jumped off and ran into a cornfield. He was caught again, and this time he was shackled in the train car and shipped east to a POW camp. Corporal George Saunders, whom hard-as-nails Manfred Gans called "the toughest guy that ever existed," was now, finally, out of commission.

Elsewhere in Normandy, as dawn broke on D-Day plus 2, Peter Masters and the men of Bicycle Troop were hunkered down on the hilly road to Sallenelles, not far from the bar where Masters and Saunders had shared a drink the previous day. Close by in Franceville-Plage, No. 45 (RM) Cdo. was still trying to take the village as part of the larger effort to capture the Merville Battery.

The road out of Sallenelles started to fill with civilians carrying bags and suitcases. Masters asked one of them what was happening, and he was told that No. 45 (RM) Cdo. was in full retreat from Franceville-Plage. Bicycle Troop was now on the new front line.

Captain Robinson had the commandos quickly dig two-man slit trenches at the crest of the road so that they could fire straight down on any advancing

Germans. As darkness fell, a volunteer who went to check on the German positions was killed by machine-gun fire. Captain Robinson continually radioed headquarters that their position was compromised and they were out of ammunition and rations. They needed to withdraw to a place where they could be resupplied. Instead, headquarters demanded a list of those who should receive medals. Infuriated, Robinson said that could wait, yelling into the radio, "If you're not busy polishing brass buttons, or making lists, or whatever else you're doing, why don't you bloody well get your arses over here and give us a hand?" He only received the order to withdraw once he had hastily drawn up and relayed his medals list. The commandos were told to dump their bikes and get away as quickly as possible.

The survivors found a deserted hayloft, and after a quick meal of dried rations they fell immediately to sleep — the first real rest they'd had since they landed. After a few hours they were awakened by the sounds of fighting. As they stumbled down the loft ladder, they discovered that the Germans were just down the road at Sallenelles.

Captain Robinson ordered the men to fix bayonets and make their way to an apple orchard. The Germans were everywhere, as No. 4 Commando was in general retreat, and the Bicycle Troopers were caught up in the maelstrom. Corporal George Thompson, who had shot the two young Austrians on D-Day and apologized, was shot in the stomach and died, "and nobody apologized to him," Masters later noted in his diary. Captain Robinson was wounded in the attack, the troop sergeant was killed, and five other men were seriously wounded. Bicycle Troop was now without any officers or senior sergeants.

The survivors were ordered to move into a gap in the No. 4 Commando line, a series of foxholes higher up on the hill road between Amfreville and Sallenelles. They were told that they had to hold the area against an even bigger German counterattack that was on its way. With little ammunition and deeply shaken by the loss of so many men, Peter and the rest of the troop moved into the foxholes.

Masters organized a watch system, but everyone kept falling asleep, so he decided to stay up himself all night. He was the senior NCO now, and he felt responsible for his comrades' welfare. At dawn mortars rained down on the two-man slit trenches. Bicycle Troop, exhausted and hungry, fired back with what ammunition they had left. The soldiers in the trenches behind them tossed them cans of "M & V" (meat and vegetable), which Masters described as "chunks of inedible, unidentifiable matter packed in what we knew to be monkey grease." The men were so hungry that they ate the food cold, straight out of the cans. The Germans pressed their attack but the line held.

That afternoon the tide began to turn again as Nos. 3 and 4 Commando, led by Lord Lovat, attacked the Germans with a concerted mortar and artillery assault. Masters and 1 Troop were moved to the other end of the line, to back up No. 6 Commando, whose headquarters was at a farm belonging to a Monsieur Saulnier situated just southeast of Amfreville. There they refilled their ammunition pouches, got food and water, and enjoyed a respite that was not nearly as long as they so achingly deserved.

Manfred Gans's unit was also struggling in the first few days after the landings. Just yards from where he was dug in on the outskirts of Lion-sur-Mer, the troop's headquarters received a direct hit when, according to No. 41 (RM) Cdo.'s war diary, "three Heinkels with spitfires on their tails suddenly swooped out of the clouds and dropped three sticks of anti-personnel bombs." Three Marines were killed and commanding officer Colonel Tim Gray was wounded. Major J. A. Taplin, the unit's adjutant, took command after the attack.

Within a few days Manfred received new orders to assist No. 41 (RM) Cdo. in taking two fortified radar stations near Douvres-la-Délivrande named Moltke and Hindenburg. This was the main Luftwaffe radar station complex, which the Germans had spent three years building, and was their most heavily fortified position on that part of the coast. Since D-Day it had been under sustained attack because the Allies wanted to set up an airfield nearby. The complex consisted not only of the radar stations themselves but also of two heavily fortified bunkers four floors deep that were connected by a series of underground passageways. The compound was surrounded by layers of twenty-foot-high barbed wire on both sides of two

1,000-foot-long minefields. There were also machine guns, mortars, and anti-tank guns, with the bunkers defended by Luftwaffe soldiers and members of the Twenty-First Panzer Division.

These were forbidding targets, but the Skipper had prepared his X Troopers exactly for such a challenge. Manfred Gans, Maurice Latimer, and their fellow X Trooper Sergeant Major Oscar O'Neill (Oskar Henschel) were given orders to sneak into the complex and gather intelligence about how many Germans were inside and what type of weapons they had. Manfred would go to the Moltke and bunker with two Marines, while Latimer and O'Neill would head to Hindenburg with four Marines.

On the night of June 11 Gans led the two Marines toward Moltke. Unfortunately the war that night had decided to be disconcertingly quiet. Outside the complex the three men quickly cut through the layers of barbed wire. They now found themselves in the first minefield, which was approximately one thousand feet across. Manfred had already worked out a plan for passing through minefields safely. As he later explained it, "Elementary physics . . . indicates that crawling is too slow to be viable." Instead, he walked hunched over with one hand on the ground feeling ahead for soft areas, since any time a mine was laid, the surface was disturbed. He mastered this method to the point that he could nearly run across a minefield, a skill that would make him much sought after for advance patrols in the weeks and months to come. Using this method at Moltke, Gans quickly led the Marines safely across the minefield.

They now came to the second dense field of barbed wire. Manfred checked that it did not hide electrified lines, and then the men cut through the wire. Moving quietly and stealthily Manfred investigated the machine-gun positions and found them unmanned, then measured the size of the bunker entrance and noted that it was protected by huge steel doors.

As he was getting the lay of the land, he heard a dog whimpering. It was coming from inside the bunker on the other side of a steel door, where it must have picked up the men's scent. Gans led the others safely back out the way they had come in, making sure to adjust the barbed wire so that it looked as if it had not been cut through.

After their safe return and report on what they had seen, the new CO of No. 41 (RM) Cdo., Lieutenant Colonel Eric Palmer, suggested that Gans lead a group of Marines back into the strongpoint so that they could try to occupy the deserted machine-gun positions.

Two nights later Gans reentered the second minefield with fifteen Marines. They went in at the same spot where Manfred had cut through the barbed wire. Gans went first as a pathfinder and noticed that new Schü-mines had been laid. They looked like cigar boxes, but inside of them was TNT, and a pin sticking out of the box would ignite the explosive inside if it was touched. Gans pointed out one of the mines by crouching and covering it with his hand; he gently laid a white handkerchief atop the second mine so the others would know the spot to avoid.

As the men moved through the minefield, Manfred heard an explosion right behind him. A Marine had set off a mine. Knowing it would likely trigger the second mine, which was under his hand, Gans quickly rolled into a ball on the ground. The mine went off and he was covered with dirt, but he was otherwise unhurt.

Since it was likely the Germans would have heard the explosions, Gans led the patrol back out to safety and then returned with a sergeant to help the Marine who had been wounded. It took nearly two hours to carry him to the edge of the minefield, where a medical orderly with a stretcher was waiting for them. The injured commando lost a foot but he survived.

Upset by this failure, Gans returned to his billet and downed a bottle of heavily alcoholic apple cider. For better or worse, the young Orthodox Jew was drinking and swearing and smoking with the best of them now.

Over the following few nights the commandos prepared for a full assault on the complex. On June 13 Maurice Latimer pushed a Bangalore torpedo across the minefield and against the wall of the Hindenburg station. The torpedo only partially exploded, and keeping his head down, Latimer relit the weapon. As he did so he set his previously injured and bandaged hand on fire. He ran back across the minefield, machine guns opening up all around him as the Bangalore exploded.

At the aid station he was told that his hand was now so badly damaged he would have to return to England. Maurice was furious, fearing that his war was over just as the fight for Europe was getting going. As it turned out he could not have been more wrong, and he would have a lot more to do once he recovered.

Back at the Saulnier farm, Peter Masters was joined by fellow X Troopers Percy Shelley and David Stewart. German forward patrols had become a lot more adventurous, and the farm was under constant assault. A Sonderkraftfahrzeug (SdKfz) 251 half-track mounting a Nebelwerfer "Moaning Minnie" mortar launcher was a particular nuisance, firing mortars at the farm and then quickly retreating out of range.

Shelley and Stewart volunteered to find and destroy it. They stalked the half-track along the Normandy bocage, zeroing in on it every time it fired its Moaning Minnies. Eventually hidden by a tall hedgerow, they got close enough to toss hand grenades at it before closing in and spraying the occupants with their tommy guns. Shelley and Stewart climbed aboard the half-track and drove it back to the Saulnier farm, where it remained for several weeks. This act of bravery and initiative were so impressive that both men received immediate battlefield commissions to second lieutenant the next day. They were among the first battlefield commissions of X Troop, but they would not be the last.

On the evening of June 12 Gerald Nichols went to the Saulnier farm, which was only half a mile from the town of Bréville, to find his good friend Peter Masters. Almost a full week after their fellow X Trooper Harry Nomburg had watched his commanding officer, Captain Alan Pyeman, take a sniper's bullet through his neck, the town still had not been wrested from its German occupiers.

High command decided that the Twelfth Parachute Battalion of the Sixth Airborne Division would be used to take Bréville instead of the commandos

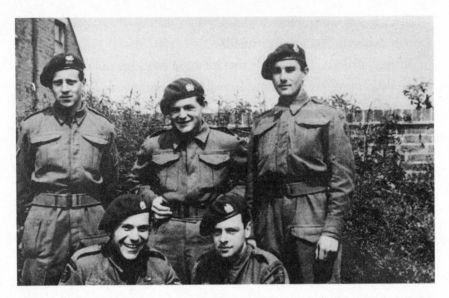

*Clockwise from top left: Percy Shelley, Richard Arlen, George Saunders, Walter Hepworth, David Stewart, 1943*

because they were the fresher force. Nichols was deeply disappointed. "Since they've taken this job away from us," he said to Masters, "let's at least go and watch them do it." When Peter found out that Brigadier Lovat and Brigadier Hugh Kindersley, the parachute battalion's brigade commander, would also be there to watch the operation, Masters agreed to go. It didn't sound dangerous because they would be on the sidelines, and surely if anything did go wrong, they would be protected by Lovat's "aura."

When night fell, Nichols and Masters found themselves with Brigadiers Lovat and Kindersley and their adjutants just outside the Saulnier farm watching the parachute battalion make its way down the leafy road to Bréville. Suddenly artillery and naval shells started to rain down on Bréville, but then, horrifically, the weapons began falling short. High-explosive shells were bursting everywhere, and the entire landscape around the farm was now filled with fire and death. It was a scene of absolute carnage.

Lovat and Kindersley were hit, and piper Bill Millin was knocked over. Men were screaming for medics and trying to take cover. Masters thought Lovat was dead, but before he had a chance to fully process what had happened, more shells came raining down. A barn exploded and splinters of wood fell down like burning arrows. Peter ran for cover in another barn. When he opened the door, he later recalled, "a gaggle of noisy geese, panicked by the shelling, emerged like white bats from out of the abyss. Hell, it seemed, had been let loose all around us." This was what war was, Peter thought. Utter confusion. Geese, dead men, dying men, shells, screaming, no one knowing what was happening.

Masters and Nichols, however, were relatively unscathed, and they knew they had to do something. They couldn't save everyone, but Lovat was special. He was their CO and their mentor. Nichols ran over to him as he lay on his back, unmoving, with blood pouring from his abdomen. Nichols picked him up, put him over his shoulder, and grabbed his walking stick. Staggering under the weight, he carried Lovat away from the shelling into a nearby field. Masters ran back to the rear, where he found a stretcher-bearer at an aid station and told him what had happened. According to Millin, who was still with the brigadier, "Lovat's face was all gray and he had a hole in his back from shrapnel into which you could get a fist — two fists. I said to myself: 'You've got no chance, sir,' and shouted to someone to get a priest to give him the last rites."

As Lovat was carried away on the stretcher he reportedly called out, "I have become a casualty but I can rely on you men to not take one step back. You are making history." Nichols told Lovat that he had his walking stick and he would make sure it would be returned to him.

Yet Nichols and Masters were not finished with their exertions.

They realized that the shells were actually coming from their own side — from a battery behind them that was firing short. Once Lovat and Kindersley were safely driven away in ambulances, they found Captain Brown, the Sixth Airborne Division's forward observation officer, who controlled the Allied artillery. Masters told him that he needed to get word to the men at the battery behind them that they had to cease fire. Brown responded that this was impossible; instead they would need to get everyone out of the way. Then to their horror Brown's jeep took a direct hit from the Germans. He and his driver were killed instantly. Nichols and Masters yelled at the survivors to get off the road.

Masters and Nichols returned to the Saulnier farm, where German prisoners were pouring in from the assault on Bréville. Masters began interrogating them as friendly fire and German artillery continued to rain down. The armory took a direct hit, and two sergeants were killed when the film intelligence unit was destroyed. Everything was on fire.

The hellish scene reminded Peter of the burning of Atlanta in *Gone with the Wind*. "Fires blazed, shell bursts ripped the air, machine gun fire rattled in the background, and the smell of smoke and gunpowder was everywhere. Bodies on stretchers, some stirring, some still, filled the farmyard." Somehow, amid all of this, Peter continued his interrogations of the German POWs. By midnight Bréville had been successfully taken from the Germans and the shelling had stopped.

There were now scores of prisoners at the farm, and they had been placed in Peter's charge. He didn't know what to do with them all, so he found himself marching forty POWs back to brigade headquarters, telling them in German, "March in line and if any of you break ranks without my permission I will shoot you."

With Lord Lovat now out of commission, his second-in-command (and close friend from their Oxford days) Lieutenant Colonel Derek Mills-Roberts was put in charge of the brigade.

Two days after Lovat was wounded, on June 14, Manfred Gans joined No. 41 (RM) Cdo. and the Seventy-Ninth Armoured Division tank battalion for a final daylight assault on the radar stations. After air bombardments from howitzers and ships offshore, the Marines attacked at 5:40 p.m.

For the full attack Sherman Crab flail tanks were used first. These tanks had a rotating roller with forty chains that detonated the mines in front of them. After the tanks came Manfred and the Marines. They ran through the cleared minefields and were now at the concrete defensive walls.

Gans noticed a periscope peeking out from the bunker that went below the Moltke station. He kicked in the periscope glass and wedged a phosphorus grenade into the hole. Then he shot at it and the grenade exploded, sending a deadly burst of white-hot phosphorus into the periscope and the bunker beneath. Immediately afterward the Germans started streaming out, clutching white flags. Approximately 150 Germans came out of the station.

Both stations were taken successfully with only one Marine killed. The British had captured 220 Germans and taken the last fortified position on that stretch of coast.

Based on the Nazi drills he had learned in his Borken high school, Gans yelled commands in German to the POWs as they were marched back to the beaches. On the way he encountered the advance force of a freshly landed British armored brigade, who were stunned to see a handful of Marines marching more than two hundred defeated German soldiers back to where they had just landed.

On June 14, the same night as the final assaults on the Moltke and Hindenburg radar stations, Peter Masters was selected by Major Bryan Hilton-Jones to go with him on a reconnaissance patrol into Varaville, five miles east of Amfreville, where the commandos were now dug in. Varaville had been the scene of intense fighting since the landings and was still being held tenaciously by the Germans. Masters and a handful of men would infiltrate three members of the French Underground into the village.

Accompanying Masters and Hilton-Jones were Harry Nomburg, Gerald Nichols, Percy Shelley, and David Stewart. Among the French partisans was a priest who spoke no English but who was carrying a huge crucifix and a tommy gun. For the mission Shelley had brought a captured German MP40 that he had gotten to like. The men were split into two groups, one with Hilton-Jones, Shelley, and Stewart, and the other with Masters, Nichols, and Nomburg.

Masters's group successfully infiltrated the partisans, but on heading back to Amfreville they were shot at by their own men. "We're British!" they yelled, as they started singing well-known songs such as "Roll Out the Barrel." After a brief, nerve-racking argument about the password (whether they were supposed to say "butter" or "breakfast" as a response to "bread"), they were let through the lines.

The Skipper's group was not so fortunate. As they approached a T-shaped hedgerow, machine-gun fire exploded all around them. Stewart, Shelley, and the partisan dispersed left and right, as the Skipper had trained them to do. The machine-gun fire was relentless and they could find no safe place to regroup. Stewart and Shelley separately made it back to British lines but were shocked to find that Hilton-Jones had not returned. It turned out he had been shot in the stomach, and when he was taken by the Germans he was so near death that a British POW was ordered to dig a grave for him.

Major Bryan Hilton-Jones was posted as "missing, presumed dead."

The X Troopers were utterly devastated by the loss of their beloved Skipper. It seemed to them impossible that their superhuman CO could have perished, and if he had died, it meant that they were all mortal. He was not only their leader but also, for many of them, a father figure of sorts, and they were to a man bereft.

# NORMANDY BREAKOUT

FOLLOWING THE SUCCESSFUL capture of the Moltke and Hindenburg radar stations, Manfred Gans decided to hitchhike the eight or so miles to St. Martin's Church in Amfreville. The church was the informal gathering spot for the X Troopers, and after the Saulnier farm had been destroyed, Gerald Nichols and Peter Masters had moved into one of its deserted wings. The other X Troopers would sometimes hang out there, share stories, and reconnect, and this was also a time when they would learn what had happened to others in their unit.

On the way to the church Gans noticed a newly dug graveyard, and he had a look around. He was shocked and heartbroken to discover the graves of X Troopers George Franklyn, Max Laddy, and Ernest Webster, all of whom had been killed during the D-Day landings. He was particularly aggrieved to notice that they had been buried under crosses and, as he later wrote, "shuddered to think that my own grave would be marked in such a fashion."

When he arrived at the church, Manfred found Peter Masters, Percy Shelley, and Dave Stewart there. The three battle-weary X Troopers were drinking wine and sharing whatever gossip they had about the other members of the troop. Peter Moody was dead. Ernest Norton was dead. Geoff Broadman was still alive.

On June 13 Sergeant Broadman, along with Lance Corporal Moody and Private Ernest Norton (Eli Nathan), had been attacked while doing reconnaissance for No. 48 (RM) Cdo. By then Broadman had become something of a legend. On D-Day he had charged headlong into the German formations, firing his tommy gun as he ran and telling surrendering Germans to make their own way to British lines while he rushed to take the next trench. Broadman was one of those mythical "unkillables," like General George Patton and — for a time — Lord Lovat: men who never flinched as the shells and mortars ripped through the sky. He called his tommy gun "his great love," and in the days following the invasion he became an artist with the submachine gun. During the attack on June 13 Moody and Norton were both killed by a German mortar, and Broadman was shot twice in the leg. He crawled to cover and was eventually rescued and taken to a casualty station, where he was expected to recover.

Gans also heard about Richard Arlen, the muscular, compact welterweight boxer from Vienna who had made it to the European Youth Finals before the Nazis came to power. Although the other X Troopers thought of Arlen as one of the toughest guys in the unit, he had told them during training that in his heart he was a poet. He had also told Masters privately, "I'm going to get myself a Victoria Cross one day, or die in the attempt." Private Arlen had been shot dead by machine-gun fire a few days after the landings while attempting to take a German pillbox at the Merville Battery.

Sergeant Didi Fuller was another terrible loss. According to fellow X Trooper Peter Terry, he "looked not unlike John Wayne and was oblivious to fear." He had been attached to No. 47 (RM) Cdo., and when they landed on D-Day under intense fire, he stood up in the landing craft and said with a huge grin on his face, "This is fantastic, just how it should be, enjoy it, boys." Also on D-Day, Fuller, a used car salesman from Vienna, talked a Nazi strongpoint into surrendering and then confiscated their weapons. On June 13, the same day Broadman was injured and Moody and Norton were killed, Fuller volunteered to hide in a farm with a radio and direct American Marauder bombers to hit a German 88 that was continually shelling the Allied-held beaches. One of the Marauder's bombs fell short and killed Fuller instantly.

At the same time, Gans was told that the Skipper was missing and presumed dead.

After digesting all the terrible news, a saddened Gans headed back to No. 41 Commando. He wrote to the administrative officer of X Troop, Lieutenant Ernst Langley (Ernst Ladau), and passed on the location of the three fresh graves. It would be Langley's duty to write to the next of kin, including Laddy's pregnant wife in Aberdovey. Manfred also wrote to his brother Theo, who was now living in an Orthodox boardinghouse in London. Using his contacts, Theo secured the promise of a rabbi who was the secretary of the Jewish Board of Governors that he would do his best to make sure that the crosses were replaced with Stars of David after the war.

The more optimistic of the Allies had assumed that the breakout from Normandy would take a week or perhaps two at the most. In fact they were bogged down just a handful of miles inland from the beaches for almost a month. The Battle for Caen was still taking place in mid-July even as troops and equipment poured in to reinforce the Allied lines. The German high command now knew that Normandy was the main front for the liberation of Europe and that Hitler had been duped into thinking the attack would come at the Pas-de-Calais. Therefore the British, Canadian, and American armies faced elite German panzer divisions, many of which had experience on the eastern front and were equipped with the latest weaponry, including the most advanced and powerful operational tank of the time: the dreaded Tiger.

During the month of stalemate in Normandy the X Troopers remained in their various commando units. As their COs had now seen how capable they were, they were continually called upon for night reconnaissance behind enemy lines and to assist in occasional skirmishes to gain more territory. While many American and British infantry soldiers found night patrols in the bocage terrifying and avoided these assignments, the X Troopers were always putting themselves forward for them. As Peter Masters recalled, "Often the pulling of straws was for who was allowed to go, not who had to go, on a dangerous mission."

The X Troopers also continued to interrogate enemy prisoners, and these were often deeply personal interviews. Corporal Andrew Turner (Oskar Pollaschek), who was seconded to No. 3 Commando, had spent two years in concentration camps before escaping. Originally from Vienna, he had first been shipped to Dachau, where he had been severely beaten and abused before being sent to Buchenwald. There, in the freezing cold, he was continually beaten and starved and witnessed fellow Jews being murdered in cold blood by sadistic SS officers. A sensitive, shy young man, he could not understand how one human being could get "delight in beating another human being." He later said that he "hated those swines and I always thought 'How can I get my own back?'" He did it by becoming a British commando. During one interrogation Turner was given the job of extracting intelligence from an SS officer: "I saw his uniform and it enraged me. Really enraged me. Of course it came back to me what had happened in the camp. And I said to him: 'Do you know that I'm a Jew?' And he didn't answer me . . . So I said to him: 'You're completely uneducated, you want to rule the world and you people are idiots who know nothing. Nothing!'"

When the X Troopers were not busy doing interrogations, their lives oscillated between those typical extremes of war: terror and utter boredom. Manfred Gans remembered this period as one of mosquitoes, mortars, gunfire, bad rations, and hair-raising night patrols. Much sought after for his field craft, Gans constantly went on reconnaissance missions. Food became a huge issue. Gans and other X Troopers would often sneak over to the American lines and swap war memorabilia and British booze for American food and cigarettes. Gans got to like the Yanks, admiring their preparation, energy, and focus.

On one of his final patrols, near Sallenelles in July with Sergeant Major Oscar O'Neill, Gans was ambushed by a German machine-gun unit. He hit the ground and rolled into a shallow ditch. He could hear the Germans looking for him and calling for the "Tommy" to give himself up. Gans buried his face in the dirt and lay as still as he possibly could. Minutes and then hours ticked by with the Germans smoking and talking nearby. Gans was cold, thirsty, hungry, and desperate to go to the toilet. He didn't want to wet himself because he thought that if he was captured, the Germans might think he had soiled himself in terror. He lay there, waiting, in the ditch, listening to the Germans discuss their actions plans.

In the middle of the night, the silence was broken by a distinct whistle. It was one of the whistles the X Troopers had distributed among themselves so they could signal to each other in the dense bocage. O'Neill was trying to find him. But there were still Germans prowling around; if he stood up now, he would be putting himself and his friend in jeopardy. Gans ignored the whistle. He also gave up holding it in any longer and urinated lying down. Manfred was horrified by how loud the noise was, but the Germans didn't seem to notice.

Just before dawn the German patrol moved out. Manfred slowly got up from the ditch and, after shaking out his limbs, jogged back to the Allied lines. As he approached the British lines, a corporal he knew waved at him. "I was expecting you," the man said. "I was told that you'd been hit and disappeared, but I said not that bloody bloke; he'll come back hale and hearty in the morning." No. 41 (RM) Cdo.'s war diary says of the patrol: "Sergeant Gray [Gans] returned early in the morning of July 2, uninjured, having lain up close to the enemy and having gained much useful information."

With Bryan Hilton-Jones now missing, Second Lieutenant Percy Shelley was temporarily put in charge of X Troop. He immediately promoted Peter Masters to full corporal and Gerald Nichols to sergeant.

At that time Masters and Nichols were still living in St. Martin's Church in Amfreville. The church became a calm and beautiful retreat, especially, as Masters later reflected, after night patrols, when the "morning light would filter in through a lovely stained glass of the local saint, Theresa, holding a bouquet of roses." The men ate bread and cheese that they obtained from a village woman in exchange for their hard "dog biscuits." Every morning that he found himself alive, Masters was surprised. Perhaps, he later recalled, it was because "St. Theresa, with her bouquet of roses had watched over me, a Jewish boy from Vienna, for many a noisy night."

One afternoon Lieutenant Stewart came to the church and told Nichols and Masters there was a new plan for the X Troopers from on high. Because they had shown themselves to be so valuable, they were to be even more strictly "rationed" than before. Whereas in the past they could head out in pairs, that would no longer be allowed so as to not risk losing two X Troopers if they were killed or captured. This meant Masters and Nichols could no longer undertake patrols together.

Shortly after that Nichols was hit by a mortar while doing a solo patrol on a bike. Incredibly he survived, but the concussion broke his jaw and knocked out some teeth, and he was sent back to England to recover. Masters, knowing that his friend had promised to return Lord Lovat's walking stick after the war, took it from Nichols's kit bag to hold it for him. He kept it until the next attack, when he had to leave it at brigade headquarters with instructions that it was the property of Lord Lovat. Brigadier Lovat eventually recovered from his severe wounds and in postwar photographs is shown with a walking stick, but it cannot be determined whether it is the one Nichols recovered in Normandy.

Toward the end of June, Masters was moved to No. 4 Commando because its X Trooper, Walter Thompson (Walter Gabriel Zadik), had been taken prisoner during a patrol and had not been seen again. Being shifted between units like this made it difficult for Masters and other X Troopers to get promoted or be given additional responsibility because, as Peter noted, with each transfer they "had to start from square one to build their reputations again."

The X Troopers' new assignments and guidelines weren't the only changes in the unit. With the Skipper gone and presumed dead, one of their fellow commandos was chosen to take his place as the acting CO of X Troop. Lieutenant James Griffith (Kurt Glaser) was named in early July. This was momentous because it meant that the higher-ups now trusted the German-speaking Jewish refugees enough to give one of them the leading role.

Griffith was the well-liked, soft-spoken, highly intelligent son of a German doctor whose family had safely immigrated to England in the 1930s. Like Maurice Latimer, Griffith had fought in the Spanish Civil War with the International Brigades. He was a medical student before the war broke out.

Griffith had been one of the handful of men selected to do the officer training course, and indeed his accreditation from the course may have been part of the reason he was chosen for this position. Though well respected by the commandos for his sincerity and for not being, in Masters's memorable words, a "parade ground bull-shitter," he nevertheless knew far less about real combat than the now battle-hardened X Troopers, since he had been training while the others had been fighting in Normandy. To his credit Griffith himself recognized that he did not have sufficient combat experience to be an effective leader, and so he started going on night patrols with Masters to learn the ropes.

Although battle fatigue was now common among the soldiers, it was less severe for the X Troopers because they were often out and about on reconnaissance missions rather than stuck in the trenches. So while the night patrols were often scary and dangerous, they at least gave the men the satisfaction that they were doing something to advance the Allied cause.

The battle-hardened commandos whom Griffith inherited from the Skipper were still spread out among a range of units in Nos. 1 and 4 Special Service Brigade. One of these units was No. 46 (RM) Cdo., and one of that unit's most distinguished fighters was Corporal Ron Gilbert. With wavy, straw-colored hair and a dry, witty demeanor, Gilbert had suffered profoundly after fleeing the Nazis and being sent to internment in Australia on the brutal HMT *Dunera*. But all that had only made Gilbert's passion for vengeance burn even stronger.

He was a tough guy among tough guys. On D-Day plus one, Gilbert was marching eleven SS prisoners along Sword Beach when they were shelled by the Germans. Everyone flung themselves onto the sand except the German officer who had commanded the captured unit. "I refuse to grovel in the dirt," the officer said in German. Not to be outdone, Gilbert also stood as the shells came pouring in. The two men faced each other, Gilbert would later recall, and "while all hell broke loose and everything was flying around we just stood there staring at each other."

Gilbert was exhilarated by the street fighting in Normandy — going house to house, clearing villages in the area around Luc-sur-Mer — but he did not enjoy the nerve-racking night patrols, when sometimes you could hear the enemy but were not able to get at them. Fighting in the bocage was personal, messy, confusing, and dangerous. Along with his X Troop friend Leslie Wallen (L. Weikersheimer), he had been involved in the battle to take the village of Rots on June 11, after No. 46 (RM) Cdo. had been placed temporarily under the command of Ninth Canadian Infantry Brigade. The Marines stormed the village, killing scores of Germans and then escaping under fire. Once safely back behind Allied lines, Gilbert found a German rifle bullet embedded in the stock of his tommy gun. "I kept that bullet throughout the war for good luck," he later said.

Gilbert's close friend in No. 46 (RM) Cdo. was Corporal Ian Harris (Hans Ludwig Hajos), another standout soldier. Fearless and determined, Harris was in his element in combat and relished fighting. With dark hair, a full handsome face, and a thin mustache, he looked like a young Clark Gable. Harris had been raised by a Viennese Jewish family that had converted to Protestantism to protect themselves from rising anti-Semitism. He had been educated in a Protestant military boarding school that had become a "hotbed" of Nazis, and he did not know he was Jewish until he was thirteen. Soon thereafter a defining moment occurred at his boarding school: "One day they all started beating up this little fellow and said 'You bloody Jew,' and I was standing there and much to my surprise all of a sudden I joined in and hit him. And he turned around and looked at me and said 'You too?' I shall never forget the face of this little fellow."

The rage that Harris felt toward the Nazis was deep. When he was eighteen he ran away from school and back to Vienna because he could no longer take the pressure of being a Jew in a school that embraced Nazism. In 1939 he made it to England and was soon chosen for X Troop. Like his friend Ron Gilbert, he became a hardened soldier. Recalling the commandos' training years later, he said, "It was miserable and quite tough. I

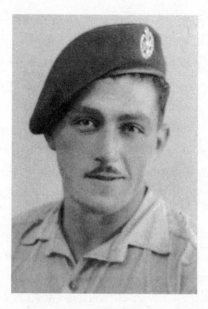

*Ian Harris*

enjoyed it immensely." As Harris described it, once he landed in Normandy he "wanted to kill as many of the bastards as I could."

Like Gans, Masters, and Broadman, Harris began to get a reputation as a man who could get things done without a lot of fuss. He could go out on a reconnaissance mission, somehow get the information that was needed, and come back without getting killed. Harris had, of course, learned his field craft from Captain Bryan Hilton-Jones in Wales, but he'd also been taught survival and patrol techniques by some of the very best Wehrmacht officers at his military boarding school in Germany. He often wondered if any of the men he was facing across the lines were his former school chums. He hoped they were.

One of Ian Harris's more memorable moments occurred on July 23, 1944. X Trooper Peter Terry had been told to lead a fighting patrol of fourteen men from B Troop, No. 47 (RM) Cdo., across enemy lines into Sallenelles to gather intelligence and capture a German officer. In Sallenelles the British and Germans had been in a virtual stalemate in different positions around the town since D-Day. Around 2 a.m. one of the Marines stepped on a mine and, as Terry later recalled, "it was like bright daylight" as flares lit up the night and made it seem as if it were daytime.

The staccato of machine-gun fire ripped through the air all around them. It was coming from a German pillbox just twenty yards away. Terry was hit by shrapnel and dived into a ditch. When Harris heard about the disaster, he kitted up and set out on his own to try to find his mate, even though the area was behind enemy lines.

Harris found the ambush location and wandered out into the fields looking for Terry. "Is anyone down there?" he said in a stage whisper.

"Yes."

Harris shined his flashlight into the ditch, and there was Terry lying spread-eagled, horribly wounded. Harris put his mate over his shoulder and carried him back to a first aid station, saving his life. Terry was sent back to Britain, where he eventually recovered. After Harris found Terry, he went back to look for other survivors, but every other member of the patrol had been killed or captured.

As part of the continuing Battle for Caen, on July 18 Field Marshal Bernard Montgomery launched Operation Goodwood, a limited attack by three armored divisions to take the southern part of the city. At the same time, the Canadians were launching Operation Atlantic to secure the rest of Caen. While the British were unable to penetrate more than seven miles into the Bourguébus Ridge southeast of the city, they kept the pressure on the Germans to keep their strongest formations directed against the British and Canadians on the eastern flank of the Normandy beachhead. This would set the stage for an American breakout on the western flank.

On July 25 Lieutenant General Omar Bradley, one of the most senior commanders in Normandy and CO of the American First Army, launched a massive offensive code-named Operation Cobra to break out of St.-Lô and the areas to the west of Caen. A huge aerial bombardment was followed by ground assaults by the First Army as they sped to the town of Avranches, the gateway to Brittany. The Germans were unable to handle the rapidity of the American advance, their defenses quickly collapsed, and they began to retreat.

The pace of the German withdrawal quickened when General George Patton, who had been kicking his heels in England waiting for a command, was given charge of the US Third Army. Beginning on August 1 Patton aggressively attacked on three fronts: south and west into Brittany, west into the "Falaise pocket," and east toward the Seine. An old cavalry officer, Patton knew how to use tanks in a way that the British generals may never have really grasped. Patton was a student of military history. He had studied Field Marshal Erwin Rommel's tactics and digested them thoroughly. Mobility and fast movement were the keys to success on the modern battlefield. Whereas Montgomery considered it a successful day if they moved the front forward a few miles with minimal casualties, on some days Patton's Third Army moved the front a hundred miles or more.

The X Troopers, who were still seconded with different units of Nos. 1 and 4 Special Service Brigade, supported these breakout operations in a variety of ways. From helping to hold bridges, to conducting information-gathering patrols across the ever-moving lines, to assisting in attacks, they drove forward along with the rest of the Allied forces, providing invaluable grease for the wheels of the Allied war machine as it surged eastward across France and toward Germany.

On August 7 Manfred Gans and the Marines of No. 41 (RM) Cdo. were ordered to assist in the push against the Germans eastward toward the Seine River. They would first make their way southeastward from Sallenelles to Troarn, then head east to Dozulé, located about eighteen miles east of Caen. As Gans later recalled, "Every day we got loaded on trucks, pushed on, dumped somewhere or another, and did another night attack. It was ten attacks in a row with the Germans on the run."

During one such movement A Troop, No. 41 (RM) Cdo., was crossing a field surrounded by thick hedgerows. Leading the men was the A Troop commanding officer, Captain Stevens. As Stevens went forward, Manfred spotted a German sniper in the hedgerows and killed him with a remarkable long-range shot. Gans never had any regrets about killing German soldiers: "On the battlefield you often don't know who shoots at you. It could be Adolf Hitler himself who is shooting at you, or it could be a fifteen-year-old boy from my hometown. If a regime is so depraved to put a fifteen-year-old boy in the front line, it's not my sin or fault that I have to shoot at him."

On August 19 Corporal Ian Harris was sent with No. 46 (RM) Cdo. to help take a hill outside the town of Dozulé. His commanding officer, Lieutenant Hardy, set out with the men at 1 a.m., but it was slow going because it was cloudy and there was no moon to light their way. Much to the dismay of Harris, who thought they should practice field craft and move stealthily, Lieutenant Hardy told them to walk up the hill single file so they wouldn't get lost. This made them easy targets. Harris knew that there were Germans hidden behind the hedgerows, and he warned Hardy about it, but the lieutenant ignored him. Hardy, Harris felt, had always treated the X Troopers as a "foreign body" because they did not speak the "King's English." As the platoon made it to the top of the hill, they were suddenly blinded as the Germans turned on aviation searchlights. Then the Germans let loose with machine guns, grenades, and mortars. Commandos began screaming and falling. It was "absolute hell" as both sides fired at each other in close quarters. Harris rallied some of his men for a flanking assault, but it was too late: the unit had been massacred. He found himself lying in a field having been hit by shrapnel. He passed out, and when he came to, he found that he was lying next to a German soldier.

"Hans, is that you?" the enemy asked in German.

"No, you bastard, I'm not Hans!" Harris replied, and grabbed the German by the throat.

"I will surrender, I am German," the soldier said.

"Yes, I'm German too," Harris replied. "Follow me."

Harris was quite badly wounded, but the German was in even worse shape. Harris helped the German get to a British aid station, and the German thanked him for saving his life by giving him his watch. Harris required surgery and was shipped back to the UK for further medical care.

• • •

Peter Masters was still with No. 4 Commando, which was also on the advance, heading from Bréville north to Bois de Bavent. The entire No. 1 Special Service Brigade was there, led by Lieutenant-Colonel Derek Mills-Roberts, and they retook the area from the Germans on August 19. Although there were a few skirmishes, the Germans retreated, perhaps put off by the realization that fifteen hundred commandos were heading straight toward them.

On August 20 No. 4 Commando came to a château outside Bois de Bavent on their drive toward the Dives River. A white flag of surrender appeared in one of the windows, but when a British party got close to the house to negotiate a truce, they were cut down by machine-gun fire. The enraged commandos immediately went on the attack, quickly capturing the château, which was filled with Germans. Masters interrogated their arrogant commander, who told him that firing on a flag of truce had been a misunderstanding and that he was "happy to have been taken prisoner by you and not by the Russians, nor even the Americans. After all, we have always liked each other . . . We call you 'Tommy'; that's almost a term of endearment. And you feel the same way about us: you call us 'Hans.'" Masters was seething and had to restrain himself from lashing out at the German officer. "No doubt he would have called me 'Saujud' (Jewish pig), had our roles been reversed and had my cover story [been] blown," wrote Masters many years later.

The following week, after nearly three months of continuous action, Masters was sent back to the UK. He was needed for a new job: training new recruits to take the place of the X Troopers who had been killed, captured, or promoted on the battlefield.

The same day that Peter Masters had interrogated the German officer in Bois de Bavent, Manfred Gans, with No. 41 (RM) Cdo., was pushing eastward from Troarn to Putot-en-Auge and then onward to Dozulé. On August 21 they got to Dozulé, which Ian Harris had helped take with No. 46 (RM) Cdo. On August 22 No. 41 (RM) Cdo. headed east toward Pont l'Évêque, where Colonel Eric Palmer asked Sergeant Gans to join him for a reconnaissance mission to the town's railroad station, where the Germans were supposed to be massing for some kind of operation.

Manfred was nervous about any reconnaissance during the day, but again a sergeant could only say so much to a colonel. As British paratroopers lobbed diversionary mortars at the Germans, the pair headed to the train station and soon came under sniper fire from a number of different positions. The whole town had also been rigged with incendiary devices, which the Germans activated from a central control point. As much of Pont l'Évêque went up in flames, Gans and Palmer retreated to the British lines while Manfred returned fire to cover their retreat. No. 41 (RM) Cdo. was ordered to withdraw to the hills that encircled the town, and the surviving townspeople were also on the move. As the citizens and soldiers retreated, the Germans directed artillery fire at them.

Manfred spotted two little girls on the road in front of him just as he heard the sound of another barrage coming in. He grabbed the girls, put them into a trench, and threw himself over them. The shell exploded but the children were safe, and he took them to a Red Cross station. By this point his fellow commandos had given up being amazed by Manfred's many exploits. He did things like that all the time and seemed impervious to enemy bullets.

After Gans and the others had moved out of Pont l'Évêque, the town was taken by No. 46 (RM) Cdo., which included X Trooper Henry Gordon (Kurt Geiser). He was sent to the German military hospital there to make sure it was free of enemy soldiers. Working his way through the corridors with his tommy gun at the ready, he found only those who were too sick to be moved.

In one ward Gordon stopped short, unable to believe his eyes. There was the Skipper, sitting up in bed with a book, looking at him.

"Private Gordon?" Major Hilton-Jones asked with typical sangfroid.

"Sir? Sir! How is this possible? We thought you were dead!"

"And yet I am not dead, Gordon, as you can see."

Hilton-Jones explained that in fact he had been well cared for by a kind German doctor, Ernst Hartmann, and that they had become friends. He had also been extremely lucky: although he had received a devastating wound in the stomach during the ambush, his surgeon specialized in stomach operations and had been able to save his life. When Hartmann received word that the British were about to liberate Pont l'Évêque, he told Hilton-Jones that he would tell his commanding officer that the Skipper couldn't be moved.

By August 29 Hilton-Jones was on his way back to England to continue his recovery at Wolverton hospital. While he was a POW, Hilton-Jones had been awarded the Military Cross in absentia. Upon his return to the UK he would spend months in recovery. Though this would mean he could not return to X Troop before the war's end, he would continue to fight for them once the war was over.

The incredible news that the Skipper was alive spread through the elated X Troopers. Manfred Gans allowed himself a moment of celebration as he continued to slog forward with No. 41 (RM) Cdo.

In the town of Duclair, Gans met with members of the French Underground, who were to arrange the unit's passage across the Seine on rafts. On August 31 Manfred's jeep was the first to cross what was the last major natural obstacle before Paris. Once across the Marines headed to Barentin, where they received a wild, rapturous reception by the locals, who packed the streets to cheer the liberating troops. There were still, however, snipers and pockets of resistance. Manfred avoided the celebrations and instead found a senior German officer, whom he grabbed by the neck. "It's very simple, chum," he explained in German. "Either I shoot you now or we go around the formation and you persuade every single German soldier to surrender. Which is it to be?"

The officer agreed to cooperate.

Manfred was ruthless, but he always preferred persuading the enemy to give up without a fight. Saving lives was better than extinguishing them, even if they were German ones.

After Barentin the commandos moved rapidly toward Belgium, stopping only to pick up and interrogate German prisoners. Manfred received notice that he was being offered a commission, but he turned it down as it would have meant going back to England for officer training. He had learned, to his horror, that his parents had been put in Bergen-Belsen, and he was "absolutely determined," he later recalled, that "I was going to see the end of the Hitler regime; nothing was going to stand in my way."

Manfred Gans's final patrol in France was at the port of Dunkirk, the infamous site from which the British Army had narrowly escaped the advancing Germans in 1940. The town had since been turned into a fortress. During one of his many reconnaissance operations around Dunkirk, Manfred's group came under attack from a much larger German force — a force too big for them to handle. As he later recalled, "The [German] fire was coming from all sides . . . There were five or six of us . . . We [ran and ran] and got ourselves to a sewage tunnel." It was Rosh Hashanah, the Jewish New Year, one of the strangest New Years Manfred had ever experienced. When morning came, the deadly game of hide-and-seek was over. Gans and his comrades managed to make their way back to the Allied lines. There Manfred showered, prayed, and showered again.

The X Troopers had performed heroically throughout the Normandy campaign, killing and capturing Germans, gathering crucial intelligence, and taking on leadership roles. They were trusted and respected, and they were highly sought after for especially hazardous undertakings. As a result they also suffered high casualty rates. Of the forty-five X Troopers who had landed in Normandy on D-Day, more than half, twenty-seven, had been killed, wounded, or taken prisoner.

# THE ADRIATIC

WHILE MANFRED GANS, Peter Masters, and their fellow commandos were mopping up in Normandy, another contingent of X Troopers were distinguishing themselves in the seemingly never-ending Italian campaign. Colin Anson, Paul Streeten, and the original four who had been sent to Sicily in July 1943 had proved so successful that eleven more X Troopers were deployed there and placed in Brigadier Tom Churchill's No. 2 Special Service Brigade.

By early September the US Fifth Army and Montgomery's Eighth Army had landed in mainland Italy, and on September 3 Italy signed an armistice with the Allies, and Mussolini was arrested. Perhaps a more nimble Allied response would have been for British and American forces to push their way up to the Alps. But it was the Wehrmacht that reacted quickly, occupying central and northern Italy, including many mountain passes and strategic bridges. This meant that the Allies had to slog their way north. After an initial optimism that Italy could indeed be, in Winston Churchill's phrase, "the soft underbelly of Europe," stalemate had descended upon the Italian theater. On September 12 Mussolini was rescued from his mountaintop prison by German paratroopers and put in charge of a collaborationist puppet state in the German-occupied northern region of the country.

In Greece, which had been fully occupied by Axis forces since June 1941, the German high command saw the writing on the wall in the summer of 1944, and a strategic withdrawal began in October. Churchill, who had long feared that the rampant Red Army would use the vacuum of the German retreat in the Balkans to drive all the way to the Adriatic Sea, was determined that the Allies should at least establish a presence in Greece before the end of the war. The X Troopers and the commandos would play a crucial part in that plan — and in so doing help determine the balance of power that would define the postwar Adriatic region for decades to come.

Colin Anson and the rest of No. 40 (RM) Cdo. had remained on the Yugoslavian island of Vis following their participation in the successful Operation Flounced, which had wrapped up the day before the D-Day landings and had allowed Tito and his partisans to escape from their hideout in Drvar. Anson kept busy conducting small raids on nearby islands and writing for the No. 2 Special Service Brigade newspaper. Then, in September 1944, he and other members of No. 40 (RM) Cdo. were sent to Albania for a much more substantial assignment: Operation Mercerised.

By the end of the summer 1944 the Allies had air and naval superiority over the Greek theater, and the Germans were relying primarily on the roads along the west coast of Greece and Albania to move men and weapons north in a general retreat that would also shorten their supply lines. The aim of Operation Mercerised was to do whatever was necessary to deny Axis forces the use of these crucial roads. Also, as part of the Allied strategy to cut the enemy off from a northward retreat, the German stronghold of Corfu needed to be captured. But first the Albanian port of Sarandë, which lay just across the Ionian Sea from Corfu and had a German garrison of approximately five hundred men, had to be taken. The plan was that the commandos would first take the high ground above the port and then attack the town from the mountains to the north.

On September 22, 1944, Anson landed with several units of the brigade in a small bay north of Sarandë. The heat was intense, and even in their tropical kit of khaki shorts and short-sleeved shirts the men were roasting.

Moving stealthily they advanced northwest up the steep hills overlooking the bay. It was hard going. The hills ranged up to two thousand feet, and the landscape was unlike anything Colin Anson had ever encountered before. Each step was tough because there were only goat paths through the terrain. The earth was covered with jagged volcanic rocks that tore up his bare legs, and thorns that cut right through his clothes and lacerated his skin.

Thinking that surprise was on their side, the Marines were dumbfounded when shells from German 88s began falling on them from Corfu, three miles across the bay. Scrambling to the top of the ridge, they dug a series of slit trenches between the rocks to provide cover. The 88s fired at the beleaguered commandos all afternoon, and then the sky opened up with torrential, monsoon-like rain. The trench Anson had dug next to a rock face quickly filled with mud. It was raining so hard that everyone expected the storm to peter out overnight, but incredibly, and horribly, it would continue for the next three weeks.

The men had no wet-weather gear, only khaki shorts, shirts, and anti-gas kits, which proved worthless against the rain, cold, and wind. According to No. 40 (RM) Cdo.'s war diary, half the commandos, more than 130 of them, were evacuated to Italy "suffering from exposure, exhaustion, and trench foot."

Anson was not one of them. By now he had thoroughly transformed into a tough, taciturn fighter. He suffered the hellish conditions without complaint: "We were all wet for three weeks, but survived. That's what we had been trained to do, survive in difficult conditions."

"Difficult conditions" is a massive understatement. The rain tore everything apart, including their boots, which disintegrated. As Brigadier Tom Churchill would later recall, "I have never seen anything like it before though I served in Burma . . . and know what monsoon rain is like."

The nights were the worst. Sleep was impossible. Anson would wrap himself in a mud-saturated blanket and lie very still in his water-filled trench. If he was lucky, the "bits of uniform" touching his skin would warm up a little. Drenched, freezing, and sleepless, the commandos also had to deal with the 88 mm shells that the Germans enjoyed firing at them from dusk till dawn. The only respite came with the regular, surprisingly good rations that were delivered from Italy at night onto the beach where they had landed. Unlike during the Normandy landings, when the men had subsisted on dried and canned meals, they now had porridge with sugar, biscuits, and tea. For lunch there was soup that would heat itself as soon it was opened. And for dinner there were set meals such as stews.

During the three weeks of nonstop rain Anson was sent northward on occasional reconnaissance missions, during which he had a knack for finding and capturing German stragglers, whom he then interrogated to get intelligence on the enemy's positions and artillery. He enjoyed working with the Albanian partisans, whose hatred of Hitler was on a par with his own, but he often had to restrain them, as he believed strongly in following the rules of war. Like Manfred Gans in Normandy, Colin savored getting the Germans to surrender without a fight. Sometimes he managed to "bag" more than just stragglers or deserters. "On one occasion," Anson later recalled, "a complete German field hospital surrendered to us and offered their services."

Since joining the Sicily campaign the previous May, Anson had developed into an extremely talented interrogator. He was fluent in Italian and German, and he exuded confidence. He'd grown a pencil mustache like the one sported by the English actor David Niven, and he'd let his hair grow a little longer, now brushing it back. Colin had always been handsome, but now he looked positively debonair, with his commando beret, brown hair, and green eyes. He'd been promoted to sergeant and enjoyed the additional responsibility. He would often joke around with the Axis prisoners, giving them cigarettes and chocolate, charming them, and getting them to share vital information before they were shipped off to POW camps.

On October 4 the rain finally broke. RAF fighter-bombers and the Royal Navy began shelling the port of Sarandë to soften up the defenses in preparation for the land attack. At 4:30 in the morning on October 8 Colin Anson and the rest of No. 40 (RM) Cdo. headed toward the town, situated on a horseshoe-shaped bay, with olive groves stretching above it. Assisting them were No. 2 Commando and a few hundred Albanian partisans. Colin's group entered from the southeastern ridge. With them was a German POW, a plumber from Saxony who had been in a punishment battalion; he had been arrested by the Nazis for giving some of his rations to an Allied POW. Anson had talked to the plumber about Hitler and the Nazis, and he had persuaded him to draw a map of the German positions and where mines were laid between the commandos and the port. Colin then laid a white tape on the ground, showing a safe path through the minefield that surrounded Sarandë, allowing the Marines to advance to the edge of the olive trees.

On the western side of town they encountered fierce resistance from German machine-gun nests and well-supplied infantry. The commandos pressed through the muddy streets, moving from house to house. As the unit's war diary described it, the attack lasted twelve hours and resulted in the capture of 725 prisoners, various artillery pieces, and a cache of diesel oil.

Once the commandos had taken the town, they discovered that there were booby traps everywhere. The German plumber helped them find and defuse a great number of them, until one went off and badly injured his leg. As he was being taken away to Italy for an operation, he said to the commandos, "You are such lovely people. Make sure you get those devils [the Nazis] and catch them for me and don't let them get away." At the end of a long day of skirmishing, Anson returned to the German officers' mess he'd found abandoned earlier and helped himself to the "Hunter" sausages and dark bread of the type he had not had since his youth. There was even lager to drink.

In a rare moment of reflection Colin thought about how much he had changed from the callow, fearful youth of only a few years earlier. Nothing seemed to bother him anymore: not the blood and gore, not the shooting, not the minefields, not the 88 mm shells. Photographs of him from this time show a man transformed. With his tommy gun on his hip, a cigarette hanging from his mouth, his pencil-thin mustache, and his charismatic grin, he looks every inch the happy warrior — a man in the right place at the right time.

Now that Sarandë had fallen, the British had to take Corfu to eliminate the Axis forces completely from that part of the Adriatic. The Germans had begun evacuating the island, but it was believed that a last-stand garrison had been left behind. Anson didn't know it, but just a few months earlier the SS and Gestapo had sent to their deaths Corfu's venerable Jewish population. Approximately eighteen hundred Jewish men, women, and children had been rounded up on June 10 and then shipped to Auschwitz-Birkenau, where they were murdered upon their arrival.

On October 13 Anson and Lieutenant Colonel Robert Sankey from No. 40 (RM) Cdo. took a gunboat across the bay to Corfu to do a reconnaissance mission and potentially capture and interrogate any remaining Germans there. When the two commandos landed on the island, they were stunned to be surrounded by, as Anson recalled, "jubilant Greeks who hadn't seen an Allied soldier in four years." The two men had assumed, naturally, that the Germans had pulled out of Corfu under cover of darkness, but after much drinking of ouzo and being kissed by young ladies and rather a lot of "bearded sea captains," Anson was informed that some of the Axis garrison was still on the island. Sobering himself up, he decided to approach the German fortifications under a flag of truce.

Anson was invited across enemy lines and taken to the garrison commander, who turned out to be a regular army officer rather than a die-hard member of the SS, and who described himself happily as the "uncrowned king of Corfu." Anson explained that there would be no honor in continuing the fight for Corfu, as thousands of British soldiers were about to land and resistance would lead to many casualties for no good reason. Anson's words were persuasive, and the officer surrendered the garrison without a shot being fired.

In the poetic symmetry of Anson's life, it is amusing to imagine that some of the men who had abused little Colin back in Hamburg were among the conscripts who surrendered to him on Corfu. Anson clearly relished playing the role of the blasé, diffident British soldier, and in oral interviews after the war he would always downplay his achievements. Talking about his role in the Adriatic, he would laugh and say that in fact he "liberated Corfu quite by accident."

# WALCHEREN

THE DUTCH COAST, November 1, 1944, 8 a.m. Winter was already here. It was raining hard and a cold wind was blowing seemingly uninterrupted all the way from the pole. As their landing ship, tank, plowed through the rough, gray waters of the North Sea, Manfred Gans, Maurice Latimer, and the other men of No. 41 (RM) Cdo. were huddled in blankets on the deck. They were in an enormous convoy comprising 182 ships and 200 amphibious vehicles. For the commandos, most of whom had landed at Sword Beach five months earlier, it seemed, according to Gans, "like D-Day all over again." They had survived the Normandy landings, the bocage, the Luftwaffe bunker attacks, crossing the Seine. As Gans later recalled, "We were battle-hardened and very experienced."

After the Normandy breakout in August 1944 the Allies had charged after the retreating Germans, but their supply lines had quickly become stretched and their pursuit had ground to a halt. All the men, fuel, weapons, and food were still coming through the Normandy beaches because the Germans were still tenaciously holding the English Channel ports in France and Belgium. Until the Allies could establish shorter supply lines, their forces in Europe would be tethered to the Normandy beachhead and their advance toward Berlin would be stymied.

On September 4, 1944, the Allies captured the largest port in Europe, Antwerp, which lay in the middle of the Low Countries. Taking Antwerp and opening the Scheldt River, which led from it to the North Sea, would cut three hundred miles off the Allied supply lines. Yet after taking Antwerp, Field Marshal Montgomery made a blunder that perhaps added months to the war. He was slow to acknowledge the importance of the nearby German-held Dutch island of Walcheren, situated at the mouth of the Scheldt, even though Ultra intelligence had shown that Hitler intended to fortify it. Approximately ten miles long and eight miles wide, Walcheren was being turned into a fortress filled with artillery that could fire on Allied ships approaching Antwerp.

Staff officers had told Montgomery what was happening in Walcheren, but he was instead focused on his disastrous, overly ambitious Operation Market Garden. The aim of the operation was to clear a route for the Allies straight into northern Germany by using airborne forces to capture and hold three bridges, including the final Dutch bridge over the Rhine at distant Arnhem, nearly sixty miles behind the German lines. The Rhine was the last obstacle before the German heartland, and if the operation had been executed with more gusto and a lot more luck, it might have worked. But Market Garden was a failure. The British paratroopers who held out heroically at Arnhem for more than a week were never relieved, and only a few thousand of them were evacuated safely. During that time Hitler managed to add ninety thousand soldiers to the islands in the Scheldt estuary, and as September rolled into October, more and more German reinforcements poured into Walcheren.

If the war was going to be won in 1945, the shipping lanes to Antwerp had to be secured. As the Allies took the Scheldt islands one by one in a series of battles, Walcheren remained impossible to subdue. British intelligence reported that most of the German Fifteenth Army, which had been so successful against the British in Operation Market Garden, had been sent to reinforce the troops in Walcheren. The shape and location of the island also made it very hard to take. The side facing the North Sea was a series of dunes, some reaching seventy feet high, which attackers might be able to scrabble up with great difficulty but where vehicles could not land. And since much of the island was below sea level, the other sides were lined with heavily fortified seawalls and dikes. There was as well the Sloedam Causeway, a little over half a mile long and fifty yards wide, connecting the east side of Walcheren to South Beveland on the mainland by a road that cut through the mudflats.

The Allied chiefs of staff now made Walcheren a priority, and a new operation, code-named Operation Infatuate, was given the go-ahead. Manfred Gans and his fellow commandos in No. 41 (RM) Cdo. wouldn't be the first to enter the fight, but they would be the ones to help finish it.

On October 3 Allied bombers began a series of raids that breached the seawall and the dikes at the village of Westkapelle, on the west side of the island, giving the landing forces access to the island's interior and causing much of the island to flood. However, because the German fortifications were above the waterline, they were still able to defend their positions. Worse, the flooding had made Walcheren's already formidable landscape even more daunting. Due to the destruction of the dikes, according to the Operation Infatuate II war diary, "the sea pouring in had transformed the center of the island into a vast lagoon, rimmed by massive dikes."

The enemy had anticipated this. As the war diary recorded, the Germans, "tunneling and boring in their usual industry and ingenuity, and employing huge masses of reinforced concrete, had turned this [Westkapelle] dike into an almost continuous fortification . . . Along this rim the Marines would have to fight their way with no room to maneuver — just a grim slog through the deep, loose sand dunes against an enemy well protected by solid concrete." The Wehrmacht had also turned the causeway on the east side from South Beveland to Walcheren into a series of machine-gun nests, with mines and anti-tank guns trained on the choke points. Brave units of the Canadian infantry had attempted to cross the causeway and been massacred.

The commandos were therefore called upon to wipe out German resistance on Walcheren by way of an ambitious amphibious operation. Infatuate I would focus on capturing Flushing in the south, and Infatuate II would aim on securing Westkapelle and the western tip of the island. Infatuate II would be commanded by Brigadier Bernard Leicester of No. 4 Special Service Brigade and would include Nos. 41, 47, 48, and 49 (RM) Cdo. Accompanying No. 41 (RM) Cdo. would be No. 10 (Inter-Allied) Commando's French, Belgian, and Norwegian troops, as well as seven X Troopers. Manfred Gans, Maurice Latimer, and their fellow commandos in No. 41 (RM) Cdo. would land on the northern shoulder of the destroyed wall and dike on the west side of the island and then demolish the German coastal batteries and capture their 220 mm and 75 mm guns. After they had accomplished that, the rest of the commandos with No. 4 Special Service Brigade would come ashore on Water Buffalo and Weasel amphibious vehicles launched from landing craft, tank.

Many of the D-Day veterans must have hoped that this time they would land on the correct stretch of beach. Ominously too this would be the first time since the catastrophe at Dieppe that a frontal assault would be attempted against beaches that were heavily mined and defended with barbed wire barriers, anti-tank defenses, and machine-gun nests. Maurice Latimer, a Dieppe and Normandy veteran, perhaps wondered if his luck would hold a third time.

"Morale was high," Manfred Gans later recalled, not only because his pal Maurice Latimer was with him but also because the commandos were battle ready. Yet from the boat's deck Gans, Latimer, and the others watched in horror as the motor launches that had sped ahead to mark the sandbanks were targeted by German artillery. Within a matter of minutes the Germans sank scores of boats. The water was filled with dead and dying men. Again. This "little D-Day," according to the Operation Infatuate II war diary, was suddenly "far more terrifying than the big one."

No. 41 (RM) Cdo. was now about to land in full daylight under heavy fire. The Royal Navy had promised to lay down a smoke screen, but the wind quickly blew the smoke away. The enemy continued to fire at the invasion force, hitting a number of ships. The sea mines just below the water's surface were also proving to be deadly.

Mere yards from shore one of the landing craft carrying the headquarters staff of No. 10 (Inter-Allied) Commando hit a mine and exploded. As the ship blew up, X Troop intelligence officer Victor Davies, who was sitting on one of the ammunition boxes, was thrown into the air. Miraculously, he landed uninjured in the freezing water. Davies swam to shore, avoiding the scores of corpses bobbing in the surf, and pulled himself onto the beach as shells landed all around him. Unlike Manfred Gans, Davies had accepted the offer to attend officer training school, causing him to miss D-Day and the subsequent Normandy operations. This was a very tough start to his first action.

Davies's fellow X Trooper Bill Watson was on the same landing craft. Watson had fought valiantly in Normandy, driven by his hatred of the Nazis, who had murdered his wife and three young children in Auschwitz-Birkenau. He also survived the explosion but had a nasty shrapnel wound in his hand. As Watson started to swim to shore, he noticed that Captain "Bunny" Emmett, the adjutant of No. 10 (Inter-Allied) Commando, was floating unconscious in the sea. Watson pulled the limp man into his arms, flagged down a boat, and bundled Emmett into it. Both men would survive the experience.

Back on Manfred Gans and Maurice Latimer's landing ship, tank, the Dieppe scenario seemed inevitable, with Germans waiting behind machine guns to simply mow them all down.

But as the landing ship, tank, juddered to a halt, a fortuitous barrage of artillery from the British craft cleared the beach directly in front of them.

The ramp lowered.

Gans, Latimer, and No. 41 (RM) Cdo. ran into the surf. They were determined not to make the same mistake as on D-Day, when No. 41 (RM) Cdo. had lost nearly half its members by being "beach happy." At first glance the shore looked every bit as inhospitable as Sword: the sand was littered

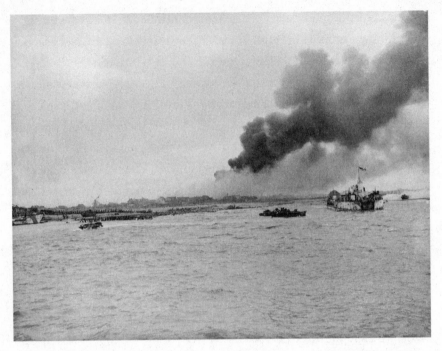

*Landing of the commandos at Westkapelle, Walcheren, November 1, 1944*

with debris and pockmarked with shell holes, and machine-gun fire was pouring down from the German positions above the beach. But Gans noticed that the enemies were aiming too high, and the men also had cover from boulders that lay along the heavily bombed dike. Moving quickly he and the other commandos made it off the beach with relatively few casualties. They moved around the German machine gunners and began making their way north to Westkapelle.

There they found a ghost town. Nearly every house had been destroyed by the RAF bombing that had preceded the landings. In this eerie, apocalyptic landscape the sound of sniper fire rang out on the eastern edge of town. There was nothing they could do about the snipers now, but at the end of the town's main street they found one of their objectives: the lighthouse, which needed to be captured immediately because the Germans

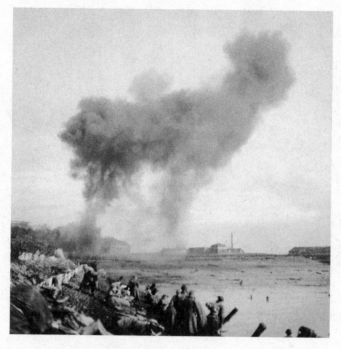

*Commandos on Walcheren, November 1, 1944*

were using it to train artillery fire on the men of Nos. 47 and 48 (RM) Cdo., who were landing farther down the coast.

Only two of the twenty-eight tanks that were supposed to support the attack had made it safely ashore. No one knew quite what to do next.

Gans decided to take immediate action. With his tommy gun on his hip he walked down the main street toward the lighthouse.

"Come out and surrender," he yelled in German, "before our tanks go into action!"

The German officer commanding the lighthouse did come out. He walked up to Gans and asked who he was. Manfred informed him that he was a British commando with half the British Army behind him. The German officer said that he saw no need for further fighting, but then he began to insist on ludicrous conditions for his position's surrender.

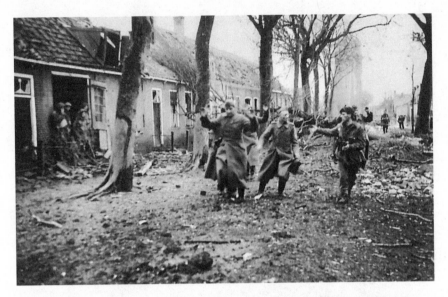

*Maurice Latimer, on right, with captured prisoners from the Westkapelle lighthouse, Walcheren, November 1, 1944*

As they were talking, Gans noticed Maurice Latimer approaching the lighthouse from the flank. A few moments later Latimer came back out, leading a disconsolate line of German prisoners of war. Manfred told the officer that he would have to surrender without any of his stupid conditions. Gans and Latimer led the prisoners back down the beach to the prisoner collection point and returned to the town.

With the seawalls destroyed, a tidal surge flooded Westkapelle just before noon. The Marines took cover on the high ground to wait for the water to recede so they could move on to their next mission: taking the German batteries between Westkapelle and Domburg. The batteries were held by a Kriegsmarine unit and were firing on the Allied troops landing there. They had already sunk three of the Royal Navy's support vessels as well as one of the landing craft, tank, causing 125 casualties.

On the upper floor of a partially destroyed house Gans, Latimer, and the other Marines huddled together for warmth while waiting for the tide to recede. When it did, the commandos were ready to head northeastward on the path that ran along the broken dike. They were going to have to take the first German strongpoint by frontal assault because the inhospitably high dunes gave them no other option. They did not know if they would be mowed down.

Nevertheless, the commandos successfully stormed their first Kriegs-marine battery, W15. Gans grabbed one of the captured sailors and got him to point out the path through the minefield to the next strongpoint. The sodden commandos continued through the dunes, the swirling sand nearly blinding them and filling their mouths, ears, and weapons with grit. Here the normally reticent tone of the Operation Infatuate II war diary be-comes atypically lyrical: "I must ask you to imagine what this fighting was like, struggling through soft, deep sand that clogged rifles and machine guns and filled your mouth, eyes, and hair." They took the second battery, which included two officers, and moved on to the third. As their com-manding officer, Colonel Eric Palmer, noted of their rapid movement, "41 (RM) Cdo. swept like wild fire along the dike."

As night began to fall, the commandos found themselves at Domburg, where they were faced with the next mission: to help take the heavily forti-fied battery there, which was also surrounded by minefields. Capturing this specific strongpoint was crucial because it was being used to fire on ships attempting to get into the Antwerp sea-lanes. Even if they couldn't take the whole island, taking this bunker would greatly assist the Allied cause.

It had been a day of extraordinary successes, and the Marines decided to press on with their advantage by doing a dusk assault on the Domburg Bat-tery. Gans was leading the others through the minefield using his terrify-ing hand-on-the-ground technique when suddenly four Allied Hurricane fighter-bombers swooped in low out of the west, dropping five-hundred-pound bombs on the Domburg fortifications. The commandos froze in the middle of the minefield, expecting at any moment to be killed by friendly fire. In the fog of war Gans had already been shelled by the Royal Artillery and the Royal Navy, and he had been bombed by the RAF. "Here we go again," he thought.

Yet again Gans was lucky. The Hurricane pilots, flying quite low, had spotted the commandos' green berets and avoided them as best they could.

None of the Marines were hurt, but the bombing had distracted the German garrison and given the commandos a narrow assault window to enter the battery.

Gans's plan was to pursue the assault the X Troop way. Heart and head. Brawn and brains. He was going to capture a senior officer and then have him convince his men to surrender. It was pitch-black as they made their way through the last of the minefields. Gans spotted a German soldier taking cover by one of the bunkers.

"You! Surrender!" Manfred called out in German.

The soldier ignored him and ran for the bunker.

Gans raised his tommy gun to shoot, but it jammed because of all the sand.

Manfred knew what to expect next: he yelled at the others to hit the deck as hand grenades exploded all around them. A bit of shrapnel hit Gans's cheek, gouging out a hole the size of a penny.

When the Germans ran out of grenades, Gans got up and ran through the no-man's-land straight into the bunker into which the German had disappeared. His amazed comrades were surprised to see him come out a few minutes later with three prisoners. He hadn't found a senior officer, however, and the pitched battle for the Domburg Battery continued throughout the night.

The commandos finally took the battery the next morning, then entered the town of Domburg itself. Gans described the ruined town as being like a scene from a painting by Hieronymus Bosch: "It was definitely the most gruesome sight I had seen in my life." Many of the RAF bombs had landed short, the town was on fire, the buildings were destroyed, and "a lot of the Dutch in their beautiful costumes were lying dead there on the street." The dead and dying included women and children. German snipers hiding in the ruins were shooting at the advancing commandos, even as the medics were trying to give first aid to the civilians. Gans later wrote that "blood was literally flowing in the streets."

As Gans and the others moved through the town, they found several detachments of German soldiers who had had enough of the war and were attempting to surrender. Gans disarmed them, interrogated them, and told them to make their own way back to the rear echelons with their arms up. Since Manfred also spoke fluent Dutch, he was in heavy demand to help the traumatized civilians.

By noon Gans was totally exhausted. He hadn't slept for two nights, and he had been fighting almost continuously since he had hit the beach the day before. He went into a house across from the temporary commando headquarters and climbed a narrow, winding staircase to a small garret bedroom. He collapsed in a heap on the bed. As a result of his shrapnel wound he was running a fever, but sleep restored him, and by the next morning he was ready to continue the battle.

Not all of his fellow X Troopers on Walcheren would be so lucky. Robert Hamilton (Salo Robert Reich), a "jolly Austrian" as Peter Masters would remember him, who had been looking forward to reuniting with his girlfriend in Brussels, had been killed during the landing at Walcheren. Victor Davies, who had survived the explosion of the No. 10 (Inter-Allied) Commando headquarters ship during the landings and was still fighting with that unit at the time of the Domburg assault, was in bad shape. He spent the first night in Domburg trying to keep a fire going in a cold, windowless schoolroom with the wind howling through the building. Eventually he passed out, and the next thing he knew he was being evacuated back to the mainland. He was later diagnosed with double pneumonia.

Gans spent the next couple of days interrogating hundreds of captured Germans to gather intelligence that would help them take the rest of the island. He was sick to death of interrogations and saw the much-feared Wehrmacht as "a pitiful lazy crowd of soldiers and dandified bullying officers," who through their arrogance and stupidity, as he later noted, had led "this world into catastrophe."

After the capture of the Domburg Battery the invading Allied troops now turned their attention to W18, a Luftwaffe-manned battery that had a commanding location on top of the dunes a bit farther along the coast northeast of Domburg. On November 4, three days after No. 41 (RM) Cdo. had

landed, they were ordered by Lieutenant Colonel Peter Laycock, commanding officer of No. 10 (Inter-Allied) Commando, to conduct a frontal attack.
Both Gans and Latimer felt this was foolhardy because there were rumors
that the battery contained an especially fierce German battalion that had
survived service on the eastern front. But orders were orders. As the commandos approached W18, the enemy saw them coming and started firing
with full force. No. 41 (RM) Cdo.'s commanding officer, Colonel Palmer,
had no choice but to order a retreat.

Palmer's second-in-command was Major Norman Peter Wood, the signaler for No. 41 (RM) Cdo. and a brilliant engineer who had risen quickly
through the unit's ranks. Together the two officers came up with a new
scheme to attack the strongpoint. Using charts that described when and
where each troop would attack and the types of weapons they would use,
the pair created a well-thought-out order of attack. By now a veteran of
many successful operations and many debacles, Gans was impressed with
the plan.

On November 5 the attack began with Hurricane fighters strafing the
target early in the afternoon. Then Colonel Palmer led the men along the
dunes toward W18 as they avoided the incoming fire. As they moved forward, Palmer realized that the timing for one of the groups to advance
was wrong, and he sent Gans to let the unit know. Before Manfred could
reach the men, he was approached by three terrified, hungry Germans who
wanted to surrender. He told them to drop their weapons and make their
way to Allied lines, then he relayed the information to the attacking unit
before running back to Palmer.

Gans was with the first wave to enter the strongpoint from the north after
getting through a minefield where one of the armored vehicles was blown
up. By late afternoon they had taken the strongpoint. Manfred helped gather
together three hundred captured Germans, keeping a particular eye on what
he labeled the "nasties" from the Luftwaffe, and marched them all back to
a temporary POW camp in Domburg.

Gans was deeply saddened to hear that two esteemed members of No. 41
(RM) Cdo., Captain Peter Haydon and his Marine orderly, Byron Moses,

had been killed in the operation. Gans knew and respected the two greatly, having led patrols with them in the bocage in Normandy, where he used to have long conversations with Moses, who was Welsh, about rugby. But his time in Wales was far in the past now, and the road ahead didn't have a clear end in sight.

On November 7 Gans and Latimer were part of the attack on the Black Hut, a bunker complex on the dunes farther northeast along the coast, which was proving hard to neutralize. It had been given the name "Black Hut" because it included two Nebelwerfer mortar launchers that delivered high-explosive shells containing either smoke (to set up screens) or, theoretically, poison gas. On November 6 Sherman tanks had destroyed the rockets for these weapons and then shot holes in the concrete embankment surrounding the bunkers. This was followed by what today would be called "shock and awe" — a full-scale attack with Typhoon bombers strafing the Black Hut with rockets and continuous shelling from 20 mm cannons and the Shermans.

There was a rumor that a high-ranking German officer was in the Black Hut, and it was hoped that if this man could be captured alive, he might be persuaded to convince the Germans in the vicinity that defeat was inevitable and they should surrender. Latimer and Gans were tasked with finding this officer during the attack.

As the Typhoons and Shermans unleashed hell on the Black Hut, the two X Troopers crossed the minefield and entered the perimeter of the bunker complex. Finding the officer seemed like a tall order amid all the chaos, but then Latimer and Gans spotted two German orderlies carrying, ludicrously, a coffeepot, mugs, and sugar.

The commandos quickly captured the orderlies and began an interrogation. "Who are you making coffee for in the middle of an attack?" they demanded. The answer was obvious. "Where is your commanding officer?" Gans asked.

The men remained silent.

"Where is he?" Gans insisted.

"We will shoot you if you don't cooperate," Latimer added, pointing his tommy gun at them.

Suddenly Gans saw a figure emerging from a door in the bunker and yelling in German, "Damn it all! Where is my coffee?"

Latimer tackled the man. Small, lithe, and ferocious, he threw the much bigger Nazi onto the sand and disarmed him. Then he and Gans took the officer back through the lines to Colonel Palmer.

The interrogation was classic good cop/bad cop. Palmer was the voice of cool English reason. Latimer, who had fought the Nazis in the Sudetenland, at Dieppe, and in Normandy, had a strong hatred of the Prussian officer class, and while he menacingly pointed his tommy gun at the prisoner, Gans translated Palmer's requests.

"Look, you're completely surrounded," Palmer said. "I think you and I should go around to these men of yours and persuade them to give up so they don't have any more casualties."

The German officer agreed. Under a flag of truce Gans, Latimer, Palmer, and Major Wood marched the captured officer to a German communications headquarters just outside the Black Hut. After a brief conversation, the surrender of all the men in the Black Hut was negotiated.

The German officer was then taken to British headquarters, where Gans, interpreting, helped negotiate the formal unconditional surrender of Walcheren at 1:15 p.m. on the afternoon of November 8, 1944. Gans would describe the moment a few days later in a letter he wrote to Leo and Luise Wislicki: "The whole garrison was assembled, several hundred [of them, who] handed over their weapons in a bunch. What a scene! Exactly seven times twenty-four hours after the first wave of the initial assault had gone in on the island. How we felt!"

For the next two days the commandos ate like they hadn't since the war started. The captured German positions around Walcheren had yielded massive hauls of eggs, cheese, meat, bread, and wine — enough for the Marines not only to feed themselves but also to set up food banks to share

their cache with the hungry locals, who were thrilled to finally be rid of
the Nazi scourge. The war diary for Operation Infatuate II describes one
memorable scene when the commandos marched through the liberated
town of Westkapelle:

> That morning a little Dutch boy in an orange sash, waving a
> large Dutch flag, stood on top of the dike at the marines shout-
> ing "Good Morning, Good morning" in a shrill treble voice.
> The Marines were a little blasé. Since D-Day, in the progress
> from the Normandy beaches, they had liberated many such
> little villages. But this little boy insisted. "Good morning," he
> shouted in his shrill pipe till at last the Marines noticed him,
> waved and shouted "Good morning" as they passed by. Where-
> upon the Dutch flag was waved wildly in the air and the little
> boy danced with glee, still shouting "Good morning, Good
> morning."

On November 9, just over a week after the initial landing, No. 41 (RM)
Cdo. joined Colonel Palmer in the Domburg movie house, where he
thanked all of the commandos for their hard work. General Dwight D.
Eisenhower would say of Operation Infatuate that it was "one of the most
gallant operations of the war." And the anonymous author of the operation's war diary would eloquently add, "This bold attack, pressed home
with fleeting air support, against formidable, concreted batteries, broke the
last bolt that held fast the door to Antwerp." Following the operation the
Scheldt was thoroughly swept by minesweepers, and by November 26 Antwerp's shipping lanes were open.

After Colonel Palmer's address to No. 41 (RM) Cdo., he called Manfred
Gans into his office. To the X Trooper's surprise Major Wood, who had
helped plan the Black Hut attack, was also standing there. "We have decided
to give you a field commission and promote you to Lieutenant," Palmer
said, shaking Gans's hand. Manfred was delighted. Field commissions

had become extremely rare because Montgomery had been actively dis-
couraging them. (He wanted a professional officer class.) Gans desired
more responsibility, but he didn't want to leave the front to go to officer
training school. A battlefield commission avoided that.

Palmer then asked the commando, coyly, what his real name was. To
his comrades he was known as Fred Gray, but Manfred now admitted that this was merely his nom de guerre. He told his story for the first
time since the war began. He was really an Orthodox Jew from Germany,
and he knew Dutch because his grandfather was originally Dutch and the
family had lived near the border. One can only imagine how surprised
Palmer and Wood must have been to learn that the diehard British commando who had been embedded in their unit since D-Day was actually a
German Jew.

That evening Manfred wrote delightedly to the Wislickis to share the
news of his commission. "I cannot help reflecting," he told them, "on the
long weary way which I have traveled from the barbed wire entanglements
of an internment camp to a king's commission in the commandos." Gans
also mentioned in his letter that he desperately wished to see his parents,
from whom no word had come since he had heard they had been put in
Bergen-Belsen concentration camp.

Palmer gave Gans two days' leave. He drove to Brussels, then in Allied
hands, and there he found a Jewish café that one of his fallen comrades,
Robert Hamilton, had told him about. While at the café he met Hamilton's
Belgian girlfriend and told her the terrible news about Robert.

On his return from his brief leave, Gans moved into the officers' mess in
Middelburg, Walcheren's provincial capital, situated near the island's center, and shortly afterward he learned that one of his closest friends from
training, Andrew Kershaw (Éndre Kirschner), would be joining him. Kershaw was originally from Budapest, where his father had been a prominent architect and his mother came from the well-known Kner publishing
family. Andrew arrived in England in 1939, was soon interned, and was
eventually chosen for X Troop. He was sent to OCTU in Morecambe along

with Tony Firth, Victor Davies, and James Griffith before D-Day, and while undergoing training he married a British woman, Hilda Mary Healey. Kershaw's arrival would mean that Gans would have a close friend with him as he transitioned to being an officer — merely the latest metamorphosis for a soldier whose life had become defined by them.

Unfortunately for the Allies, Hitler too realized the importance of Antwerp, and on December 16, 1944, he initiated what would become known as the Battle of the Bulge. Hitler rolled the dice on a massive surprise attack to retake the port through the heavily forested Ardennes region of eastern Belgium, northern France, and Luxembourg. This, Hitler thought, would split the four Allied armies and perhaps even force them to the negotiating table. After some early German successes, the Allies quickly reinforced their weakened lines and tenaciously fought back. By gambling everything on the attack on Antwerp and the Ardennes, Hitler lost his best reserves of tanks and men and weakened the western front because there were few crack German divisions left to defend the Rhine.

During the Battle of the Bulge, Gans worked with intelligence officers to interrogate captured German soldiers, discovering a hitherto unknown German plan to use torpedo boats on the Scheldt to destroy Allied ships. By the end of January 1945 the Germans had been gradually pushed back in the Ardennes, and it was clear to most neutral observers that this had been the Reich's last stand and the war was coming to an end.

During these months Manfred continued to write regularly to Joan Gerry in New York using his nom de guerre, Fred Gray. In early February 1945 a letter arrived from her that was handwritten in light blue pen. This was unusual because most of her letters were typed. While Joan's previous correspondence had been flawlessly written, this letter was filled with crossed-out words and misspellings, suggesting that it had been written under a great deal of stress.

She wanted to come clean. She was not really Joan Gerry of New York City. In fact she was Anita Lamm from Berlin, the first girl Manfred had

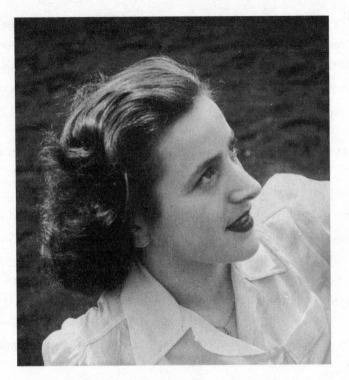

*Anita Lamm*

kissed and the one whose family his father had helped escape to America when the Nazis came to power. She had hidden her true identity because she thought that Manfred wouldn't respond to her letters if she used her real name. She thought he was still angry at her for having ended their correspondence in 1939 at her mother's insistence. Anita wrote that she had "often wondered how you were and what had become of you," adding, "When war broke out I was most anxious to hear that you were well." She also figured that since she had been dropping a lot of hints about her true identity, Gans would figure out it was her, or at least she hoped he would. Anita wrote, "I hope that you will not judge me too severely although I am rather afraid of your verdict." She signed the letter "Yours Jo, or rather Anita."

One can only imagine how Manfred must have felt to have it confirmed that "Joan" was really his childhood sweetheart from Germany. This was a tangible and direct connection to his past that the Nazis hadn't managed to wipe out. Also, it must have been amusing to him that they were both operating under false names and identities. In any case, Manfred did not, as Anita feared, judge her too harshly.

Manfred wrote back immediately. His first words were "My Dear Anita," followed by "Well I'm glad you have given up the bluff at last." He wrote that he had, in fact, suspected she was really Anita because she had gone to such lengths to hide her handwriting by typing all of her letters. He added that she really hadn't had to hide who she was; he had held no grudge against her for stopping their correspondence. In fact he had "just very pleasant memories of her." He signed the letter "Love, Manfred." From then on their letters became even more intimate than before and their synergy was clear. They began planning to meet after the war, in either the UK or the United States.

Anita's was not the only revelation that Manfred received in the mail as 1944 gave way to 1945 and the war's end edged closer. Manfred also received startling news from New York informing him that his parents were still alive.

Not only that, his uncle wrote, but they had been transferred from Bergen-Belsen to Theresienstadt concentration camp. Heinrich Himmler had recently released twelve hundred prisoners from Theresienstadt in exchange for 5 million Swiss francs collected by Jewish organizations. One of the released prisoners from the camp had written to Manfred's uncle telling him that Manfred's parents were being held there. He then conveyed this news to Gans at the Wislickis', his cover address in Manchester.

On learning of this, Gans wrote to the Wislickis that he was "burning to get going to find my parents, but there is no chance as of yet, as longer leaves can't be granted at this moment." The Battle of the Bulge was still raging, and the Allies were still locked in what for Germany had become an existential struggle. Every able-bodied soldier would be needed to bring Hitler to his knees.

First Belgium, then Holland, then the bridges over the Rhine, and then, if he was very lucky, he would try to find his parents somewhere in the ruins of the Thousand-Year Reich.

# CROSSING THE RHINE

PETER MASTERS HAD thought his war was over until January 7, 1945, when on a brief leave visiting his mother in London, he received a telegram that ordered him and sixteen other original X Troopers, including the unit's commanding officer, James Griffith, and Sergeant Harry Nomburg, to board a ship immediately for Holland. They were to go to Antwerp as a possible last-ditch line of defense in case the German "bulge" managed to reach the vital port city. Masters was elated; all he wanted was to be back in the heat of things fighting the Nazis. He had been in Eastbourne for more than six months, since the previous August, instructing new commando recruits to replace the men X Troop had lost during the Normandy campaign. Using the Skipper as his model, Masters trained them as rigorously as he had been trained.

The X Troopers sailed from Tilbury across the Channel to Ostend, Belgium, and then took a train east to Helmond, in Holland. In freezing rain, Lieutenant Colonel Derek Mills-Roberts, commanding officer of No. 1 Special Service Brigade, met the new arrivals and told them that the German advance to Antwerp had been halted when General Patton's Third Army had smashed through the enemy's southern flank, forcing the enemy to retreat.

It was one of those curious moments of war when men who are trained to fight see the fight taken away from them. Masters and the other X Troopers were disappointed at Mills-Roberts's news. They were happy to learn that the Germans had been stopped, of course, but they wanted to be part of the action.

The X Troopers' disappointment didn't last long. Mills-Roberts told the commandos that he would instead use them to help take German-held positions between the Meuse and Rhine Rivers. Although the Wehrmacht was in retreat, there were still pockets of fanatical resistance that had to be destroyed before the Allies' full-scale crossing of the Rhine, the last natural boundary before their assault into Germany.

The X Troopers now had a stellar reputation among the commandos, and because of this they were given the honor of leading the very first search and destroy missions across the Meuse. These operations were particularly difficult not only because the commandos were up against desperate defenders but also because of heavy snowfall and historically low temperatures. Also, unlike the Germans who were equipped with white gear, the commandos were still wearing khaki camouflage, which made their attempts at field craft extremely difficult.

Like Masters, Harry Nomburg was glad to be back on the continent. He had been sent home to England to recover from his wounds during the Normandy campaign. Now he wanted nothing more than to fight the enemy that had caused his parents to disappear without a trace after they had left him at the Berlin train station just a few years earlier.

During one of Nomburg's patrols he led a group of commandos in two rubber dinghies across the Meuse on an unusually mild night. His mission was to capture Germans and bring them back for interrogation. They crossed without incident, but as Nomburg climbed the embankment on the other side he heard "Achtung! Halt!"

Nomburg responded in German, "Hasn't the Signal Section informed you that there'll be a patrol out tonight?"

"We've heard nothing," the Germans answered.

"Show yourselves immediately!" he yelled back.

They came out obediently. Harry took them all prisoner and marched them to the dinghies.

As they paddled back across the river, German machine guns started firing at the boats. Nomburg barely made it back in his damaged dinghy with his terrified prisoners of war.

By March of 1945 the Allies had regained their momentum after the setbacks at Arnhem and the Ardennes, and the Germans had retreated to a defensive line closer to the Rhine. Yet the optimistic feeling of the summer of 1944 was gone; faced with fierce German resistance, the Allied commanders feared that the war was not going to be over soon. The first step would be another amphibious invasion: the crossing of the Rhine.

For the supreme Allied commander, General Dwight D. Eisenhower, a deliberate but brilliant military tactician, the best way to do this was with a cautious set of strategic river crossings. General Patton and the French Army would attempt to cross in the southern sector, from Switzerland to Luxembourg, and the British would attempt to cross in the northern sector. Once these forces were across, the plan was to encircle the Ruhr, Germany's industrial heartland, strangling its military production. After this was achieved, the British and Americans would head east and meet up with the Red Army somewhere near the Elbe River, which runs right through the heart of Germany, and effectively smash what was left of the Third Reich between two pincers.

To prepare for the attack, the British had begun laying down smoke screens, and the Americans had set up dummy regiments in their sector. The smoke was so thick it was hard to breathe, and many commandos became sick. Peter Masters and others climbed to the tops of trees to try to get some fresh air, but with German spotter planes flying overhead, the men were ordered to turn their green berets inside out to conceal their identity.

Operation Plunder began at 5:30 p.m. on March 23, with hundreds of RAF Lancasters obliterating the town of Wesel, the chief communications hub of the German Second Army. The commandos ate biscuits, drank rum, and watched the bombing like a picture show from the western bank of the Rhine. The artillery opened up next, focusing on Grav Island, a swampy area a few miles downstream from Wesel.

The plan was for elements of No. 1 Special Service Brigade, the Canadian First Army, the British Second Army, and the US Ninth Army, with additional support from the First Allied Airborne Army, to attempt to cross the Rhine along a twenty-two-mile front in the vicinity of Wesel. No. 46 (RM) Cdo. was to land at Grav Island, push into town, and secure the bridgehead. No. 45 (RM) Cdo. would then cross the river and head northeast to seize the factory zone. Peter Masters and Ian Harris were with No. 45 (RM) Cdo.; X Troopers Robbie Villiers, the lock picker who had trained the men in Aberdovey, and Herbert Seymour (H. P. Sachs) were with No. 46 (RM) Cdo.

The evening was clear as the Marines packed themselves onto Water Buffalo amphibious vehicles, which had also been used in the assault on Walcheren the previous November. The vehicles looked like tanks but lacked protective armor, having only high tin sides to shield the men inside. The commandos were in camouflage gear with blackened faces, and again they wore their berets with pride rather than "metal hats."

The Germans recovered quickly from the advance bombing and began firing on the Water Buffalos as they crossed the river. The boat next to Masters caught fire and stalled. He didn't know it then, but the two X Troopers aboard that craft, Villiers and Seymour, were both killed. As the men of No. 45 (RM) Cdo. scrambled up the far bank, a young lieutenant whom Masters had been asked to look after told him frantically that he had lost the map with the routes and battle plan. Unable to find it on either the Water Buffalo or the riverbank, Masters tracked down an officer in No. 46 (RM) Cdo. and with a practiced hand quickly copied his map.

The commandos ran up the embankment into the beating heart of Germany. For Peter Masters, a native of Vienna, there was no special joy at being back in the Third Reich. Masters's friend and fellow Viennese, Ian Harris, was, however, elated because crossing the Rhine was what he had been dreaming about since the start of the war. He loved every minute of it. "I really felt I was finally getting my own back," he later recalled, "and I was having a tremendous time."

By the following day, March 24, the British commandos had taken most of Wesel, with the support of the airborne army. Masters and Harris were plying their trade in the basement of one of the town's hotels, interrogating three German engineers who had been captured that morning. Engineers were generally sent to blow things up, and Masters needed to know what their exact mission was.

"Tell us what unit you are with," Masters demanded in German.

"We are not part of any division or battalion," one of the men responded arrogantly.

Peter had kept scrupulous notebooks during his commando training, and he had an illustrator's memory for detail. He reviewed in his mind his drawings focusing on German ad hoc regiments and compared them with the shoulder flashes and sleeves of the captured soldiers. He suspected that they were part of a hastily put together ZBV (*zur Besonderen Verwendung*, "for special deployment") unit that came from the Luftwaffe.

"So you are part of the ZBV then? Luftwaffe men shoved into the front lines?" Peter asked the Nazi.

The man gasped, stunned. "H-how do you know this?" he stuttered.

"Oh, we know everything about you," Peter said. "You cannot hide anything. Now tell us about your plans and your mission."

The information began to stream out of the three men. They explained that they had been sent to Wesel to ascertain whether the town's bridges had been demolished properly when the Wehrmacht had retreated. Harris and Masters took turns interrogating the POWs, who crumbled relatively quickly and gave up the German positions east and north of the town.

Harris remained with the POWs while Masters went to find Lieutenant Colonel Nichol Gray, Colonel Tim Gray's elder brother, who had taken command of the unit after Lieutenant Colonel N. C. Reis had been wounded during the Normandy landings. Earlier that morning Gray and Masters had been talking over mission plans on a street corner in Wesel when a huge blast knocked both men off their feet. They had been shot at by a Panzerfaust, an anti-tank weapon that was held on the shoulder. The colonel was hit by shrapnel, and two men from headquarters were killed.

As Masters headed to Gray's office, he passed the signaler crouched in another room in the basement who was in touch with Allied artillery. When Masters asked what targets they were firing at, the signaler replied that they were only being given routine targets. "In that case I've got a good one for you," Masters said, and asked how big a barrage he could call for.

"Whatever we want, including Uncle and Victory targets," he replied, meaning that every available artillery piece could be trained on the targets. Masters gave him the six-figure map reference of a village that he and Harris had coerced out of the engineers. This village, they suspected, was where command headquarters and German reinforcements were gathered. Masters then hurried on to Gray's office to make sure his CO approved of the barrage.

Peter found the colonel slumped in a chair, his upper arm and shoulder covered with dressings drenched in blood from the wound he had suffered earlier in the day. As Masters entered the room, he saw an orderly pour cold water on Gray's head to wake him from a faint. Once Gray came to, Masters shared the news that he had found where the Germans were concentrating for a possible counterattack.

"Splendid," Gray responded, and told Masters to give the signaler the grid reference immediately.

"I've already done that," Masters answered.

As Peter uttered those words, he heard the sky above start to rumble and then the "long, drawn-out whistle of a great many shells streaking overhead, culminating in a crescendo of explosions." The ground began to shake beneath them. Using the intelligence Masters had gathered, the full force of the Allied attack was underway and the Germans were being pummeled.

For Masters this moment was immensely satisfying.

After Masters and Harris had successfully interrogated the Luftwaffe engineers, they helped round up more German prisoners, persuading pockets of them to surrender rather than fight on pointlessly. Within a few days an American airborne infantry division arrived and brought with it SS men to interrogate as well. At one point Harris lost his cool and hit one of the prisoners in the mouth. Masters was shocked by this breach of protocol. "Why did you do that?" he asked.

"The Germans have lost the war," Harris seethed, "but the Nazis [are] still killing people . . . and when I saw that shitload of silver braid on that sergeant's epaulettes I just lost my temper." Masters got it. He knew that anger was a typical response among the X Troopers to the terrors the Nazis had inflicted on them, their families, and their friends.

After a few days of hard resistance from the Germans, the Allies broke through the enemy's defensive lines on the eastern side of the Rhine and began heading across northern Germany. By March 28 the twelve bridges crossing the river had been secured, and there was now an Allied bridgehead thirty-five miles wide. In the southern sector Patton's Third Army had pushed even farther into Germany.

Shortly after Wesel was captured, Masters was summoned to the mess of X Troop's CO, James Griffith, who had been recently promoted to captain. He gave Peter the surprising news that he was being sent back to England for officer training. Masters refused to go; he didn't want to leave the front lines when the war was nearly over to attend a "bullshit school" where, as he told Griffith, he would be "up to my ears in pamphlets." Griffith explained that the orders had come down from Montgomery's staff and that Masters had to accept the transfer. New X Troopers had to be trained, and they needed officers to do it.

With a heavy heart Peter agreed. As he did so he thought that perhaps Griffith was sending him home because he wanted to make sure he was not killed in the final days of the war after he had survived so much. By early April Peter was back in England to attend officer training school. For him the war was over — again.

When Peter Masters returned to England, Ian Harris became the sole surviving X Trooper with No. 45 (RM) Cdo. He was known among the men as being focused on one thing and one thing only: killing and capturing Nazis for all the evil they had done.

After capturing Wesel, the Marines moved rapidly northeastward across Germany. For the first thirty miles to Erle they were on foot, but whenever possible they also used improvised transport such as bicycles, civilian cars, and handcarts. Once in Erle the commandos were put in trucks for the nineteen-mile ride over pitted roads to Osnabrück, where they would assist the Sixth Airborne Division in taking the city.

After the long, uncomfortable journey the commandos marched into town on the afternoon of April 4. There they found that the Germans had mostly retreated to sniper positions. For the rest of the day and throughout the night they fought street to street, taking the town by the following morning. At the end of the battle four commandos were dead and twenty-nine were wounded.

The SS had set up a satellite concentration camp for slave laborers in Osnabrück. Harris took a jeep and went to the camp, where he came across a group of soldiers — presumably German, although his later remembrances were vague on this point — who were beating Jewish prisoners. Harris rescued the Jews and got them medical attention. "This was one of the better things I did in those days," he later recalled. "They were immensely grateful. I didn't say who I was or what I was. I just saved them."

After this Harris was even more determined to help get the war over as quickly as possible. On the outskirts of Osnabrück he found a lost Hungarian soldier who told him that many of the Axis forces outside the town wanted to give themselves up. The two drove into a German headquarters area with only Harris's tommy gun for protection. Harris was expecting to find a few stragglers there and was shocked to discover an entire SS battalion.

A German major came out, saluted Harris, and asked him, "What do you want?" The major was obviously confused because Harris's uniform had no rank insignias.

"I've come to accept your surrender," Harris replied.

Harris knew that he was in a terrible position. They could kill him outright or take him prisoner. To distract the Nazi major, who was trying to remove his pistol, Harris pulled a packet of Gold Flake cigarettes out of his breast pocket.

"Gold Flake? Is that a Gold Flake?" the major asked, inhaling deeply. "I always smoked Gold Flakes before the war!"

The ice was broken, and Harris threw him the packet. "Here you go, this is for you, old boy," he said casually.

"What rank are you?" the German asked.

"Major," Harris replied (although he was really a corporal at this point).

The officer happily smoked a cigarette. "Perhaps you will have dinner with me and we will negotiate the terms of the surrender?"

"Yes," Harris said.

While they ate a meal of war rations, the officer asked, "Why should we surrender to you?"

"Well, there are more of us than you and our weapons are better," Harris replied.

"Nonsense! The Luger is the best gun in the world. I'll show you. We'll have a shooting competition. My Luger against your machine gun," the major responded.

They went back outside, and the major had one of his junior officers put ten bottles against a wall. The German shot three of them. Then it was Harris's turn. Ten more bottles were lined up. He shot them all with his tommy gun.

The major had seen enough. He told Harris, "We will give up if you guarantee we will be POWs and be sent to America, not Russia." For Germans, the Red Army represented a terrifying force that did not follow the Geneva Conventions, while the Americans were considered to be trustworthy captors.

Harris agreed.

He climbed into his jeep and slowly drove back to Allied headquarters with hundreds of POWs marching behind him.

Harris had single-handedly taken the entire garrison. The sight of Harris with hundreds of POWs was so compelling that a film crew captured the moment. This footage was then broadcast on newsreels throughout the

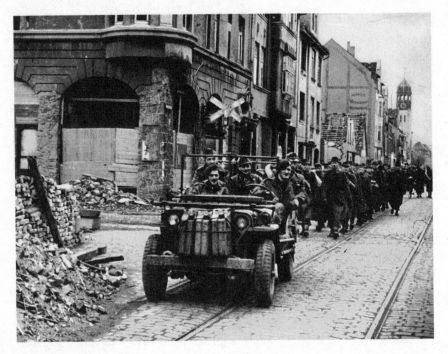

*Ian Harris leading captured German prisoners, Osnabrück, April 1945*

world as a fine example of a British officer taking the initiative. Of course Harris was neither British nor an officer, but he certainly knew an opportunity when he saw one.

As the commandos pushed on from Osnabrück, the next major barrier was the Weser River, where an ad hoc training battalion of the formidable Twelfth SS Panzer Division Hitlerjugend (Hitler Youth) was dug in on the right bank. To get there, the commandos got back in the trucks and headed fifty miles northwest to the town of Stolzenau, where the British faced a ferocious response from entrenched German positions.

It was a scene of utter confusion. Some of the Germans were attacking; others were trying desperately to surrender. Harris ran along the riverbank, capturing those who wanted to surrender and ordering them to the rear. As he approached one of the men, the German tried to blow himself up with a grenade. Harris smashed his tommy gun into the man's teeth, then threw him into the river.

Harris realized that he had overrun a series of German trenches filled with soldiers and he had to act immediately. He ran straight at the enemy firing his Thompson submachine gun from the hip.

He killed several men and grabbed others, throwing them down the riverbank.

Two more Germans rushed at him, but he was out of ammunition and it became a hand-to-hand melee. Harris clubbed one man with his tommy gun and kicked and stabbed the other.

Harris was not done fighting. He saw a terrified British private lugging a Bren light machine gun. "What the hell are you waiting for, man? Give me your Bren!" Harris yelled.

The gunner knew that this lunatic would kill him with his bare hands if he didn't do as he was told. Firing the Bren on the run, Harris charged the remaining German defenders. He couldn't quite understand why they hadn't surrendered by this point. Most of the Wehrmacht infantry he had come across so far certainly would have, but these were SS Hitler Youth, fanatical and fearless teenagers. The young men fell left and right under the Bren gun as other commandos arrived to help him.

Harris's beret fell off his head. He found it, picked it up, and put it back on. Just as he did, the magazine of his overheating gun was hit by a bullet and exploded. Harris's head snapped back, as he later recalled, with a "tremendous feeling of whiplash, rather as if one had been sideswiped by a bus." A piece of shrapnel had hit him in the eye.

Harris rolled down the riverbank, alive but seriously wounded.

Harris was loaded onto a dinghy and ferried back across the river for medical care. There was blood all over his body and he could barely see, except to notice that the prisoner rowing the boat was the one whose teeth he had smashed in. He had no regrets at all about those he had killed and wounded that day. As he later said, "These were the SS and some might have been my former classmates. I knew all about them and I felt so proud that I had accomplished what I had set out to do—to get my own back."

Harris survived, although he lost his eye and wore, with considerable dash, an eye patch for the rest of his life. For his acts of bravery he was awarded the Military Medal for gallantry under fire. The citation for his award was signed by Field Marshal Montgomery. It read: "The courage of this NCO has seldom been surpassed and he undoubtedly saved the lives of many of his comrades by his spontaneous action. His unceasing determination to get at the enemy will always be an inspiration to all."

Some in X Troop grumbled that if Harris had been an officer or a "proper" Englishman, he would have been awarded the Victoria Cross for this action. But Harris was deeply moved by the recognition. As he would later put it, "There weren't many medals going around for refugee boys from Vienna."

A few days after Harris's injury, on April 11, 1945, X Troop's CO, Captain James Griffith, was killed by a German sniper during the advance to cross the Aller River just outside Essel.

Griffith was buried in the woods near where he was killed. Brigadier Derek Mills-Roberts later wrote movingly of Griffith's death and burial:

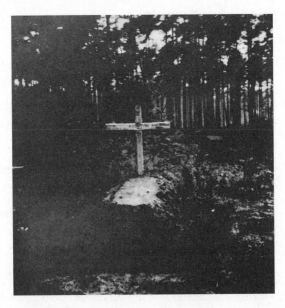

*James Griffith's makeshift grave, Essel, Germany, April 1945*

"This German — who had allied himself to our cause — was a great favorite with everyone and we were very sad to lose him. We lifted James into his grave at the same time as the Medium Regiment fired for the last time—it was a real soldier's funeral." Griffith was interred under a cross, since no one knew that he was really Kurt Glaser, an enemy alien and German Jew.

Griffith was twenty-six when he was killed. He had trained with Tony Firth at OCTU, and later Firth would write of him that he was the "best, most highly skilled, and bravest soldier" he had ever met. That he was killed in one of the final days of the war only added to the tragedy.

# THE FINAL PUSH

THE LOSSES SUSTAINED by X Troop in the liberation of Europe had diminished the strength of the unit just as it was becoming most vital to the Allied war effort. German speakers were needed to help the Allies grapple with the ruined nation that lay before them as they pushed closer to their final victory. More commandos like James Griffith and Ian Harris were required, and fast.

In mid-November 1944 Colin Anson was sent from freshly liberated Corfu to Monopoli, in southern Italy, where No. 2 Special Service Brigade had its headquarters. On December 31 Lieutenant Ken Bartlett, Colin's good friend from Aberdovey — whom he had accidentally shot during training — arrived with interesting news. He had been sent there to organize a new "half troop" of German speakers from British colonial units from North Africa, Jewish refugees from Palestine, and the French Foreign Legion, and he needed Anson's help.

The creation of this new, supplemental commando force coincided with a broader push by the British War Office to enlist more Jewish refugees in the fight against the Nazis. In September 1944 the War Office had created a brigade made up of Jewish recruits from Palestine commanded by Jewish British officers. This hastily assembled formation assisted the British

Eighth Army in several campaigns in Italy in March and April 1945, but ultimately the Jewish Brigade represented something of a missed opportunity. If the British had begun their recruitment earlier in the war and had trained the Jewish Brigade to the level to which the X Troopers had been trained, perhaps it could have become another elite fighting unit that might have altered the course of the war in the Italian theater.

Bartlett would be the CO of the new half troop, with Percy Shelley his second-in-command. David Stewart and Colin Anson would be the two section officers. Colin was overjoyed to be working side by side with X Troopers he had not seen since Aberdovey.

The week after Anson's old friend arrived in Monopoli, in early January 1945, Bartlett and Shelley drove to Caserta, just north of Naples, and interviewed thirty potential recruits, selecting fifteen of them for training. As with the original group, they all had to take on fake names and regiments. The training for the half troop was held in the small hilltop village of Minervino Murge, near Bari, which was also the new location of No. 2 Special Service Brigade's headquarters. The recruits were housed in an empty school on the town's main square, and every morning Anson would wake them up by reading them the news and giving them the day's orders over the school's loudspeaker.

Colin Anson had transformed into a man as fit as the Skipper, and he relished teaching the recruits based on Hilton-Jones's principles. From mid-February through mid-March 1945 Anson and the others trained the men on the hills and plains around Minervino Murge. They mimicked their experiences in Wales but at times added their own creative touches. For instance, to teach the recruits to recognize the sounds of different weapons, Shelley fired a range of guns above their heads in a ravine near the town. With only a month to whip the men into shape, everything was done at an accelerated rate: weapons, speed marches, cross-country marches, field craft, and navigation.

After the training was completed in mid-March, Anson was given a two-week leave in Rome. There he fell in love for the first time, with a beautiful dark-haired woman named Livia. He spotted her at a piazza and approached her — something the shy young man he had been before his military service would never have done. After an initial conversation, he ended up renting a room in her mother's apartment. They had a passionate affair, and he would return to see her later in the spring during his next leave.

On April 4, 1945, the new half troop received orders to assist No. 2 Special Service Brigade in the Battle of the Argenta Gap, the last push to drive the Germans out of northern Italy. The weeklong fight, April 12–19, took place between the British Eighth Army and the German Tenth Army on the muddy plane around Lake Comacchio, in the northeast corner of Italy. Instead of taking part in the battle itself, the half troop was used for the interrogation of thousands of captured Germans. During these interrogations, one of the new X Troopers, according to Anson, went crazy when he realized that one of the prisoners was in fact an SS guard from the concentration camp where he had suffered the torments of hell before escaping to England. Anson calmed the man down, and the X Troopers turned the SS guard over to the military police on suspicion of committing war crimes.

Anson had little time to shave or bathe during this time of nonstop interrogations, and instead of a uniform with a badge showing his rank, he wore a coverall jacket called a Denison smock. One afternoon a column of German open-topped cars drove into the POW holding area, their occupants wishing to surrender to the British. In the front car sat a general who gradually became more enraged as no one rushed to attend to him, and his face turned red with fury. "What's the matter here?" he yelled. "Is there no camp commandant? I'm a general!"

Anson approached and told him that he would have to wait until his men were seen to first. The general was, according to Colin, "horrified and indignant" to be spoken to in German by this man in a Denison smock with a day's worth of stubble on his face. The general bellowed at a German private to carry his luggage, but Anson told the private to do no such thing; the general was a POW now, and he would carry his own bags.

The next day Anson escorted the general and other high-ranking Nazi officials to Bologna. He delivered them to the military police and then found a barber for a much-needed shave and haircut. From Bologna he

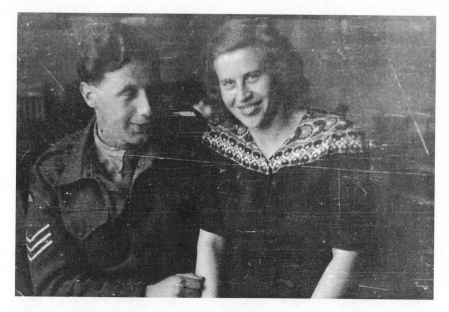

*Ron Gilbert reuniting with his sister, Lilo, in Paris, Fall 1944*

headed west to Ravenna to assist in the interrogation of captured members of a Waffen-SS unit. As he rode his motorcycle west, he came across some British soldiers escorting female prison guards. Colin overheard one of the women say that their escorts were going to lynch them from telegraph poles. Anson told her that no, they were not like the SS — they did not hang people. For Colin it was satisfying to contrast the British treatment of prisoners with that of the Germans, who often operated with barbaric cruelty.

Ron Gilbert had been shot in the leg in the final stages of the Normandy campaign but had refused to return to England. He remained with No. 46 (RM) Cdo. when they went to Dunkirk to fight the Germans in late September 1944. While there Gilbert received news that his sister, Lilo, who had been hiding in France with her young daughter and husband, was still alive. Gilbert had lost his parents, so this was extraordinary news. He knew that Lilo and her family were somewhere in Paris, having moved there from their hiding spot in the South of France following the liberation of the city in late August.

Gilbert went to his CO and explained the situation: "I need to get to Paris to try and find my sister. She is the only one left in my family."

Gilbert was given a jeep and a one-week leave. He drove straight to the city and following a few days' search located them. After a heartwarming reunion they shared a meal.

An elated Gilbert returned to his unit. His story circulated among the X Troopers. Some Jews were still alive in the Third Reich, and if they could end the war quickly, maybe more survivors would be found.

Manfred Gans had not been able to participate in Operation Plunder because he was stuck on desk duty in Walcheren. He wrote of his frustration to Anita Lamm on the night of March 23: "I could just sit down and cry. There is the British 2nd Army driving into my home country (Borken fell yesterday) and here I am sitting in a so called 'quiet sector' doing just about nothing."

The following day Gans received permission to take a jeep to his hometown of Borken with his fellow X Trooper and close friend Andrew Kershaw. Gans felt deep satisfaction at seeing the leveled German towns they drove through, as he wrote in a letter to the Wislickis in Manchester: "On the way there we passed through all these places where such heavy fighting has been lately. Hardly any of them still stand. I'd like to take a photo of one of these completely flat German 'towns' and write underneath it 'Germany, 1945 style.' I think they have had their lesson."

Gans and Kershaw arrived in Borken a few days before Easter and a day and a half after the town's occupation by the Allies. This was Manfred's first time back since he had fled as a youth.

They parked their jeep at the gymnasium, and then he and Kershaw walked around the town. Gans spotted a number of the people who had been so cruel to him and his family. He didn't know if they recognized him now, wearing the uniform of the enemy, and he didn't care. The town had been fanatically defended by the Nazis and reduced to rubble, and he

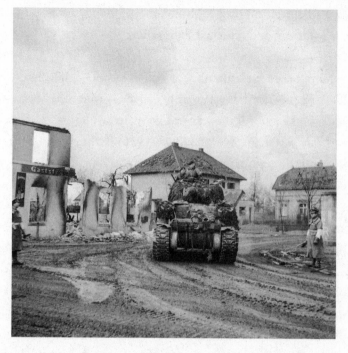

*Sherman tank in Borken, March 1945*

was heartbroken to see that the synagogue where he'd had his Bar Mitzvah had been destroyed.

Remarkably, the Gans family home at Bocholter Strasse 48, on the outskirts of town, was in nearly perfect shape. It had been used as Gestapo headquarters during the war, a place where the feared German secret police had held dissidents and tortured prisoners. Now it was used by the Allied military to house their government staff. When Manfred went inside, his former home still stank of the so-called master race's cigars, brandy, and cruelty.

After their day in Borken, Gans and Kershaw were returning to base when they encountered Field Marshal Montgomery. The British commander had overseen the successful crossing of the Rhine and quick capture of much of northwest Germany, and had established his headquarters in an estate just outside town. The X Troopers got out of their jeep and saluted the most senior British officer in Europe. Montgomery stopped his jeep as well, got out, smiled warmly, and returned their salute.

By early May there were rumors that Hitler was dead, but fierce fighting was still taking place, and huge areas of Germany were still unoccupied by the Allies. No one knew if the war was going to last hours, days, or weeks. The Soviet flag was flying over the Reichstag in Berlin, but in Hitler's Götterdämmerung thousands of fanatical Nazis in allegiance to the Führer were determined than ever to fight to the death and destroy everything.

Manfred Gans had no idea if his parents were still alive in Theresienstadt concentration camp. There was news leaking out that as the war was coming to an end, the SS was massacring Jews by the tens of thousands. They were gassing and machine-gunning and marching them to death because they knew that the game was up and they wanted to wipe out any living evidence of the war crimes they had committed. Every minute was now precious.

On May 6, 1945, Manfred felt he could delay no longer. There were stories circulating that the Germans were about to formally surrender. He went to his commanding officer, Major Norman Peter Wood, and explained the situation. Gans asked if he could take a jeep, a driver, a machine gun, and some cans of gasoline for the four-hundred-mile trek across Germany to Theresienstadt.

Major Wood replied that this was madness, as the war was not even officially over yet. Even though surrender seemed to be imminent, thousands of SS troops in particular had sworn to defy the high command and fight to the death. Manfred was undeterred and Wood eventually relented.

If the Germans wanted to fight, he would give them the death they wanted. Manfred was willing to battle through the heart of the Reich, all the way to the literal gates of hell, if that's what it would take to discover whether his parents were alive or dead.

# INTO THE ABYSS

SUNRISE OVER THE dams, marshes, and wheat fields of Zuid-Beveland, Holland. Lieutenant Manfred Gans of X Troop puts on his uniform, cleans his tommy gun and his .45, and fills a bag with grenades and rations. He finds his driver, a young private from London named Bob, and they get their jeep from the headquarters of No. 41 (RM) Cdo. They load more ammunition and rations and collect transit papers that will permit them to get through roadblocks and receive "all possible assistance" from Allied troops along the way. May 7, 1945, is a warm spring morning, and both men roll up their sleeves. As they pull out of the parking lot, Bob turns to Manfred and says, "I hate to tell you this, mate, but the brakes aren't working properly on this jeep."

"That's OK," Manfred says. "We'll get them fixed on the way."

They drive into the still-rising sun. They don't know it yet, but today will be the last day of the war in Europe. A war that has seen as many as forty million killed, including six million of the continent's Jewish civilian population murdered by the Nazis.

The landscape is flat, green, and speckled with farms and small scenic towns. Tulips are coming up. If "April is the cruellest month, breeding / Lilacs out of the dead land," May is definitely giving it a run for its money in terms of spring flowers, death, and irony. The calm, dark-blue Scheldt runs peacefully by the road. Timber and debris are floating down the river into the North Sea. As they drive east, Holland begins to awake. Adults are out looking for food, children wave as they go by, and some kids can be seen scavenging bits and pieces from a crashed aircraft. The roads have been cleared by Royal Engineer bulldozers, and travel is surprisingly easy. Outside Roosendaal they pick up two hitchhiking Canadian soldiers who want a lift into Germany.

As they come into the town of Tilburg, it is clear the jeep needs to be repaired, so they find a motor pool. No one wants to do any work, as the war is ending and the day is hot. But Manfred is a lieutenant now, and he gets the mechanic to at least try to fix the brakes. They finally continue on, but after a few miles it is obvious that the brakes still aren't working properly.

They cross the border into Germany. The RAF and US Army Air Forces (USAAF) have been busy here. Bob is appalled by the flattened towns, but the hardened Canadian soldiers crack jokes about Nazi Germany and its denizens. Manfred knows this area well and remembers some of the lovely days he had here before the rise of Hitler. His boyhood homeland has been completely transformed by war.

He tells Bob to slow down as they drive through Borken. The Allied military government has set up its headquarters in his old home at Bocholter Strasse 48. American and British flags are flying next to his bedroom window. Most of the other houses in Borken have been pulverized, but his house is in good repair. "It looks very impressive and I am glad. That'll teach the Jerrys."

They continue to the city of Münster along a road that young Manfred had traveled a hundred times. When he was last here, he was wearing the peaked cap of a German schoolboy. Now he is wearing the green beret of a British commando.

Gans and his driver cross into the American lines, where they exchange a few cigarettes for some eggs at a local farmhouse. They spend the night in a barracks the Americans have taken over from the German military. As Manfred lies down to sleep, he thinks of the times he used to stand outside these particular barracks "enviously watching German soldiers drilling." Little did he know that "one day he would be sleeping in the officers' quarters together with the Yanks."

He does not yet allow himself to think about the fate of his parents, who were last sighted east of here at a sinister place called Theresienstadt, in the medieval garrison town of Terezín, Czechoslovakia.

Theresienstadt concentration camp was founded by the SS in November 1941 in a eighteenth-century fortress in Terezín. The camp would serve three main functions: as a transit camp for Czech Jews to the German extermination camps in eastern Europe; as a holding camp and ghetto for elderly and "cultured" Jews; and as a "model camp" to show the world that the Jews were being treated well by the Nazis. As part of this hoax, in June 1944 Adolf Eichmann brought the Red Cross to visit the "spa town"' of Theresienstadt, where elderly and cultured Jews supposedly lived in dignity and comfort. In what is one of the great moral disgraces of the war, the at best willfully naïve Red Cross delegates passively accepted the Nazis' Potemkin village and passed on the propaganda. They saw charming cafés and shops, clean buildings, uncrowded conditions, inmates in new clothes. The delegation even attended a performance of Verdi's *Requiem* conducted by the inmate and well-known Czech composer and pianist Rafael Schächter.

The Red Cross delegation was duped, and photos of the visit were widely disseminated by the Nazis.

The reality was that in preparation for the visit, 7,503 Jews were deported to Auschwitz-Birkenau to lessen the overcrowding; the buildings were freshly painted; the cafés and shops were fake; the new clothing was taken away after the visit; and Rafael Schächter and most of the musicians in the orchestra were later deported to Auschwitz-Birkenau, where they were murdered.

Daily life in Theresienstadt was horrific (as in all the camps holding Jews), and even though it was not an actual extermination camp, 33,000 men, women, and children died there from hunger, disease, and sickness. The winters in the camp were particularly brutal because of the freezing weather and lack of warm clothing, and the overcrowding was another factor in the high death rate.

Approximately 15,000 children passed through Theresienstadt on their way to the extermination camps. To give them moments of normalcy and freedom before their inevitable deaths, the well-known avant-garde artist Friedl Dicker-Brandeis taught them art and collected and hid their paintings and drawings. Before Dicker-Brandeis was sent to Auschwitz-Birkenau, she hid more than 4,000 pieces of their artwork in suitcases that miraculously survived the war. A cache of poetry written by children and young adults there also survived, including the poem "I Never Saw Another Butterfly" by Pavel Friedmann. Born in Prague in 1921, Friedmann was put in Theresienstadt in 1942 and was later sent to Auschwitz-Birkenau, where he was gassed on September 29, 1944. In the poem he writes of living in Theresienstadt: "I never saw another butterfly . . . Butterflies don't live in here."

In the concentration camp, intellectuals, artists, musicians, and actors gave lectures, staged plays and art shows, and performed concerts. Yet tragically nearly every important cultural figure was deported to Auschwitz-Birkenau for that camp's final round of gassings in October 1944. Those murdered included the composer Viktor Ullmann, who in Theresienstadt staged his play *Der Kaiser von Atlantis, oder Der Tod dankt ob (The Emperor of Atlantis, or Death Abdicates);* the pianist and composer Carlo S. Taube; the cartoonist and satirist Bedřich Fritta; the poet and artist Peter Kien; and the artist who collected the children's artwork, Friedl Dicker-Brandeis.

By the end of 1944 the only remaining inmates were approximately 11,000 women and the elderly, whom the SS meant to kill but did not have time to because the Red Army was advancing too rapidly. By April of 1945 more than 13,000 new inmates had arrived in Theresienstadt. The Nazis had marched these people westward before the advancing Red Army could reach their camps. Most were close to death from the march. Dressed in light cotton pajamas, they had received no food or water for hundreds of miles, and many were sick with typhoid fever, which quickly spread through Theresienstadt.

As the great Italian chemist and intellectual Primo Levi made clear, to survive in a concentration camp was not a matter of being strong or being smart. It was a matter of luck. In Auschwitz-Birkenau, where Levi was held, stronger and cleverer people than him were shot or gassed. Manfred would soon find out if either of his parents had somehow had the extraordinary good luck to survive the Holocaust, where approximately 63 percent of all European Jews had been murdered.

The morning after their night in Münster, Manfred and Bob bid farewell to the Canadian hitchhikers and return to the highway. Now it is daylight and they see that Münster is nothing but a "heap of rubble."

They are heading for Paderborn. The roads are becoming more and more clogged with people "pushing handcarts, baby carriages, carrying rucksacks, cycling. Everybody trying to get home: Poles, Russians, Dutchmen, Belgians, French, Yugoslavs and German evacuees." There are many beautiful farms on either side of the road, and Manfred notes that the reason the fields are in excellent shape is that the Germans used slave labor to maintain them.

Soon they are nearly out of gasoline, but they are able to refill the tank with the help of an American fuel truck. In Paderborn nearly every house has been leveled. They drive southeast toward Kassel, home of the Brothers Grimm.

The landscape is striking. Rolling tree-covered hills, scenic villages that are mostly intact, wooded areas. Kassel, which was the headquarters of the local German military district, is, however, nearly flattened. The town housed a slave labor camp that provided workers for a Henschel factory that manufactured Tiger tanks. When the Allies repeatedly bombed the factory, it was repaired by slaves, many of whom were literally worked to death.

On the road east out of Kassel, a spring goes in the jeep's suspension. Luckily they run into an American ordnance shop, where Manfred convinces a reluctant mechanic to fix it. He does it quickly and efficiently, and then they pull onto the autobahn, which is packed with American trucks.

They continue due east toward the Czechoslovakian border. At one point they are pulled over by some American military police, who check their papers; the Yanks are surprised to see any British soldiers this deep into the American sector of the front. They drive on toward the town of Chemnitz and see dazed civilians everywhere, many heading west with all their belongings. The Red Army is close, and white flags have been hung from windows. There are a few German soldiers in full uniform milling about the square. Has the war ended or not? Has this place been taken by the Allies? Manfred isn't sure what to do. They seem close to the Allied front lines, and the Germans look at them with complete amazement. There is the sound of vehicles in the distance, and suddenly Russian soldiers begin flooding into the town from the south and east. Manfred is surrounded by greatcoated Red Army soldiers waving their "papasha" submachine guns.

Two Soviet officers ride over on horses to find out what's going on. Manfred gets out of the jeep, and the officers dismount. "They look grim. Silently they shake hands with us." Manfred knows little Russian, and the Russians don't seem to understand his English or French. Wait a minute, Manfred thinks. "Seien Sie ein Yid?" he asks. Are you Jewish?

"A Yid, a Yid!" the officer nods in agreement.

Manfred explains in German (which the Yiddish-speaking Russian can understand) that they are trying to get to Czechoslovakia. The officer tells him that he's going to have to go back to the American lines and try to enter the country from there, as he can't possibly progress right through the front of the entire Red Army. The men salute each other, and Manfred and Bob leave.

They recross to the American lines. They need to find someone in charge to issue them a formal letter allowing for their passage through the Russian area and on to Terezín. At the local army headquarters they find the American CO, Colonel Blatt, who assures Manfred that he will get them a letter for their safe passage and invites them to spend the night while they wait. The three of them listen to the BBC and hear Churchill's speech stating that the Germans unconditionally surrendered at 2:41 in the morning on May 7.

For most Allied soldiers this announcement means that the war is over and they will soon be going home. But for Manfred Gans and all the X Troopers, VE Day is only the start of a new battle to try to locate any surviving remnants of their families in war-ravaged Europe and to get them to safety. Like Gans, most have heard rumors about Nazi death camps, but the truth would be far, far worse than they ever imagined. The so-called civilized Germans and Austrians they had gone to school with had, in a few short years, become the least civilized people to ever walk the earth.

Early on the morning of May 9, after a bath and a "Yankee breakfast," Manfred and Bob set out again. They are going to backtrack southwest toward the town of Aue, where they hope to find a clear road heading east to Terezín. The jeep is filled with petrol and days of rations given to them by Colonel Blatt. They drive through crowds of German civilians yelling that they want help getting their property back from the Russians, who have been taking whatever they can find as they capture the towns. They are the first British soldiers to appear in this area, and the civilians and soldiers alike stare at them, amazed.

Manfred and Bob reach the mining town of Aue that afternoon after a slight delay due to a flat tire. Located in the mountains, Aue was too far east to be hit by British and American bombers and is still under German administration. As Gans would later describe it, "This was Germany the way it had been during the war, it was relatively untouched . . . Everything was fine and dandy, still the way it had been under the Nazis."

German soldiers and civilians crowd around them, pummeling them with questions. "Are you coming or are the Russians? Can you take our surrender?" The people look bitter, hard, and sinister. For the first time in Manfred's years of fighting on the front lines of major battles, he feels scared as he is surrounded once again by angry, frightened Germans. There is a lynch mob atmosphere. Manfred urges his driver forward.

The jeep speeds out of town and winds through spectacular mountains, and Manfred is awed by the landscape around them. Fir trees line the road, and little rivers come down the hillsides. In the distance he can see civilians cutting wood or tilling their fields as though nothing has happened.

They reach Schwarzenberg and cross the old Czech border into the Sudetenland. The Sudeten Germans, whom Hitler "liberated" after the

Munich Agreement in 1938, are overwhelmingly pro-Nazi and anti-Czech, and the towns are largely untouched by Allied bombers.

They drive into a small village in the Ore Mountains, where Manfred finds thousands of German soldiers unsure of what they are supposed to do. When the soldiers spot his British uniform, they yell out, "Can you take us prisoner? Can you take us to the American lines?"

"You've been fighting the Russians and you have to surrender to them," Manfred tells the soldiers who are waiting there with thousands of fleeing Sudeten German civilians.

"Please, you have to protect us. We cannot live under the Russians; they will rob us," a German woman begs him.

"Your soldiers have done far worse in Poland, Russia, and Holland," Manfred replies icily.

The crowd surrounds the jeep in supplication. Manfred doesn't tell them who he is or why he is there, saying only, "I have to push on. I have a mission."

They continue eastward through the Sudetenland, where they spot some British POWs walking along the road. Gans shares cigarettes and rations with them and gives them directions to Karlsbad. Some of the POWs are mere skeletons. All of their stories end with the same stomach-turning refrain: "You ought to see what they did to the Jews."

The roads are packed with civilians, British and Russian POWs, Wehrmacht soldiers. It's utter chaos. Eventually they start to come across Russian vanguard units that "had never met an officer in a vehicle . . . These were the ordinary men who had survived battles like Stalingrad and were almost at the end of their road. We were the first Allied troops they had run into. They were beside themselves with joy." For the Red Army soldiers who have been relying on propaganda from the Soviets that the war is over, meeting a British officer in a jeep is direct proof that this is indeed the case.

Finally at nightfall on May 9, three days after they set out from the Netherlands, Manfred and Bob reach the garrison town of Terezín. They pick up some Czech Resistance fighters, who show them the way to the camp, which, typical of many Nazi ghettos, is located right in the town itself, set behind heavy barbed wire. They find out that the Red Army arrived here only that morning.

As the jeep approaches the gates of Theresienstadt concentration camp, Manfred remains stoic. He has spent years suppressing his emotions and focusing only on the battle at hand, and it has served him extremely well as a commando. On this journey to Theresienstadt his focus has been on one thing: getting to the camp to find his parents. "At this moment I am pretty cool now, only that queer feeling in the pit of the stomach which I would get before a parachute jump."

The Soviet guards at the camp gates are astounded to see a British officer and ask him what he is doing here.

"I have come here to find my parents," Manfred explains.

They agree to let them in.

The gates open and they drive into a nightmare.

Hundreds of starving Jews crowd around the jeep. Thousands more are crammed into huts. Typhoid fever and starvation are rampant, and the dead are lying everywhere. The Soviets have not begun organized relief. Men and women wrapped in blankets or rags, with oh so familiar Jewish faces, reach out to Manfred. He hears Yiddish, German, French, Czech, Romanian, Dutch, Polish. They are too sick to string together coherent sentences. They are living skeletons.

Manfred stops the jeep and moves into the crowd.

It is a scene worse than he ever imagined. The rumors of Nazi savagery were all true.

"How do I find my parents?" Manfred asks someone.

"There is a central register. You should go there."

Like all the German camps, Theresienstadt is efficiently organized, with carefully cataloged data on the living, dying, and dead. Manfred finds the registration office, the Meldestelle, and is stunned that there is actually someone working there, a lone young Jewish woman.

"Ich suche nach Moritz Gans und Else Gans," he says.

The stupefied woman starts looking through an endless roster of names.

Suddenly she looks up in amazement and starts crying with joy. She responds in English, "I think you are lucky. I think they are still here. They are here."

"Please take me to them," he says.

Manfred and the young woman get in the jeep, and Bob drives them along more roads filled with dying people. They pass buildings and through the windows Manfred sees stacks of bunk beds with two or three people lying on each of them.

They reach a house in the so-called Dutch Colony section of the camp. His parents were put here, he later learns, because they were originally taken by the SS when they were hiding on a Dutch farm.

"Your parents should be in here," the young woman says.

"Please find them and tell them that their son is here," Manfred says, worried that the shock of seeing him will be too much for them.

The woman goes into the house and after a few minutes returns and says that she has found his parents and told them the news. She leads him inside the building and up the packed staircase to the apartment where his parents have been living.

Manfred's diary records the reunion: "The next minutes are indescribable. I suddenly find myself in their arms. They are both crying wildly. It sounds like the crying of despair. I look at Father and in spite of having prepared myself for a lot, I have to bite my teeth together not to show my shock. He is hardly recognizable. Completely starved and wrecked."

Manfred later said, "If I had met him on the street I wouldn't have recognized him."

His father is at first too overwhelmed to speak.

Quickly the news gets out in the camp: The impossible has happened. A son has returned to seek his parents and has found them. Not all the Jews in the world have been killed. The Nazis have not triumphed everywhere.

Outside the packed house where Moritz and Else have been living, the mute, broken masses of Jews start reacting with joy and disbelief to the news of the Ganses' reunion with their son. Yells of "Mazel tov" fill the air from the street below. As word spreads, people from the camp come and offer congratulations and gaze in wonder at this German Jewish British commando.

Manfred remembers that his driver is still outside, having eaten nothing since early that morning. He calls Bob in, and to celebrate someone produces some matzoh that they have somehow saved from Passover.

While Bob sleeps, Manfred sits with his parents and they talk. He realizes that his father's spirit seems unbroken. They discuss their former lives in Borken and Manfred's brothers, one in the UK and one in Israel. And they contemplate the unthinkable — their future.

It is now very late, and Manfred promised the Soviet guards that they would leave the camp. But he can't bear to part from his parents, so he goes to the office of the Russian camp commandant and gives him the letter asking that all assistance be given to him.

"I came here to find my parents, Moritz and Else Gans," Manfred explains.

The Russian seems shaken by this and gently asks, "Did you find them?"

"Yes."

"Look, I have to close both eyes. I can't leave you here. There is typhoid in the camp and you'll carry it to the British Army. I'm going to close my eyes but you have to be out of here by eight tomorrow morning, when we are closing the camp completely to stop the typhoid epidemic from spreading."

Manfred agrees that he will leave in the morning. He knows that his parents are far too weak to take them back on roads that are getting more and more dangerous as the Sudeten Germans are becoming increasingly panicked. And he knows the Soviet guards will not let him take them out. He returns to his parents and they spend the rest of the night talking on the apartment's balcony. "There are stars in the sky and it is warm. Many people sleep in the open. My parents and I talk and talk."

His parents tell him the horrific details of their lives in Bergen-Belsen, where hundreds of thousands of Jews passed through on their way to be gassed. They tell of the order when all the girls under the age of fourteen were murdered. They speak of watching a six-year-old nephew of theirs get taken to the gas chamber and then of the murder of Moritz's dear sister and her new husband.

They talk about twice being packed into cattle cars and nearly dying of thirst and hunger as they were shipped first to Bergen-Belsen and then from there, on January 29, 1944, all the way to Theresienstadt. The trip took days. There was no air for the fifty-nine Jews stuffed inside the car, and as they began to suffocate, Moritz was able to punch an air hole in the wooden slats large enough to save them.

When they got to Theresienstadt, the Czech guards and the SS forced them to take off all their clothes to make sure they were not hiding any valuables.

Manfred asks how they survived.

Else had the amazing good luck of getting a job in the SS kitchen, where she would occasionally steal potatoes. Moritz was a high-value prisoner whom the SS might have wanted to use as a bargaining chip near the end of the war: he had been the head of the *League for War Injured, War Orphans, and War Widows* in Borken, and he kept a recommendation from the organization in his wooden leg. The potatoes that Else stole kept them alive during the freezing-cold winter, when so many others died of hunger and disease. For the last month they had been living on nothing but two slices of bread a day.

Moritz and Else ask Manfred about himself and are not surprised to hear that their focused, capable son is a British commando officer. That he knows how to jump out of airplanes. That he has killed and captured innumerable Nazis. He tells them that he was "in a unit that largely consisted of German and Austrian Jews," and he talks about "D-Day, the heavy fighting in France, Walcheren, the endless winter in Holland, the complete ruin that was Germany."

As Manfred talks, one of the prisoners in the camp takes notes so that he can write this incredible story for the camp newspaper.

After Manfred describes the German surrender, his dad says to him, "We can never get adequate revenge for this, because we can't be that cruel."

At four in the morning his parents doze off, but Manfred remains awake, feeling that "I could cry all night." He thinks about all the Jews in the camp: What will their fate be? Will the British take them? Or will their home countries? Will some be able to get to Palestine?

When dawn comes, Manfred gives his parents hundreds of cigarettes, a prized currency for trading in the camps, as well as the huge box of war rations the Americans gave him. As he gets ready to go, the desperate inmates give him hundreds and hundreds of letters to pass on to the Red Cross to send to any surviving family members.

Before Manfred leaves, he meets with the leader of the Dutch Jews, a former judge, to figure out a plan to get his parents and the others out of the camp. They decide that he will try to contact Princess Juliana of the Netherlands and present a letter to her written by the judge describing the situation in the camp. Princess Juliana has just returned from exile in Canada to set up a temporary Dutch government now that the Germans have been defeated.

Manfred tells his parents he has to leave but he will get them out as soon as possible. They share a heartfelt and moving goodbye. As they part, Moritz and Else tell their son that seeing him has given them the will to live.

Manfred and Bob leave Theresienstadt and drive back toward the American lines. On the return journey they pick up as many Allied POWs as they can carry. They somehow manage to squeeze in close to a dozen men, prioritizing those in the worst shape. Many of the men who pile into the jeep are just skeletons, and "one American is a bundle of bones in rags of a uniform."

By 3 p.m. on the afternoon of May 10 they arrive in Karlsbad, where they hand over their charges. Within two days Manfred and Bob are back at No. 41 (RM) Cdo. headquarters in the Netherlands. Manfred gets the letters from those in Theresienstadt to the Red Cross. Then he catches a ride to Breda, the new home of the Dutch government, and makes his way to the Repatriation Department. There he meets a sympathetic young woman, and he describes the situation at Theresienstadt and gives her the letter from the judge who is the head of the Dutch Colony in the camp. As usual Manfred is extremely persuasive, and the woman offers to arrange a private meeting with Princess Juliana. The two of them drive in an open jeep to the royal estate, which is just outside town. He meets the princess, hands over the judge's letter, and describes the situation of his parents and the others in the camp. She promises that she will get the Dutch Jews out.

Shortly thereafter his parents and the others in the Dutch Colony are flown back to the Netherlands, where they temporarily settle in Eindhoven, just a few hours east of Walcheren. They live in a house with a young Jewish woman named Loewenstein, who knew the Gans family from Borken and was successfully hidden throughout the war.

Once back in Walcheren, Manfred receives new orders that he is being sent to Borken to help with the denazification efforts there.

He allows himself an afternoon off before heading back to Germany to resume his duties. He makes a cup of tea, eats his army rations, and goes to bed early, knowing that his parents are safe now. Against all odds, he would later reflect, he had won his own private war.

# DENAZIFICATION

ON MAY 8, 1945, Sergeant Colin Anson was in Italy interrogating Nazi POWs when he heard Winston Churchill's statement over the wireless that the war was now officially over. His response was different than he had imagined it would be. "It was expected that everyone would celebrate and go wild," Anson later recalled. "What happened was quite the opposite. We were all very subdued and rather depressed. It was as though the firm you had worked for, for the last six years had gone bankrupt. I went for a lonely walk."

For the past five years he and the other X Troopers, displaced exiles, had found a brotherhood. Now, with the end of the war, they had to get their bearings without the kind of support others had. Demobilized British soldiers had homes to return to and families and friends to help them, and often they received financial and emotional assistance as they transitioned to civilian life. The X Troopers had no homes to go to, and many of their families had been murdered. They also were not naturalized citizens of Britain, which meant their futures were still uncertain, despite the fact that they had played an important role in the Allies' success.

According to the X Troop war diary, eighty-seven men served in the unit before No. 10 (Inter-Allied) Commando was formally disbanded in

September 1945. Twenty-two were killed in action and another twenty-two were seriously injured, with seven of them, including Paul Streeten, so critically wounded that they were not able to return to battle. Eighteen X Troopers were commissioned during the war, with four, including Manfred Gans, receiving battlefield commissions (an extremely high number for any unit).

When many British soldiers were getting sent home, most of the X Troopers were being handpicked to lead the Allies' denazification campaign in Germany. In the summer of 1945 the Allies found themselves in the midst of a ruined continent, with millions of refugees and concentration camp survivors to be fed and cared for. Berlin and many other cities were in utter ruin, and jump-starting the continent's economy was now the responsibility of the same men and women whose goal during the war had been to wreck the enemy's industrial infrastructure. Germany had been partitioned into different administrative zones run by each of the Allies. The Soviets, in their zone of control, were dismantling factories and moving them east, and refugees were pouring into the Allied sector, adding to the difficulties.

Six million Jews, at least a million of whom were children, had been murdered by the Nazis with the often enthusiastic assistance of the civilian populations. The Allies, therefore, had to sort out how to run Germany and Austria when there were still hundreds of thousands of Nazis and their sympathizers still around. As part of this process of restoring Germany and Austria to democratic nationhood, these countries had to be cleared of Nazism. The denazification campaign would focus on eliminating Nazis from the higher echelons of civilian government and gathering detailed information on their crimes so that they could be brought to justice. In the Trial of the Major War Criminals which ran from November 14, 1945, to October 1, 1946, the highest-ranking and most influential Nazis and their sympathizers were prosecuted by the Allies for war crimes and genocide.

X Troopers, with their fluent German, local knowledge, and intelligence training, ended up playing crucial roles hunting down and capturing Nazis, interrogating them, and preparing documents for the Nuremberg trials. To do this they were transferred into the British Army of the Rhine (BAOR); the Control Commission in the British occupation zone; or field security units which were focused solely on hunting down Nazis.

In this new capacity many of the X Troopers would stay in Germany or Austria for at least a year, sometimes much longer, before being demobilized. Most would use their time back in their original home countries to try to find missing family members, while also hunting down Germans and Austrians who had been directly responsible for destroying their old lives. The war may have been over, but X Troop and its missions, public and private, were not.

Like many X Troopers, Colin Anson was reassigned to the British Control Commission in Germany to help with denazification efforts there. Since his main goal was to get to Frankfurt to try to find out if his mother was still alive, he requested that his first posting be there. His request was accepted, and he was sent to the American sector of Höchst, just outside the city, to work with Field Intelligence Agency Technical (FIAT), which sought to exploit German advances in sciences and technology for postwar aims while also gathering information from the industrial centers about possible war crimes.

Colin tried to find his mother in a city that was nearly unrecognizable. As he walked the bombed-out streets of his childhood, the double identity he had been living with for years as a German Jewish exile and a British soldier disoriented him and caused deep psychological stress. As he later described it, with each step walking ahead of him in Frankfurt was the "ghost of a German schoolboy . . . with whom I had absolutely nothing in common anymore." He was now, for better or worse, Colin Anson, British commando and member of the Church of England, and he would remain that person for the rest of his life. He was British through and through.

Colin managed to locate his mother's apartment on Hermann Strasse. The building had miraculously survived, although everything around it was in ruins. This was the moment he had been waiting for since being sent to England in the Kindertransport while still a teenager. As he later described it, "I started up the stairs and called her name and heard my mother coming down from the top floor . . . I rushed up and embraced her. And she said 'Nanu' (Good Lord! What's all this!)." At first she didn't recognize her own son, who now looked like the British officer he was, but once she realized it was him, they hugged, cried, and talked all night. She told Colin that she had suffered profoundly not knowing where he was, and that she was still heartbroken over the murder of her beloved husband in Dachau. She described the cruelty with which she had been treated by coworkers and friends for not having divorced her Jewish husband after he was arrested. She was comforted, however, to have her son back and living so close by.

Colin's job at FIAT included translating German documents related to industry and science. He also went to Berlin two days a week to translate and review documents from Albert Speer's Ministry of Armaments and War Production, and his research would later be used in Speer's war crimes trial.

When not working or visiting with his mother, Anson spent any free time he had trying to find the person who had denounced his father to the Gestapo. He used his contacts in the Frankfurt police to receive permission to go through his father's arrest file, where he learned that his father had been betrayed by a man named Henkel, a lockkeeper on the Main River. Anson located Henkel and for a morning considered shooting him in cold blood, but after much soul-searching he simply reported him to the denazification office. Anson later said, "I hated the Nazis, but I could not enact revenge on Herr Henkel for the death of my father. It was not my place to take another life in revenge."

Just before Anson was demobilized in August 1946, he received a recommendation from the Skipper. Colin kept the cherished letter for the rest of his life. In it Hilton-Jones wrote that Anson had "shown himself throughout to be an extremely capable and effective soldier" who always approached his work with "readiness and enthusiasm." In conclusion, he wrote, Anson had "made himself one of the most valuable members of a unit whose standard happened to be exceptionally high." One can only imagine how extraordinarily gratifying it must have been for Anson to read these words from his much-loved Skipper, validating his transformation from an awkward, accident-prone young man into a tough, battle-hardened commando.

Unlike Colin Anson, who had a mother in Germany, Sergeant Ron Gilbert had lost both his parents to the Nazis. With no immediate family left in the country, his aim was different: to root out the Nazis who had destroyed his old life.

Gilbert was sent to Essen to help find and capture Nazis as part of a team led by Major Kenneth Wright, previously the intelligence officer of No. 4 Commando. On one mission soon after VE Day in Hildesheim, Gilbert drove a car filled with pro-Nazi members of the Werewolf movement, which sought to violently resist the Allied occupation of Germany. He was pretending to be a sympathetic member of the group. The vehicle's trunk was filled with weapons that the group had just retrieved from a hiding spot in the woods near Hildesheim. They were going to use these weapons to mount an armed attack on the British occupiers. Little did they know that the man who was driving the car — and who had arranged for the weapons to be hidden in the woods — was an undercover British commando turned Nazi hunter.

As they drove through the night, they came upon a military roadblock.

"I have to stop," Gilbert said.

In the back seat, one of the Werewolves pulled out a pistol and shoved it into Gilbert's neck.

"Drive through," he snarled in his ear.

Gilbert hit the gas and drove straight through the roadblock at full speed. The military police pursued them and within moments managed to surround the car. All the men inside were arrested, and the weapons in the trunk were confiscated. Within hours of his arrest Gilbert was quietly released, with the rest of the group unaware that he had in fact set up the whole sting. In addition to infiltrating the Werewolf group and arranging the weapons pickup, Gilbert had arranged for the roadblock in advance and put his foot on the clutch to slow down the car so that the police could catch it. Thanks to him, a major cell and its weapons had been captured.

After unmasking the cell Gilbert infiltrated another one led by an ex–Luftwaffe pilot, Peter Gross. Gross asked Gilbert to go with him to Bremen to meet a group of men who were planning to use explosives placed on small boats to blow up Allied ships. However, something alarmed Gross, and he jumped onto a tram. Gilbert shot at him, but he managed to escape, although Gilbert and the police were able to capture the rest of the cell. Gilbert interrogated Gross's girlfriend and got her to tell him about the ex-pilot's safe house, where Gross was subsequently arrested.

For another mission Gilbert was sent to infiltrate an insane asylum outside Münster where it was rumored that a number of former SS members were hiding by pretending to be patients. Gilbert spent a few days at the asylum, speaking with all the patients. One of them did the interview while sitting on a stool completely naked except for a large hat with a feather in it. The man proved not to be a Nazi, but Gilbert did manage to discover several fakers, including some who served in the SS.

Gilbert also oversaw the distribution of ration books to civilians, whom he required to watch movies about the concentration camps before they received them. He was demobilized on June 28, 1947, and working for British intelligence was made head of station in Düsseldorf.

For most X Troopers it was deeply satisfying to find and bring to justice the Nazis who had wrought so much evil. Sergeant Geoff Broadman, the ex-boxer, was sent back to Austria to work as an interrogator and interpreter for the joint Allied administration. He was also given the task of locating and capturing Nazis in the British occupation zone of Vienna. He would later recall, "We found them, got them, and brought them down. It was like a detective job." He would also end up working on the United Nations War Crimes Commission, collecting and interpreting material for the Nuremberg trials. Lieutenant Tony Firth, who had spent much of the war in officer training school, was posted to the military police in Iserlohn. Having worked as a film extra in London before being interned and sent to Australia, Firth was soon given a job with the police censoring films for any pro-Nazi content.

Captain Gerald Nichols, who saved Lord Lovat's life after the shelling in Normandy but had been sent back to the UK after suffering a serious injury, became a member of the team pursuing Heinrich Himmler, one of the central architects of the Holocaust, who had gone into hiding after the German surrender. Nichols tracked him down to a farmhouse but arrived about twenty minutes after Himmler had fled. However, due in part to the intelligence Nichols gathered interrogating the servants in the farmhouse, Himmler was soon captured. He committed suicide shortly thereafter.

Some of the X Troopers involved in the denazification process found this work profoundly troubling because it brought them into contact with Nazis who had been personally responsible for killing members of their own families. For instance, Fred Jackson (Peter Levy) had to interrogate Rudolf Höss, the notorious commander of Auschwitz-Birkenau, the death camp where Jackson's mother had died. Höss had been in charge of perfecting the means of mass extermination, including the use of Zyklon B gas, which enabled his camp to murder 4,000 Jewish men, women, and children per hour. He also oversaw Operation Höss, in which 420,000 Hungarian Jews were sent to Auschwitz-Birkenau to be murdered in fifty-six days beginning in May 1944. This was one of the most horrific atrocities of the Nazi regime, as the mass murder was conducted despite it being evident to most high-ranking Nazis that they were likely to lose the war. Following the German surrender, Höss escaped to a farmhouse, where he hid for nearly a year before being captured on March 11, 1946, by a group that included a number of German Jews working in various branches of the British military.

Fred Jackson found interrogating Höss so disturbing that, he recalled, "I got drunk for a week. I just could not live with myself. He was the man who had killed my mother." Höss was unrepentant about what he had done, and his callousness and hypocrisy were evident to the whole world a few months later during the Nuremberg trials.

Many other X Troopers were involved in denazification efforts. Sergeant Major Oscar O'Neill assisted in bringing the war criminal Irma Grese, "the Beast of Bergen-Belsen," to justice. Another X Trooper, Geoffrey Dickson

(Max Dobriner), interrogated industrialists who had run slave labor factories. It was a remarkable turnaround in the X Troopers' fortunes, from being
victims of the Nazis to bringing their evil to light and making sure that the
Nazis were punished for what they had done.

After the war Manfred Gans was assigned to Borken, where he had previously lived as a "despised untermensch," as he called it. Manfred was aware
of the irony of his new reality as a British occupier: he was billeted in one of
the town's "most beautiful patrician houses, homes to which Jews would
never have been invited, even in pre-Hitler times"; he did his weapon prac-
tices on the soccer field where Jews had been banned as both spectators
and participants by the mid-1930s; his military drills took place in the
woods outside the town, which had been off-limits to Jews; and he swam
in the town pool, which also had previously excluded Jews. When German
inhabitants protested the loss of their houses, Gans and the others pulled
out pictures of the concentration camp horrors to silence them.

Many of the civilians recognized Manfred from before the war. In his
discussions with the townspeople he found that most had not changed at
all and that he was getting lots of dirty looks on the street. As he wrote in a
letter to Anita Lamm, they were "still filled up to the brim with Nazi propaganda." As an insider with local knowledge, he knew who deserved help:
the math teacher who had looked after his Jewish students; the county
executive who had protected Jews during Kristallnacht. But Manfred also
knew who had been Nazis and Nazi sympathizers, and he had these people
arrested. This included his biology teacher, Dr. Damen, who had been in
the SS and had introduced anti-Semitic initiatives in his school and in the
town.

Manfred spent his days off during the denazification period visiting
his parents in Eindhoven, just over the border in Holland, and his grandmother, who was still in Friesland. He also reunited with his younger
brother, Theo, who had spent much of the war working on a farm in Yorkshire, and his older brother, Gershon, who had served with the Jewish Brigade in Italy. He slowly learned that many members of his extended family

in Holland and Germany had been murdered by the Nazis, including many young children. When he met with the German administrator responsible for rebuilding Borken, he was told of plans to rebuild the synagogue. Manfred told the man that "none of us will ever come back."

In May of 1945 Manfred Gans and Andrew Kershaw were given strong recommendations for their applications to be "considered for military government duties" in Germany. In the late summer of 1945 Manfred was sent to a camp outside Recklinghausen, north of Essen, to interrogate the former SS guards imprisoned there. As he wrote to Anita, most of the inmates assured him that "they have never been Nazis at all." He found the extermination camp functionaries soulless and rather stupid individuals. "When these fellows have been beheaded one will have to tell them that they are dead, otherwise they won't know," he commented to Anita. He found it a strange reversal of fortune that he was now in control of the people who "once were our greatest and seemingly most secure oppressors."

In the fall of 1945, No. 41 (RM) Cdo. was redeployed to the Far East, but Gans was encouraged to remain in Germany and work for the military government. Manfred was promoted to captain and given the responsibility of helping run the town of Gladbeck, just a few towns south of Borken. Part of this work included purging the local government of Nazis while helping to establish a public health system there. Manfred also took it upon himself to help arrange religious services for the few remaining Jewish survivors found in the surrounding towns. After the services survivors would often recount the horrors they had suffered, with the Polish Jews telling their stories in Yiddish.

In Gladbeck, Manfred became friends with a survivor named Kahn, who, remarkably, already knew of Manfred. He had heard the rumor that a German Jewish British officer had rescued his parents from Theresienstadt. The story had spread like wildfire among survivors in the area, and months later when Manfred was visiting a camp of Jewish refugees in Kaunitz, he was heralded as "the soldier from Theresienstadt."

"Is there anything I can get for you? Any way I can help?" Manfred had asked Kahn soon after they became friends.

"I'd like a tallis and tefillin [Jewish prayer shawls and phylacteries]," his friend answered. Manfred had Leo and Luise Wislicki send these to him. In the coming months Gans would often arrange for the Wislickis to send him Jewish religious objects that survivors could use as they tried to rebuild their destroyed communities. Manfred spent many sabbaths with Kahn and his wife. Bit by bit the soldier formerly known as Fred Gray was publicly reclaiming his former identity.

In September 1945, the same month that No. 10 (Inter-Allied) Commando was formally disbanded, the British government decided that those who had been labeled enemy aliens, which meant nearly all of X Troop, could no longer serve as military government officials. Suddenly these men who had dedicated their lives to the British cause found themselves rejected yet again.

Manfred feared becoming one such castoff. In a November 30, 1945, letter to Anita Lamm he mentioned that his "German parentage" had been discovered, and now it was likely he would lose his job in the military government in Gladbeck. Yet Manfred needn't have worried. He made himself indispensable, stayed under the radar, and kept his job in the government until the spring of 1946. At that time he was given an even more important role when he became deputy commander of the intelligence section, tasked with interrogating high-ranking Nazi officials imprisoned at Paderborn. The camp was just over a hundred miles east of Borken. Manfred would run interrogations there every day from 8:15 a.m. to 9 p.m. Each interrogation would begin with him typing the Nazi's answers to a set list of questions, followed by him homing in on the Nazi's nefarious activities during the war. Prisoners at the camp included the notorious German industrialist and Nazi Party member Alfried Krupp, who had run slave labor factories that made weapons for the Nazis. His slaves included thousands of Jewish girls in their early teens, most of whom he worked to death. The deputy commandant of Auschwitz-Birkenau, Hans Aumeier, was also under Manfred's command in the camp. When some of the high-ranking Nazis in the prison claimed that the death camps were a lie, Manfred made Aumeier give them a lecture on how the exterminations were conducted at Auschwitz-Birkenau. Aumeier described how he would get the Jews to enter the gas chambers by pretending that they were going to take a shower and then would have all of them suffocated with Zyklon B, including hundreds of thousands of children. As Manfred later remembered, the impact of Aumeier's lecture was devastating to those listening, as they were forced to finally confront their monstrous behavior.

Manfred interviewed some Nazi generals who claimed that they had been part of the effort to kill Hitler, known as Operation Valkyrie. When Manfred realized how easily this could have been done if they had just had the nerve to shoot the Führer, he was incensed. "You were not willing to take the risks which we soldiers on the field had to take," he exclaimed. "It would have been so easy for you to take out a pistol and shoot [Hitler] in the head. Get rid of him, and get rid of the war."

During his months at the camp Manfred collected evidence that would be used in the Nuremberg trials. When he was demobilized in August 1946, he returned to England to prepare to take the entrance examinations to study engineering at the University of Manchester.

As for Peter Masters, when the war ended he was transferred to the Oxfordshire and Buckinghamshire Light Infantry. He was delighted to be put in the unit that had performed so admirably at Pegasus Bridge on D-Day.

Although Masters knew he could opt for denazification work, he did not have any desire to return to Germany or Austria, where, he felt, all the locals would claim that they had "no inkling of what had been perpetrated under their noses." He also wanted to travel and see more of the world, and he was happy to be dispatched to Ghana, in West Africa, to train Ghanaian troops there.

After a year overseas he was officially released from military duty on August 28, 1946, and returned to London with the intention of attending art school. Depressingly, Peter learned that as a civilian he had to report to the police every month because he was technically still an enemy alien. This indignity was galling, given all that Masters and his fellow X Troopers had done for their adopted country. But another hard-earned victory lay ahead.

At the same time that the X Troopers were working to capture and indict Nazis, Major Bryan Hilton-Jones was fighting to get his men naturalized. By September 1945 he had recovered fully from his war wounds and had accepted a post in the Foreign Office as the third secretary in the German Department.

Throughout the war he had frequently pleaded with the government that his men be made British subjects. These requests were repeatedly refused, despite other units, such as the Polish and French troops of No. 10 (Inter-Allied) Commando, receiving their naturalization papers during the war. On December 20, 1944, the Home Office, which was responsible for immigration issues, had authorized Act 1658, which stated, "No promise of any kind about future policy on naturalization has been given or can be given now, generally or with regards to any particular class of applicant." That being the case, the Home Office would "not consider the question of naturalization until after the war was over."

Yet once the war ended, the X Troopers still were not naturalized, even though doing so would have made it easier for the government to transition them to their new military roles in Germany and Austria. In an April 24, 1945, letter to Anita Lamm, Manfred Gans wrote that he and the others were so frustrated by this that the officers among them were considering resigning their commissions in protest.

During this time Britain was still darkened by a pervasive distrust of enemy aliens — even those who had risked everything to help the Allies win the war. Hilton-Jones's former second-in-command found this out the hard way. George Lane, who had been imprisoned at Oflag IX AH in Spangenberg Castle since shortly after his improbable meeting with Field Marshal Erwin Rommel, finally escaped in the waning days of the war and made his way to Paris to the apartment of Miriam Rothschild's brother, Victor. Victor immediately called Miriam to tell her the good news that

George was alive and safe. The following day Lane flew to England — where he was arrested because of his German accent and held in prison for one night, until Major General Robert Laycock, chief of Combined Operations, intervened and got him released. In such an atmosphere it was no wonder that the X Troopers had a hard time getting naturalized.

On December 7, 1945, a top secret meeting was held on the topic of the commandos' naturalization. Sir Alexander Maxwell, permanent undersecretary of the Home Office, made a formal plea to Major General Pigott, director of recruiting and demobilization at the War Office, that these men be given priority to naturalize. Pigott refused the request. Instead, a process for naturalization of all "aliens" (not just former enemy aliens) in the British military was hashed out, where priority would be given based on length of service. Other factors would also come into play. For instance, the commanding officers of such aliens would write their recommendations based on criteria including how well the applicant had "assimilated himself to the British way of life." By March 1946 applications for naturalization were being processed, and the time frame to receive one's new status was a few weeks.

However, the X Troopers were at a distinct disadvantage in the newly instituted process for naturalization. Since most of them were now serving in a range of units in postwar Germany and Austria, their new COs did not know them well enough to write recommendations. To fix this problem, in May 1946 it was decided that all applicants would now be required to have in-person interviews with the Inter-service Naturalisation Board. As a result the time frame was pushed back from a few weeks to many months.

In April 1946 Major Hilton-Jones finished his appendix to the X Troop war diary, which concluded with yet another plea for the men's naturalization: "These men are now, almost without exception, eager to become naturalized British citizens, and to set up their lives in this country. It seems their right that, having been deemed good enough to serve in what is admitted to be an elite corps of the British army, and having passed the test of this service successfully, they should be able to point to their time with the

Commandos as an adequate reason for receiving prompt and sympathetic consideration [of] their claims."

In July of 1946 the War Office finally agreed to reconsider the expediated naturalization of the X Troopers. By then the matter had been brought up in Parliament, and it seemed public opinion was on the men's side. A detailed memorandum was drawn up that presented what was considered to be a very strong case. The X Troopers' risks had been much greater than others', and their bravery and exemplary service in the war had been unimpeachable. Almost a quarter of the original eighty-seven commandos had become officers, an extremely high rate, which surely showed their worth. The statement concluded that rejecting the X Troopers for accelerated naturalization would be "extremely unfair on men who by their standards of intelligence and education and their proved eagerness to serve in an exacting role are qualified to do valuable national work."

The following month a top secret brief from Major R. G. S. Hobbs, chief of staff for Combined Operations, noted that the Home Office had offered to give the commandos preference and admit them "en bloc" if the War Office agreed to this. Major General Pigott, however, continued to refuse, stating that "the commandos have no better claim than anybody else." Because of this the War Office would "oppose any preference being given to them."

The brief from Hobbs ended by stating that they could either accept the extremely long delay for the men's naturalization or have the adjutant general intervene and overrule Pigott. On September 13, 1946, Major General Robert Laycock, who was still chief of Combined Operations, sent Pigott the full list of all the X Troopers seeking naturalization. It seems that Pigott had finally been overruled. From this moment forward the commandos were naturalized at an accelerated rate.

Many of the X Troopers were bitter about how long it had taken for them as compared with other units of No. 10 (Inter-Allied) Commando. The drawn-out process also had real human costs. For instance, when commandos such as Didi Fuller were put forth for posthumous awards such as the Victoria Cross, which would entitle their widows to a higher pension, the applications were denied because they were not British citizens.

Miriam Rothschild, for one, railed against the government for years about the hypocrisy that the X Troopers had been sent to fight for the Crown but were not given full rights as British subjects until several years after the war ended.

In spite of the obstacles the X Troopers faced in getting naturalized, to a man they felt extremely proud of their roles in the war. All of them had been deeply traumatized by the Nazis; they had lost family, friends, and homes. They had arrived in England as teenagers, mostly alone. They had been locked behind barbed wire, and many had undergone horrific abuse by the British in Canada and Australia. They had had to reinvent themselves as British commandos with new names and new personas. But then they had been given the opportunity to fight back.

As Ian Harris later said: "For this I'm ever grateful to this country: they gave you a tommy gun, they gave you ammunition, they gave you grenades, and then they said nothing more. Just let this idiot go on and do his own thing. And that's what I did. I never had that chance again."

By serving as commandos the men of X Troop not only had played crucial roles in the Allied effort, but they also had been able to feel a sense of agency — and eventually personal victory — over those who had destroyed their childhoods. As refugees they had been subject to the whims of history. As X Troopers they had helped shape it.

Time and again the X Troopers had seized the initiative, using strength and guile to penetrate German lines, to capture prisoners, to interrogate them on the spot, and to help the Allies advance. As Lord Mountbatten would explain at a banquet in October 1946, when he finally told the world about this "hush hush troop," as he called it: "They were fine soldiers and I was so proud of these men."

As the X Troopers transformed their trauma into a mission to beat the Nazis, they played vital roles in the Allies' successes. George Lane gathered crucial information about German mines that helped the D-Day invasion to go on as planned. He shared the location of Rommel's headquarters, which led to the attack on his car that severely wounded him. Colin Anson was at the forefront of many of the most important battles in the Italian and

Adriatic campaigns, and even used his negotiating skills to obtain the surrender of Corfu without a shot being fired. Peter Masters took a leadership
role within Bicycle Troop, helped capture a machine-gun nest, and gathered crucial intel for the Rhine operation. Manfred Gans led the way on
D-Day and beyond during the capture of the crucial radar station Moltke,
and then was central to the Allies' success at Walcheren. And Ian Harris
single-handedly got hundreds of the enemy to surrender in Osnabrück and
killed a number of Nazis during his attack on the SS Hitler Youth during
the Rhine crossings. After the war as well, they were crucial to the capture
and prosecution of many Nazis.

These, of course, are just some of the extraordinary things done by the
handful of men I have focused on in this book. Each X Trooper had an
incredible personal narrative that deserves to be uncovered, and I hope
that future historians will delve deep into the archives as I have done to tell
these other stories. Bryan Hilton-Jones wrote that X Troop had proved itself the "most worth-while" of all the troops in No. 10 (Inter-Allied) Commando. The manner in which the X Troopers dealt with the Nazi scourge
showed that a group of young, scared outcasts could escape death and help
turn the tide against their fellow countrymen, whose perverted vision of
a Thousand-Year Reich would have ensured a permanent midnight upon
the world.

# Afterword: The Legacy of X Troop

ON A BALMY afternoon in July 2018 I caught an Uber from Reagan National Airport to Bethesda, Maryland, to meet Peter Masters's widow, Alice Masters, and their son, Tim. I had spent the last few months going through archival material on X Troop at the United States Holocaust Memorial Museum in Washington, DC, the Imperial War Museum London, and The National Archives in Kew, England. I had found a wealth of material already, but this was the first time I would meet the family of one of the commandos.

Peter Masters had received one of the first Fulbright fellowships to study art in the United States, originally at the Parsons School of Design and later at Yale. After he relocated from London to New York City to attend Parsons, he met Alice Eberstarkova. Originally from Trstená, Czechoslovakia (now Slovakia), she had been sent on a Kindertransport to London, where she and her two sisters survived the war. Her parents were murdered at Majdanek extermination camp. In 1949, when Alice was working at the International Monetary Fund in Washington, she visited New York City and while there met with Peter to drop off a book from her then boyfriend, Gerald Nichols.

A few weeks after their initial meeting Peter and Alice were engaged. The two married on April 6, 1950, and never looked back. In celebration

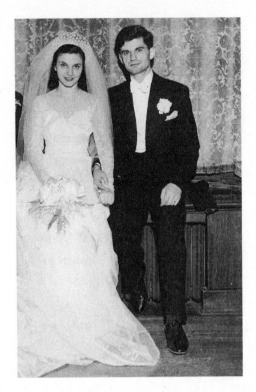

*Peter and Alice Masters on their wedding day, April 6, 1950*

of Alice's seventieth birthday, Peter wrote in his birthday card to her, "Married now for forty-five years of splendid happiness."

Peter passed away in 2005 at the age of eighty-five, but Alice still lived in their family home on a quiet suburban street in Washington. As I entered the house, I realized this was no ordinary DC commuter home. Every inch of the walls was covered with Peter Masters's stunning art: paintings and drawings from D-Day, the Normandy campaign, his prewar life in Vienna, and his postwar life in America. I spent the day with Alice and Tim listening to stories about Peter and looking through his personal archive of material saved from the war. This material included letters to him from Lord Lovat and Miriam Rothschild, notes for his book *Striking Back: A Jewish Commando's War Against the Nazis,* and his annotated datebooks from the war. They also shared with me a collection of the striking and often very funny birthday cards he had made for his three children, Tim, Kim, and Anne, along with an exquisite children's book he had written for them.

Alice and Tim both spoke of their deep love for Peter and told me that he was one of the most ethical and creative people they had ever known. "A one in a trillion," Alice said. I already knew a lot about Lieutenant Peter Masters, having gone through his donated papers at the United States Holocaust Memorial Museum, read his book, and listened to the many oral interviews that were conducted with him. As we wrapped up the visit, Alice and Tim shared one more story with me.

One evening in 1960 Peter was driving home to Bethesda from a late night working in Washington designing the *Profiles of Poverty* exhibit for the Smithsonian. On his car radio he heard about a contest for the Italian film *La Dolce Vita*. Participants had to write a poem, fifty words or less, describing what "the sweet life" meant to them and submit it by midnight. Masters raced to the main post office in Washington and submitted a poem he composed on the way.

I asked Alice and Tim if they had a copy of the poem. They recited it in unison, from heart:

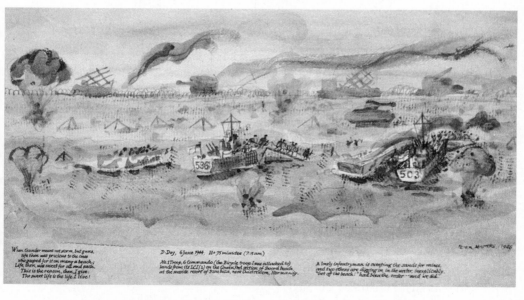

*Peter Masters's painting of D-Day with his poem "The Sweet Life"*

*When thunder meant not storm, but guns,*
*life then was precious to the ones,*
*who gasped for it on many a beach;*
*Life, then, was sweet for all and each.*
*This is the reason, then, I give:*
*The sweet life is the life I live!*

Masters won the contest, and he and Alice had an all-expenses-paid trip to Italy.

At the end of the day I hugged Alice and Tim and thanked them for showing me Peter's art and personal material related to the war, including an extraordinary hand-painted book titled "The French Window: A Scrapbook from Normandy." As I left their home, I carried with me a newfound awareness that the story of X Troop was unlike any other that had been told about World War Two and the Holocaust. This was a true tale about a group of extraordinary men set on fighting the evils of Nazism and determined to make the world sweet again.

Over the coming months I made contact with the children of many former X Troopers who invited me into their lives to talk about their dads. Several of them remembered their fathers as mysterious men who had served in the war but who did not want to speak about it or about their prewar childhoods in Germany and Austria. Others, such as the children of Peter Masters and Manfred Gans, were raised on their fathers' stories of life before and during the war.

When a few months later I spoke with Daniel Gans, son of Manfred Gans and Anita Lamm, who Manfred had married soon after the war, I saw in him the determination and devotion to truth and goodness that I was so familiar with from my research about his father. Daniel's profound love for his father was so palpable that it was almost as if the departed X Trooper was sitting in the room with us.

Most of the interviews I conducted were similarly emotional. These children all struggled to express the grief they carried — the pain of having lost their heroes and of knowing what those men had endured. I had one particularly moving conversation in a quiet pub on the outskirts of London with Geoff Broadman's son Ladi, who, like his father, had spent his life in the British military. I asked him the question I always asked: "Do you know what happened to your dad's family during the Holocaust?" He suddenly broke down, overwhelmed with grief. We sat there silently as he cried. It seemed to me as if this was a terrible burden he had carried for years.

After some time Ladi explained to me that his father had always refused to discuss his prewar life, so this had been a huge mystery for him growing up. One afternoon after his father died, Ladi was with his own children at a playground when he received a phone call from his wife, Sue, who was in Berlin and had discovered the family's fate. She told Ladi that his grandparents, Victor and Emilie Sruh, had been moved by train from Vienna to the Lodz ghetto on October 23, 1941. They were never heard from again. Geoff had never known what had happened to his parents, and now his son was discovering their terrible fate.

After I interviewed Ladi Broadman, I realized that the story of X Troop was also the story of the intergenerational trauma caused by the Holocaust. The book that I was writing would, of necessity, be about more than a group of commandos during World War Two. It would depict the manner in which the Holocaust nearly destroyed the families of even those who survived it; about the Germans and Austrians who turned on local Jewish children and forced their parents to make the impossible decision to send them alone on trains to England in an attempt to save them. It was about how those same refugees turned the tables and fought back, overturning the anti-Semitic stereotype that Jews were the passive victims of the Nazis. Yet it was also about the hundreds of thousands of equally precious, intelligent, gifted young men and women who did not manage to get out on Kindertransport, but instead fell into the warped clutches of evil Nazi bureaucrats and prison guards and were murdered in the bloom of youth.

Peter Masters and Manfred Gans were very much the exceptions — among the few X Troopers whose parents had not been murdered by the Nazis. They were also unusual for their openness with their children about their experiences before and during the war. I suspect this may have been not only because their parents had survived, but also because both X Troopers had immigrated to the United States. Most of the commandos who had stayed in the UK, by contrast, wanted desperately to embrace their new lives as Brits and avoided talking much about the past. They also frequently raised their children as Anglicans — a fact that surprised me when I first learned it, but that I have come to believe is an essential and revealing part of the story.

In many of the interviews that I conducted with the children of X Troopers, I discovered that these men and women often had no idea that their fathers were Jewish until some chance occurrence revealed that fact. For instance, a distant cousin might have a Bar Mitzvah, and the event would lead to a broader inquiry about how they had a Jewish cousin.

Some of these X Troop veterans, themselves survivors of anti-Semitic terror, may have been motivated by a desire to protect their children from the dangers that could befall them if they were perceived as being Jewish. Others simply felt such gratitude to the country that had saved them and let them fight the Nazis, that they chose to raise their children "more British than the British," as Colin Anson's daughter Barbara put it to me.

Tellingly, too, most of the children I met had the same last names that their commando dads had chosen during those stressful minutes when they were told to shed their old selves and construct a new British persona. As far as I have been able to determine, only Manfred Gans and Harry Nomburg (who also immigrated to the United States) reverted to their birth names after the war.

Maybe the other X Troopers kept their noms de guerre because they were more comfortable with their soldier selves. Perhaps their birth names reminded them too much of their losses. Or possibly they identified more closely with the names and identities they became just as they were turning into adults, and it may have felt strange to revert to their childhood selves. The decision to keep their British, Anglican personas also suggests that many X Troop veterans may have felt insecure about their Jewishness. Having been through the Holocaust and also having undergone naturalization struggles in the UK, the more secure choice may have been to fully embrace their new lives as Brits. And since many of the men had been raised in assimilated homes where their parents downplayed their own Jewish roots, it may have made sense to shed that past to move on. Anson's and many of the other X Troopers' full embrace of their new personas is part of a long history of immigrants to Britain adopting anglicized, middle-class norms as a means to be fully accepted into society.

In any case, by essentially maintaining their wartime cover identities for the rest of their lives, these X Troopers were reinventing themselves, much as many European refugees who settled in Israel during and after World War Two did. Many of those immigrants also changed their German- and eastern European–sounding names as a way, in part, to get some distance from the Holocaust. They, like the X Troopers, found their own ways to cope with the unfathomable losses they had endured.

These questions about identity spilled over in 1999 when some of the surviving commandos decided to commission and erect a memorial to X Troop in a beautiful park overlooking the harbor in Aberdovey (now called Aberdyfi), the village in Wales where they had done their training. The group erecting the memorial was led by Brian Grant, now a prominent British judge. He and several of the X Troopers living in Britain were opposed to the word "Jewish" being put on the memorial. The arguments were varied: the X Troopers weren't *all* Jewish (although it seems that at least eighty-two of the eighty-seven were); putting a reference to their Jewishness on the memorial might make it more likely to be vandalized; they didn't want to "rub it in the face" of the Welsh villagers with whom they had billeted (an idea that suggests lingering anti-Semitism); many of them hadn't told their friends and families of their Jewish roots and had no intention of doing so now; they were soldiers first and foremost; most were not religious; and so on.

In furious opposition to this negation of their Jewishness were Peter Masters and Manfred Gans—both of whom were living in the United

States and raising their children as Jews — and Miriam Rothschild, ex-wife of George Lane. Rothschild felt that the X Troopers' reluctance to put the word "Jewish" on the memorial was in part a form of internalized anti-Semitism. For Masters and Gans, putting the word "Jewish" on the memorial was simply a matter of telling the truth: the X Troopers had been a primarily Jewish unit, and this fact needed to be acknowledged. Even if a small handful of them hadn't been Jewish, 95 percent of them *had*. Moreover, the X Troopers' Jewish roots meant that they had fought and served differently than the standard British soldiers of World War Two. The commandos' Jewish heritage was an inextricable part of their unit's history and of their extraordinary motivation to defeat Hitler.

In the end, despite many letters from Masters and Rothschild, Brian Grant won out, and the beautiful gray slate memorial in Aberdovey (Aberdyfi) does not include the word "Jewish." Instead it says (somewhat confusingly): "For the members of 3 Troop 10 (1A) Commando who were warmly welcomed in Aberdyfi while training for special duties in battle 1942–1943[.] Twenty were killed in action." Set into the seawall of the park is a plaque that refers to the troop as "eighty-six German-speaking refugees from Nazi oppression." Again no mention that they were overwhelmingly Jewish. And the pamphlet produced for the unveiling of the memorial, *The Story Behind the Monument: Penhelyg Park, Aberdovey,* seems to go out of its way to avoid using the word "Jewish," instead describing the unit as a hodgepodge of Germans, Austrians, and others of various backgrounds.

Despite these disagreements, on May 15, 1999, twenty-three of the surviving commandos, including Manfred Gans, Peter Masters, Victor Davies, and Ian Harris, went back to Aberdovey with their families for a moving tribute and ceremony. The event was covered by the BBC.

The dispute over the memorial continues to this day. Over the years Martin Sugarman, former archivist of the Jewish War Veterans of the UK (AJEX, or Association of Jewish Ex-Servicemen and Women) and author of the book *Fighting Back: British Jewry's Military Contribution in the Second World War,* wrote numerous letters to the Aberdyfi Community Council about this topic. He pointed out the Jewish nature of X Troop and asked

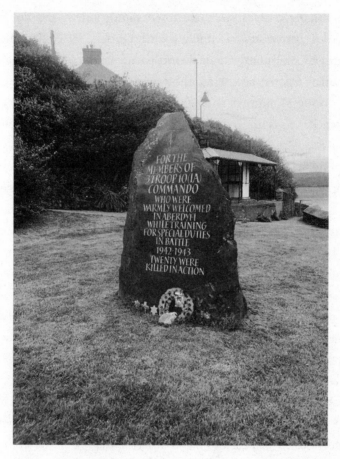

*Memorial to X Troop in Aberdovey, Wales*

that the word "Jewish" be added to the slate memorial as well to the plaque set into the seawall. In 1999 and again in 2018 the council rejected his request, stating that they would not make the change because they wanted to honor "the original intentions of this memorial—to recognize the incalculable sacrifice of all those who were proud to be part of a unique and selfless group of individuals from all over Europe, regardless of race, colour, creed or religion." And even though the troop was, as we have seen, 95 percent Jewish, the letter mistakenly claimed that the unit "represented a broad mixture of different social and religious backgrounds." Sugarman persisted, also noting that the problematic pamphlet *The Story Behind the Monument,* which is still given to visitors to the town, should at least mention that the commandos were overwhelmingly Jewish. On July 23, 2020, the clerk to the Aberdyfi Community Council emailed Sugarman yet again saying that "the Council wishes to reiterate their original decision not to make any changes to the Monument in Penhelig Parc . . . and as far as the Council is concerned, this is the end of the matter." Perhaps the publication of this book will encourage the council to revisit its position.

The controversy over the Aberdovey memorial also has been repeated, in less dramatic fashion, in the cemeteries where fallen X Troopers are buried. All of them were interred under a cross, and during the war Manfred Gans dreamed of someday getting that Christian symbol replaced with a Star of David. It seems that his brother Theo, working with the Jewish Board of Governors, did manage to change a few crosses to Stars of David. But despite recent attempts by Martin Sugarman and AJEX to change the remaining ones, this has not come to pass. Many X Troop veterans and their families — at least those who are aware of the tension between their ancestors' birth identities and assumed identities — have preferred to let the crosses stand.

The challenges of remembrance highlight the conflicted status of many of the X Troopers: they were given arms but not naturalized; they faced profound internal insecurities about whether they could be both British and Jewish; they came from mostly secular backgrounds, and many had one non-Jewish parent; some of their parents converted their children to Christianity to try to keep them safe during the rise of Nazism.

In addition to spending much time with the descendants of the men who populate this book, I also had the extraordinary good luck to interview two living X Troopers. One of them was Paul Streeten, who fought heroically in Italy until a shrapnel wound ended his active duty. After the war he went on to become a world-famous economist.

I tracked Streeten down, and in September 2018 his daughter Tish generously agreed to ask him questions on my behalf because he was too unwell to meet me in person. As a stateless internee in 1940, her father described how he had been very lost: "You really felt without any friends in the world which was a very unpleasant and unkindly feeling." X Troop was a means for him, and for all the men, to have roots again. The men of X Troop became a surrogate family or, to borrow from Prince Hal and Stephen Ambrose, a "band of brothers." The fellowship changed them for the better. One of Streeten's answers to my questions summed up how X Troop transformed him and many of his friends: "The troop made me tougher, on the inside and on the outside, against weather, nature. It made me better equipped and more self-reliant. It made me more considerate, even though it was war, considerate of people who were suffering, the oppressed. It made me tougher but also more gentle." Paul Streeten passed away on January 6, 2019, while I was still writing this book. His family mourned not only a war hero but also an amazing father and grandfather.

About a year into my writing, in early 2019, I discovered that there was another living commando, whom I call Victor Davies in this book. After we exchanged letters and emails, he kindly agreed to speak with me, so I flew out to meet him on the West Coast of the United States. He had spent his life living under his nom de guerre and had never made public the fact that he had been a child refugee from Germany whose parents had "disappeared without a trace" after they had gotten him safely to England. I agreed to honor his decision to keep his story private, which is why I do not use either his birth name or his nom de guerre in this book.

I spent a glorious day in Victor's art-filled home interviewing him and looking through the papers and photographs he had saved from the war. When he and his gracious wife served me lunch, it included the same type of German potato salad that I had been served several times before by other descendants of the X Troopers.

I listened to Victor's accounts of his life before and during the war. Though ninety-seven years old, he was vivacious and full of energy. His singsong voice, which still had a heavy German accent, darkened only when he described prewar life in Germany or the good friends he lost during the conflict. When Victor spoke of the X Troopers who were killed during the war, he did so with the tenderness, sadness, and profound feeling of loss usually reserved for one's family members. (As Peter Masters's son, Tim, put it to me, the most meaningful relationships that his father had besides his family were with his commando buddies.) Yet Davies also visibly seethed, his hands shaking with anger, when he recounted how the guards on the *Dunera* had forced Jewish refugees to walk over broken glass — a story I relate in chapter 2, thanks to his painful disclosure.

At one point during our meeting Victor shared with me a copy of the Skipper's glowing, four-page, handwritten recommendation letter for him from April 5, 1946. As I read Bryan Hilton-Jones's words "recommending him most highly as both a man and as a soldier," I understood the impact the Skipper had had on these men. Most of them, having lost their parents to the Nazis, found a proxy father in their commanding officer. Hilton-Jones's admiration for and devotion to these refugees must have helped assuage some of the grief they felt.

Like so many veterans of X Troop, Victor filled his life after the war with art, culture, and learning. He published books of poetry and short stories — he even had a new collection on the way when we talked — and hiked and traveled around the world with his beloved wife. At the time of this writing he is still undertaking new adventures.

Meeting with, researching, and writing about the men of X Troop has had an indelible impact on me both as a historian and as a person. As I was completing the first full draft of the manuscript, I received word that my own father was in the hospital, having been diagnosed with stage four cancer. While writing the book and hearing all the children of the X Troopers speak about their dads, and while drafting a manuscript drawing from their recollections, I had continually reflected on my often troubled relationship with my father. Sitting with him during his final days while he mostly slept in the oncology unit at Massachusetts General Hospital, I found that one way I could cope with my own monumental loss was to work on this book, which is so much about the legacies that fathers give to their children. After my father died, writing the book continued to be a form of solace for me.

The story of Jewish servicemen was one I was familiar with from my own family: my grandfather Abraham Klein served in the Medical Corps in General George Patton's Third Army; my great-uncles Jake and Sig Lichterman also served in the Medical Corps, in Europe and the Pacific. My previous book, *Young Lions: How Jewish Authors Reinvented the American War Novel*, is about the manner in which Jewish servicemen such as Herman Wouk, Joseph Heller, Norman Mailer, and Leon Uris taught Americans about World War Two and the Holocaust through their best-selling novels.

Yet for X Troop the larger lessons were different from those of their American counterparts. Their story reflects the at times uncomfortable relationship between Britain and its Jewish refugees, but also the remarkable chances that Britain gave these men to get their own back. Through their exemplary and courageous service, their story challenges the idea that only in Israel did the Jews become armed warriors who fought to try to establish a safe life for themselves and their families.

These men often came from educated and cultured backgrounds, and as fighters they relied as much on their brains as on their brawn. Most of them were rooted in a Jewish intellectual tradition that prized ethical behavior, and we see how this spilled over into their service. As Manfred Gans, the efficient and steely warrior, would reflect after the war, he was most proud of getting literally thousands of Germans to surrender without anyone getting hurt.

Whenever possible, the X Troopers used their intelligence to outmaneuver the Nazis and to capture them before a shot was fired. In this regard the X Troopers were the opposite of Quentin Tarantino's vengeful Jews in his film *Inglourious Basterds*. Rather than wreaking personal revenge on the Germans, they followed the rules of war. They coolly collected battlefield intelligence from the enemy and outwitted them using their intellect rather than brute force. And even in extreme instances, such as when Colin Anson confronted the man who had been responsible for his own father's death, they refused to compromise their own moral standards.

When the X Troopers were called on to fight and shoot and kill, they did so both bravely and extremely effectively. They gathered crucial intelligence in the heat of battle, and their interrogations of captured Germans uncovered important information on what the enemy was doing and had done. As both fearsome commandos and masterful interrogators, the X Troopers were central to the Allies' success during the war and later to their denazification efforts.

It was clear to me from speaking with their children that after the war the X Troopers devoted themselves to being good fathers with the same energy they had brought to their military service. Their new families, built on the ashes of their old world, would be places of hope and healing and happiness.

One afternoon in August 2019 I took the train from London to Woodley, near Reading, to interview Ian Harris's son Mark about his father. When I got there, Mark's two sons had prepared a barbecue (with German potato salad, of course), and we spent the afternoon talking about Ian, looking at a trove of photos, and watching videos of him. It was clear that Ian's grandsons were as much in awe of their grandfather as their father was.

We talked about Ian's amazing capture of hundreds of POWs in Osnabrück, and we watched a newsreel showing him riding in a jeep with the captured men walking behind him. We discussed Harris's role in the assault on the Rhine, when he attacked and killed a number of Germans. Mark showed me the Military Medal that Ian received for this action.

Toward the end of the day, as we stood in the kitchen looking at Ian's many medals lovingly laid out on the table, Mark told me the story of his father's funeral. Before Ian died, he had made Mark promise to say a particular phrase at his funeral service. It was a phrase that he had learned in England but that wasn't really appropriate for a British funeral ceremony. Mark assured his dad that he would carry out his wishes to the letter.

Ian Harris passed away in 2012 at the age of ninety-two. At the closing of the funeral service, a Royal Marine bugler played the "Last Post" and then silence descended on the packed congregation.

Mark stood up, looked at the crowd, grinned, raised the two-fingered salute his dad had learned in Aberdovey, and shouted his father's words:

"Up yours, Adolf!"

# Acknowledgments

First and foremost I want to the thank the extraordinary families of the X Troopers. They generously welcomed me into their lives and shared with me the personal stories of their beloved husbands, fathers, and grandfathers.

Because it was impossible for me to tell the full tales of all eighty-seven commandos, early on I made the decision to focus much of my attention on three who I hoped would represent the others: Manfred Gans, Peter Masters, and Colin Anson. Their families were enormously helpful to me in all stages of writing this book. Daniel Gans and Aviva Gans Rosenberg were always there with suggestions and ideas; they read and commented on the first full draft of the manuscript; and they met with me and shared priceless personal material about their family. Alice Masters invited me into her home to discuss Peter and look at his amazing artwork; Kim Masters shared very helpful comments on the manuscript; and Tim Masters met with me and helped me organize the photos for the book. Barbara Wiseman, Colin Anson's daughter, let me interview her about her dad and shared a cache of private audiotapes and photos with me.

*X Troop* also focuses on many other men, of course, and their families were incredibly generous in their assistance with this project: sitting for interviews with me; sharing family photos, private memoirs, unheard audio- and videotapes; and responding to my constant email queries as I wrote the book. A huge thank-you to Mark, Samson, and Leon Harris; Tish Streeten and Jay Palmer; Ladi and Ander Broadman; Kathryn Firth; Stephen and Michael Gilbert and Liliane Grèze; Ursula Hilton-Jones; Elizabeth Lane; Annabel and Juliet Kershaw and Susan Kirschner; Patricia Humphrey; Beno Zeiner; and Jodee Culver Evans.

I was extremely lucky to have two surviving X Troopers to interview. My deepest gratitude to Paul Streeten, who answered my questions through his daughter Tish before he passed away, and Victor Davies, who invited me into his home and shared his personal artifacts and memories of his wartime service.

My most profound thanks go to the great military historian Ian Dear. He conducted interviews with many of the X Troopers for his groundbreaking book *10 Commando*. Without those interviews, the material he donated to the Imperial War Museum, and his book, I would never have been able to write this one. But more than this, Ian Dear has been a total mensch: always answering my queries and helping me to unpack the story of the unit, being supportive of the project, and even carefully reading the first full draft of the manuscript and offering suggestions for improvement (although, of course, any and all errors are mine alone).

I have the nicest and most diligent editor in the world, Alexander Littlefield, who was passionate about the project and offered guidance and support through all stages of the writing. Thank you as well to my amazingly thorough copyeditor, Barbara Jatkola, and my helpful and diligent production editor, Beth Burleigh Fuller. Huge thanks as well to my wonderful UK editor at Chatto (Penguin Random House), Poppy Hampson. And thank you as well to Greg Clowes and Ryan Bowes at Chatto (Penguin Random House) and Olivia Bartz at Houghton Mifflin Harcourt for all their hard work on the book.

To my supportive, funny, and cool as shit agent, Geri Thoma, of Writers House — thank you for believing in me and this project and for being there every step of the way. Thank you as well to Geri's assistant, Andrea Morrison, for her great suggestions regarding the original book proposal.

I could not have written this book without all the groundwork that was laid by other historians. Martin Sugarman has tirelessly fought to tell the stories of Jewish servicemen in the UK generally and X Troop in particular. Helen Fry has published extensively on Jewish soldiers, and her biography of Colin Anson, *German Schoolboy, British Commando: Churchill's Secret Soldier*, was invaluable to me.

Steven Karras, who filmed and produced the documentary *About Face: Jewish Refugees in the Allied Forces*, generously shared all his videotaped interviews of the X Troopers with me. The work of other historians has been crucial, and all of the following helped me with different sections of the manuscript: Nick van der Bijl, Ion Patrick Francis Drew, and David O'Keefe. And thank you to Mark Hickman, who runs the amazing Pegasus Archive, for his assistance finding online commando war diaries.

In graduate school I was fortunate to study Yiddish, Hebrew, and German and to be trained in archival research. I want to thank all my teachers along the way for making me work so hard at gaining the fundamentals for this kind of historical research.

A special thanks to Shane Salerno and Don Winslow for all they have done for our family. If you are ever in a tight spot, you would be so lucky to have either of these gentlemen in your corner. Thank you as well to Nancy Buirski and Jonathan Segal for their guidance during the early stages of this project.

The archives of the commandos are located all over the world, and the librarians at a number of institutions went beyond the call of duty to help me find material: Richard Hughes, John Delaney, Andrew Webb, Anthony Richards, Simon Offord, Jane Fish, and Jane Rosen of the Imperial War Museum; Loran McNamara of the Jewish Museum of Australia; Judith Cohen, James Gilmore, Megan Lewis, and Caroline Waddell Koehler at the United States Holocaust Memorial Museum; Joey Balfour at the National WWII Museum; Kathrin Pieren at the Jewish Museum London; and Neil

Cobbett, Colin Williams, and the Record Copy Team at The National Archives of the UK.

Thank you to my research assistant, Simon Cawthorne, who was like a detective hot on the trail of leads in the Kew archives, and to Aaron Welt, who helped with the final edits. And my very deepest thanks to the military historian Adam Seipp for kindly reading and commenting on the manuscript.

I moved back to New York City a few years ago to run the Jewish Studies Center at Hunter College, City University of New York, and I have found Hunter to be an extraordinarily supportive home. I am proud to be part of an institution that is so devoted to its remarkably diverse and interesting students, many of whom are the first in their families to attend college. Even during the devastation of the COVID-19 pandemic, the college, led by the great Jennifer Raab, was focused on providing care: food banks, housing, and psychological help to our students. It is a remarkable institution, and I am so grateful to have found a home here. Thank you not only to President Raab, who has been incredibly encouraging of me and my work at Hunter, but also to the Department of Classical and Oriental Studies and the programs in Jewish and Hebrew studies where I have been a much-welcomed new faculty member. Thank you as well to Andrew Polsky, Lon Kaufman, Malkie Schwartz, Anna Stein, and my friends at Hunter in a range of departments — Robert Koehl, Barbara Sproul, Sangeeta Pratap, Yasha Klots, Vivian Louie, Benjamin Hett, Harold Holzer, and Mary Roldán — not only for receiving me so warmly but also for their passionate focus on social justice and the education of our extraordinary students.

Thank you to Mette and Bettina — I honestly don't know what I would do without your constant love, support, and guidance over the many years. During the pandemic lockdown, my regular lunches with Hasia Diner kept me grounded and hopeful for better days.

I lost my dear friend Linda Russell while writing this book. I'm glad for the time I had with her and the great advice she always gave me. She is deeply missed.

Thank you to my husband's family, the McKintys. I was so lucky to marry into this warm, smart, and hilarious family.

My mother, Susan Vladeck, has been my greatest cheerleader and an enthusiastic reader of the manuscript. I'm extremely grateful to her, as well as to my brothers, Aaron, Josh, and Hung, especially during this tough year when our father died.

To Arwynn and Sophie—I love you more than anything in the world. And to Adrian, thank you for patiently reading and commenting on multiple drafts of the manuscript.

And finally, thank you to the X Troopers. You have been an inspiration to me, and I am so grateful that I got to share your story with the world.

Appendix

# PRINCIPAL FIGURES

## Colin Anson (Claus Ascher)

Sergeant Colin Anson landed with the commando forces in Sicily. After recovering in Egypt from a serious head wound, he returned to Italy and fought on to Corfu, which he almost single-handedly liberated. In 1945–1946 he worked on denazification efforts in Frankfurt.

Anson was demobilized in August 1946 and soon thereafter met Alice Gross in a London café. Alice had been a Jewish refugee from Austria who had come to England via the Kindertransport program when she was fourteen. Like Colin, Alice had done crucial work during the war. She was one of the only refugee women accepted into the Women's Auxiliary Air Force (WAAF). Working in the photographic section of RAF Bomber Command, she processed and analyzed the photos taken by reconnaissance target cameras. In one instance her group pinpointed sites of German V-1 flying bombs — the "V for vengeance weapons" — which were then attacked by the RAF. Colin and Alice married in 1951.

After the war Colin worked for a range of companies and as a traveling salesman. He spent his free time flying two-seat vintage gliders, eventually becoming a flying instructor. In 2010 the historian Helen Fry published a loving biography of Anson titled *German Schoolboy, British Commando: Churchill's Secret Soldier.* Colin and Alice had three children, Barbara, Diana, and Edward, and seven grandchildren.

## Geoff Broadman (Gottfried Conrad Sruh)

Sergeant Geoff Broadman helped train the X Troopers in Wales, landed in Normandy on D-Day with No. 48 (RM) Cdo., and fought his way through France until he was injured. Geoff worked for the United Nations War Crimes Commission in Germany after the war.

Broadman spent his working life in the British Army, joining the West Yorkshire Regiment as a battalion ski instructor and also winning interservice ski championships. He was one of the founders of the Army Outward Bound School in Wales, using there many of the methods he'd learned from the Skipper during his own training. He continued to be an avid mountain climber throughout his life. He had two sons, Ladi and Pete, and five grandchildren.

## Tony Firth (Hans Fürth)

Lieutenant Tony Firth was sent to Australia on the *Dunera* and interned there. He was selected for officer training school before D-Day and was later sent to Holland with No. 4 Commando as an assistant intelligence officer. After working on the Allies' denazification efforts, Firth was demobilized and returned to the UK.

In 1954 Firth immigrated to Canada, where he worked in public relations and advertising until his retirement. He was a lifelong avid skier and won a gold medal in Canada in the over-seventy category of the Canadian Masters Championships. He had one daughter, Kathryn, and one grandson.

## Manfred Gans (Fred Gray)

Manfred Gans landed with No. 41 (RM) Cdo. at Normandy, fought his way through France, and was part of the Walcheren operation in Holland, where he received a battlefield commission. In the final days of the war he commandeered a jeep and drove across occupied Europe to rescue his parents from Theresienstadt concentration camp. During the Allies' denazification efforts Gans led multiple successful interrogations of high-ranking Nazis that were used in the Nuremberg trials. He was promoted to captain in 1945.

When he was demobilized in August 1946, he officially switched back from his nom de guerre, Fred Gray, to his birth name, Manfred Gans. He sat for the highly competitive entrance exams for engineering at the University of Manchester, was accepted, and began his undergraduate studies a few months later. In the spring of 1947 he invited his childhood sweetheart and letter correspondent, Anita Lamm, who was living in New York, to visit during the university's Easter break. They went to Holland together to celebrate Passover with his parents and his brother Theo, and became engaged on Shavuot, May 25, 1947. His former landlords in Manchester, Leo and Luise Wislicki, threw them an engagement party. In July 1948 he and Anita were married in New York City, and after their honeymoon traveling around New England, they returned to the UK so he could complete his studies. During this time Manfred's parents fought for restitution for their stolen property and possessions, as well as payments for the slave labor they had to endure in the camps. Eventually they received some compensation from Germany, although not the return of their home. With their sons Gershon and Theo now living permanently in Israel, Moritz and Else immigrated there in 1954.

After Manfred completed his chemical engineering degree in June of 1950, he and Anita moved to Boston so that he could pursue a master's degree in chemical engineering at MIT. Once he completed his degree, the couple moved to New York, where Manfred was hired by the Scientific Design Company. He devoted his professional career to the invention, development, and commercialization of new chemical processes. He rose

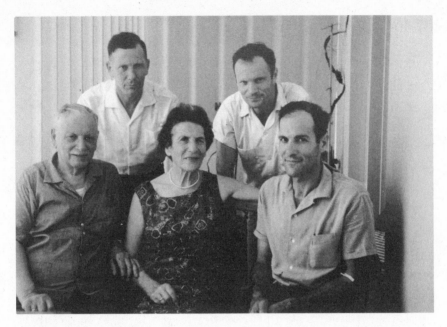

*Gans family in Israel, 1958. Clockwise from top left: Gershon, Manfred, Theo, Else, Moritz.*

to senior vice president, consulted for the United Nations, had numerous patents in his name, and authored fifteen technical papers. Manfred's work also brought him frequently to Washington, DC, where he often would spend time with Peter and Alice Masters.

In 1985 Manfred retired from the Scientific Design Company and began his own chemical engineering business with Anita as the administrative assistant. Both he and Anita volunteered for numerous organizations, and Manfred became president of his synagogue, Congregation Sons of Israel, in Leonia, New Jersey.

In 1988 Manfred traveled to Borken to help the town commemorate the fiftieth anniversary of Kristallnacht, and he returned yearly to lecture local high school students on the Holocaust. In 2009 he published his autobiography, *Life Gave Me a Chance.* Manfred and Anita had two children, Daniel and Aviva, and three grandchildren. His parents, whom he rescued from Theresienstadt, lived long and full lives in Israel, as did his brothers.

## Ron Gilbert (Hans Julius Guttmann)

Sergeant Ron Gilbert was sent to Australia on the *Dunera* and interned there. He landed with No. 46 (RM) Cdo. on D-Day and fought in the Normandy campaign, in the Battle of the Bulge, and in the Rhine crossings. During the postwar occupation of Germany he led a number of successful operations capturing Nazis and their sympathizers.

After Gilbert was demobilized in June 1947, he joined British intelligence and was employed as the head of station in Düsseldorf. He worked there with politicians, the police, and intelligence agents until he retired. On January 1, 1965, he was named a Member of the Most Excellent Order of the British Empire (MBE). He had two sons, Stephen and Michael, and three grandchildren.

## Ian Harris (Hans Ludwig Hajos)

Sergeant Ian Harris fought on D-Day with No. 46 (RM) Cdo. and then throughout France until he was wounded. He joined No. 45 (RM) Cdo. after his recovery and single-handedly convinced hundreds of Germans to surrender in Osnabrück. In the Battle for the Rhine he killed and captured numerous Nazis in hand-to-hand fighting and lost an eye. He received the Military Medal for his gallantry there.

Harris became a chartered accountant after the war. When he met Queen Elizabeth as chairman of the Commando Association, he joked with her that he had been naturalized on the same day as her husband. He was an avid skier, water-skier, and chess player. He had two sons, Mark and John, and four grandchildren.

## Bryan Hilton-Jones

Major Bryan Hilton-Jones was the commanding officer of X Troop. He received a Military Cross for Operation Tarbrush, which gathered intelligence on the German mines planted on the Normandy beaches. Hilton-Jones was severely wounded in the stomach and captured during the Normandy campaign and was presumed dead. Later discovered in a prison hospital abandoned by the Germans, he continued in recovery until the end of the war.

After the war Hilton-Jones worked for the Foreign Office as the third secretary in the German Department and then as the continental manager for Imperial Chemical Industries in Spain. He continued to be an avid and extremely competent mountain climber and in 1952 helped train the British team that would be the first to reach the summit of Mount Everest the following year.

On New Year's Eve 1969 he and two of his daughters were killed in a car accident outside Barcelona. The survivors included his wife, Edwina; his daughter Nerys; and his son Gavin. His untimely death sent a huge wave of grief through all of the X Troopers. To commemorate his life George Lane and Miriam Rothschild dedicated an area of woodland on Miriam's North Hampshire estate to Major Hilton-Jones and X Troop.

## Andrew Kershaw (Éndre Kirschner)

Lieutenant Andrew Kershaw attended officer training school before D-Day. Afterward he was sent to No. 41 (RM) Cdo. in Belgium, where he worked closely with Manfred Gans training Dutch recruits and overseeing intelligence operations.

After the war Kershaw immigrated to Canada, where he became the chairman of one of the world's largest advertising firms, Ogilvy & Mather. He had two daughters, Annabel and Juliet, and five grandchildren.

## George Lane (Lanyi György)

Lieutenant George Lane was awarded the Military Cross for his efforts in Operation Tarbrush. After the war he joined his wife, Miriam Rothschild, on her family estate, Ashton Wold, and helped run it. They had three daughters and a son and were divorced amicably in 1957. In 1963 he married Elizabeth Heald, whose father, Sir Lionel Heald, had been attorney general in Winston Churchill's government. Elizabeth was employed as a director at Christie's. George worked for an American stockbroker setting up offices in locations around Europe.

## Maurice Latimer (Moritz Levy)

Maurice Latimer fought in the International Brigades in the Spanish Civil War and engaged in guerrilla warfare against the Nazis in his homeland, the Sudetenland, before escaping to the UK. He was plucked from the Special Operations Executive (SOE) to be part of the Dieppe Raid and was the only member of X Troop to return from the botched operation uninjured. He landed in Normandy with No. 41 (RM) Cdo. and fought his way through France. During the Walcheren operation he was responsible for capturing hundreds of Germans. After the war, Maurice Latimer led a calm life working as an assistant in a pharmacy in London. He married and had one son, Norman, and three grandchildren.

## Peter Masters (Peter Arany)

Lieutenant Peter Masters landed in Normandy on D-Day with Bicycle Troop, helped save Lord Lovat's life, and fought his way through France. He was selected for officer training school after the Rhine assault, during which he gathered crucial intelligence, and later was chosen to train new recruits.

Following the war Masters was sent to Ghana to train Ghanaian forces. After he was demobilized, he attended art school in London and then New York. He married Alice Eberstarkova and moved to Washington, DC, where she was working for the International Monetary Fund. There he got a job designing sets for *Face the Nation* and other TV shows. In 1964 Peter worked for the federal government creating logos for President Lyndon

Johnson's antipoverty programs, such as Head Start and the Job Corps. The following year he helped design the groundbreaking *Profiles of Poverty* exhibit at the Smithsonian. When Richard Nixon became president, Peter was moved to the General Services Administration, where he created signs for federal buildings. He was president of the Art Directors Club of Metropolitan Washington and did volunteer work to help integrate local neighborhoods. He retired in 1984.

In 1997 he published his excellent autobiographical account of X Troop, *Striking Back: A Jewish Commando's War Against the Nazis.* Masters organized regular X Troop reunions and kept in touch with many members throughout his life. He had three children, Tim, Kim, and Anne, and seven grandchildren.

## Gerald Nichols (Heinz Herman)

Captain Gerald Nichols landed in Normandy on D-Day with the headquarters section of No. 6 Commando. He rescued Lord Lovat after he was wounded on June 12, 1944, and went on to receive a battlefield commission. Nichols was wounded during the Normandy campaign but after his recovery returned to fight in Germany. After the war he helped capture Heinrich Himmler.

Nichols later became a successful businessman in London, married the actress Jane Griffiths, and had two children.

## Harry Nomburg (Harry Drew)

Sergeant Harry Nomburg landed with No. 6 Commando at Normandy's Sword Beach (where he touched Lord Lovat's belt for luck) and fought through the bocage until he was wounded. After recovering, he fought in Holland and then in Germany. In 1948 he immigrated to the United States and dropped his nom de guerre, returning to his birth name of Nomburg. He joined the Eighty-Second Airborne Division and served as a US paratrooper until he was demobilized in 1952. He became a mailman in New York City and lived a long and happy life. His *New York Times* obituary said, "He bettered the lives of all he touched."

## Miriam Rothschild

Miriam Rothschild deserves her own book.

She came from the famous animal- and nature-loving side of the Rothschild family and during the war worked at Bletchley Park on the Enigma code-breaking campaign. After she married George Lane, she moved to Wales, where she became known as "the Lady of X Troop." Following the war Rothschild became one of the world's foremost authorities on fleas and one of Britain's leading naturalists. She published books and hundreds of articles, and her work is held in the Rothschild Collection at the Natural History Museum in London. She also founded the Schizophrenia Research Fund and was a pioneer of art therapy. Rothschild was appointed a dame by Queen Elizabeth in 2000. She received honorary doctorates from eight universities, including Oxford and Cambridge, and was named a fellow of the Royal Society — all despite having no formal academic training.

Rothschild was a liberal moral crusader who campaigned tirelessly for causes she believed in. She was a fierce advocate for Jewish refugees and fought to have their monies and property returned to them after the war. Rothschild also fought for equal rights legislation and the legalization of homosexuality in the UK. She had four children with George Lane.

## George Saunders (George Salochin)

Lance Corporal George Saunders fought with No. 45 (RM) Cdo. at Normandy until he was captured carrying wounded men in an ambulance across enemy lines. He escaped and was captured again. He was finally sent to a POW labor camp in Sagan, in western Poland. He escaped twice, the second time successfully. He headed east, hoping to reach safety behind the

Russian lines. He made his way to Odessa, where he talked a British ship captain into giving him a lift back to the UK.

When the war ended, Saunders moved to Moulsford, Oxfordshire, where he was a businessman and became an avid horse rider and sportsman.

## Paul Streeten (Paul Hornig)

Sergeant Paul Streeten landed in Sicily with No. 41 (RM) Cdo. and received serious shrapnel wounds while trying to set up a bridgehead outside Catania. He recovered in Egypt and then in the UK. He was eventually able to walk again, although the left side of his body and his arm remained weak, which meant he never again enjoyed his cherished pastimes of rock climbing, skiing, and long-distance running.

After the war Streeten studied economics at Oxford, becoming a fellow of Balliol College, and then became a professor at the University of Sussex. He was a senior economic adviser to the World Bank on issues related to the basic needs of poor populations. Streeten played a central role in the United Nations Development Programme's annual Human Development Report and was the founding editor of the journal *World Development*. He moved to Boston University in the 1970s, eventually becoming a professor emeritus there. He was also the director of the World Institute for Development Economics Research. He had three children, Tish, Judith, and Jay, and two grandchildren.

## Bill Watson (Otto Wassermann)

Private Bill Watson landed in Normandy on D-Day, fought through France, and participated in the operation at Walcheren, where he was wounded and saved the life of Captain "Bunny" Emmett.

Watson had been raised in a Jewish family in Berlin and married an Orthodox Jewish woman named Inge. On Kristallnacht his business was destroyed by the Nazis, and he and his brother were soon sent to Dachau.

They arrived in late November 1938. At night, without blankets, the Jews slept packed together "like sardines" trying to get warm, and in the morning they had to stand for hours in thin cotton pajamas in the bitter cold while the names of the twenty thousand or so men were checked. His work was chipping and carrying large stones, and if anyone was too ill or cold to keep up, he was kicked and beaten. As Watson later wrote in his unpublished memoir, he saw many men hurl themselves "against the electrified wire fencing. They would rather meet a terrible but instant death, than face any more of the heinousness meted out by the SS."

On one particularly horrific day, the SS decided to punish all the men because one of them had gone missing. They were forced to stand in the freezing cold from six that night until noon the following day while the previously missing man was beaten to death "like an animal before our eyes." Many of the men, including Bill's brother Bruno, caught pneumonia. When Bill desperately tried to get him checked into the hospital, his petitions were refused because Bruno was deemed healthy enough to continue working. Bruno died at just twenty-two years of age. A few days after his brother's death, in March 1939, Bill was told during the morning roll call that he and his brother were being released. He informed his captors that his brother had died.

A heartbroken Bill returned to his wife and two young children in Berlin, where he was required to report twice daily to the police. An uncle in the United States sent Bill an affidavit of support, and he was issued a transit visa for the UK. The plan was that he would earn money in the UK and find a way to send for his wife and children. He knew that if he remained in Berlin, he would be arrested again. He later recalled, "I can still see them! Inge my wife and our two children standing at the door and waving goodbye to me. We were in tears. I felt so low having to walk away from them."

In England, Bill lived at the Kitchener Camp in Sandwich. He picked up work as a tailor, bought himself a bike, and spent every spare minute begging shopkeepers in the neighboring town to give his wife in Berlin an offer of employment. He finally found a shopkeeper who was willing to employ his wife and give her a work visa. By August 1939 he had managed to secure tickets, visas, and passports for his wife and children to join him in England. Ecstatic, he put the documents in the mail.

War broke out one week later. In desperation Bill volunteered for the only unit available to him, the Pioneer Corps. In January 1940 he received a letter from the Red Cross telling him that Inge, who was now in a concentration camp with their two children, was pregnant with their third child. On January 30, 1940, Inge gave birth to a son, named Danny. After Bill was selected for X Troop, he heard that his wife and their three children, Ursula, Jackie, and Danny, had all been murdered in Auschwitz-Birkenau.

Watson married a British woman and had two daughters, Robin and Susan. After the war he returned to being a tailor and opened a shop. His second wife died when he was just forty-one and their children were thirteen and eight. He married a third time and was survived by his daughters and three grandchildren. Watson wrote in his memoir, "When everything was dark, England with her great compassion, offered me a helping hand, the chance to fight and the chance to start again."

# Notes

page

xi    *three weeks before D-Day:* Information on this encounter can be found in Roy Wooldridge letter, Records of the Ministry of Defence (hereafter cited as DEFE) 2/612, The National Archives of the UK (hereafter cited as TNA); WO 106_4343, TNA. George Lane gave multiple interviews about his experiences, as found in the following sources: Audio interviews with George Lane (13307 and 28406), Imperial War Museum (hereafter cited as IWM); George Lane, interview for BBC show on Aberdovey memorial unveiling, May 1999; Ian Dear, *10 Commando* (Barnsley, UK: Pen and Sword Military, 2011), pp. 86–91; Janusz Piekalkiewicz, *Secret Agents, Spies, and Saboteurs* (New York: William Morrow, 1971), pp. 392–397. I have the tapes for the George Lane interview for the BBC show on the Aberdovey memorial unveiling and for the other interviews for the show cited in the notes, but I don't have any additional information about the program. For information on Operation Tarbrush and Lane's role in it, see Hilary St. George Saunders, *The Green Beret: The Story of the Commandos* (London: Michael Joseph, 1949), pp. 216–217; James Owen, *Commando: Winning World War II Behind Enemy Lines* (London: Little, Brown, 2009), pp. 260–270. For Roy Wooldridge's account, see "Rommel Saved Me from Being Shot as a Spy and Even Served Me Cigarettes and Beer," *Daily Mail*, November 20, 2014. Information about the operation also comes from my phone interview with George Lane's wife, Elizabeth Lane, July 28, 2020. After Lane and Wooldridge were taken away, Rommel wrote to his wife about his "extraordinary interview with 'a sensible British officer.'" As quoted in Giles Milton, *Soldier, Sailor, Frogman, Spy, Airman, Gangster, Kill or Die: How the Allies Won on D-Day* (New York: Henry Holt, 2019), p. 20. The information on the Rommel meeting can be found on pp. 9–21.

xii    *a Kriegsmarine lieutenant shouts:* The Kriegsmarine was the German navy.

*Rommel has chosen this spot:* Anthony Beevor, *D-Day: The Battle for Normandy* (London: Penguin Books, 2010), p. 34.

xiii  *his Welsh accent is terrible:* Lane noticed that one of the Germans spoke flawless English, and he was worried that if he spoke with an English accent, the German would notice it was fake. Instead he used a singsong Welsh accent to try to hide his Hungarian origins.

xiv  *during his interrogation:* Wooldridge later recounted the full details of his interaction with Rommel in "Rommel Saved Me from Being Shot as a Spy."

*the Gestapo or the SS:* Rommel was so taken with Lane's "charm and bravado" that he made sure his life was spared, as found in Rommel's letter to his wife, as quoted in Milton, *Soldier, Sailor,* p. 20.

### Introduction

3  *Special Service Brigade:* The Special Service Brigade would be renamed the Commando Brigade during the war, but to avoid confusion, I use Special Service Brigade throughout.

*At least eighty-seven volunteers:* Depending on the source, the total number varies between 87 and 142, including a half troop that was put together in the final days of the war. The X Troop war diary ("The History of 46 [RM] Commando August 1943–June 1944 and Activities of No. 10 [Inter-Allied] Commando, June 1942–October 1944," DEFE 2/977, TNA) and most secondary sources put the number at 87, which is the number I use in this book. Martin Sugarman has compiled a working list in "World War II: No. 3 (Jewish) Troop of the No. 10 Commando," Jewish Virtual Library, n.d., https://www.jewishvirtuallibrary.org/no-3-jewish-troop-of-the-no-10-commando. There is also a list with the volunteers' original names and noms de guerre, along with some brief biographical information, in Martin Sugarman, *Fighting Back: British Jewry's Military Contribution in the Second World War* (London: Vallentine Mitchell, 2010), pp. 325–339.

4  *"seemingly insurmountable odds":* Peter Masters, *Striking Back: A Jewish Commando's War Against the Nazis* (Novato, CA: Presidio Press, 1997), p. xii.

*"all the killing":* Peter Terry, interview by Steven Karras for his documentary *About Face: Jewish Refugees in the Allied Forces* (Xenon Pictures, 2019). Karras kindly shared all his interview reels with me.

### Chapter 1: Exile

5  *the young man who would become Colin Anson:* Much of the information on Colin Anson in this chapter comes from Helen Fry, *German Schoolboy, British Commando: Churchill's Secret Soldier* (Cheltenham, UK: History Press, 2010). Additional information comes from the following interviews: Audio interviews with Colin Anson (30188 and 11883), IWM; Audio interview with Colin Anson (484), Jewish Museum London (hereafter cited as JML); Audio interviews with Colin Anson, privately recorded, 1988 and 2014, in family collection; Colin Anson, interview, BBC Radio 5 Live, September 2007; Colin Anson, interview, *Saturday Live,* BBC, November 10, 2007; Colin Anson, interview for *Churchill's German Army,* directed by Mark McMullen (True North Productions, 2009); Colin Anson, interview, *Remembrance Week,* BBC, 2013; Colin Anson, interview, "German Soldier Who Fought for Britain in World War II,"

*Magazine,* BBC News, April 30, 2010. Anson was also interviewed in "Churchill's Secret Commandos," newspaper article, Private Papers of Brian Grant (263), IWM.

7   *"first and foremost a German":* Fry, *German Schoolboy,* p. 14.

8   *"My father's ashes":* Fry, *German Schoolboy,* p. 38.

    *"leather-bound pocket editions":* Audio interview with Colin Anson (484), JML.

9   *an easy target:* Audio interview with Colin Anson (484), JML.

    *"I'll die here":* Anson interview, BBC Radio 5 Live.

10  *"a peasant in a Sunday suit":* Fry, *German Schoolboy,* p. 31.

11  *things he thought he might need:* A photograph of this list appears in Fry, *German Schoolboy,* photo insert.

    *"Get out of this train now":* Fry, *German Schoolboy,* p. 47.

12  *an excited sixteen-year-old:* Much of the information on Peter Masters in this chapter comes from his autobiography, Peter Masters, *Striking Back: A Jewish Commando's War Against the Nazis* (Novato, CA: Presidio Press, 1997). Additional information comes from the following sources: Audio recording of Peter Masters lecture (20786), IWM; Peter Masters, interview by Steven Karras for his documentary *About Face: Jewish Refugees in the Allied Forces* (Xenon Pictures, 2019); Peter Masters, Oral History Interview conducted by Esther Finder, August 7, 1998, File 1998.A.0190, RG-50.106.0110, United States Holocaust Memorial Museum, Washington, DC; Peter Masters, Oral History Interview conducted by Joshua Gray, April 19 and 23, 1996, File 996.A.0125, RG-50.106.0024, United States Holocaust Memorial Museum, Washington, DC; Peter Masters, Oral History of D-Day, Eisenhower Center, Peter Kalikow WWII-Era Collection, National WWII Museum, New Orleans. Masters's discussion of the soccer game is found in his April 1996 interview with the United States Holocaust Memorial Museum. His daughter Kim Masters also supplied biographical information to the author.

    *going to the World Cup:* For information on this game, see Kevin E. Simpson, *Soccer Under the Swastika: Stories of Survival and Resistance During the Holocaust* (London: Rowman and Littlefield, 2016), pp. 118–119.

13  *"Österreich! Österreich! Österreich!":* Within ten months, the greatest footballer in the world, Matthias Sindelar, would be dead in an apparent suicide.

    *came to power in 1933:* For a discussion of Hitler's takeover of Austria and the Anschluss, see Ian Kershaw, *Hitler: 1936–1945 Nemesis* (New York: W. W. Norton, 2000), chap. 2.

14  *"You should just cast":* Masters, *Striking Back,* p. 6.

16  *"somebody your own size":* Masters, *Striking Back,* p. 5.

18  *Manfred Gans had just turned:* Much of the information on Manfred Gans in this chapter comes from his autobiography, *Life Gave Me a Chance* (self-published, 2009). Additional information comes from the following sources: Audio interview with Fred Gray (Manfred Gans) (30192), IWM; Manfred Gans, interview by Steven Karras for his documentary *About Face: Jewish Refugees in the Allied Forces* (Xenon Pictures, 2019); Manfred Gans, interview for BBC show on Aberdovey memorial unveiling, May 1999; *One Less Fight,* directed by Jennifer Hahn (Bridgeseeker Productions, 2017); Manfred Gans, Oral History Interview conducted by Amy Ruben, November 11, 2004, File 2004.563, RG-50.030.0489, United States Holocaust Memorial Museum, Washington, DC. Manfred Gans's children, Aviva Gans Rosenberg and Daniel Gans, also supplied biographical information to the author.

20 *Gershon:* He was originally called Carl.

22 *"having grown up as an Orthodox Jew":* Gans, *Life Gave Me a Chance,* p. 13.

*"the thought of a free society":* Gans, *Life Gave Me a Chance,* p. 31.

*"allowed to return home":* Gans, *Life Gave Me a Chance,* p. 31.

### Chapter 2: Behind the Wire

23 *fellow passengers were smiling:* Fry, *German Schoolboy,* p. 48.

24 *"honest, willing and obliging":* Fry, *German Schoolboy,* p. 50.

*"without fear of being arrested":* Gans, interview for *About Face.*

*The subsequent Munich Agreement:* For an overview of the Munich Agreement, see Kershaw, *Hitler,* pp. 113–123; David Faber, *Munich, 1938: Appeasement and World War II* (New York: Simon and Schuster, 2010).

25 *following the Jewish laws:* Daniel Gans, interview with author, October 16, 2018.

26 *"enemy alien":* For discussions of the history of alien internment in Britain, see Peter Gillman and Leni Gillman, *Collar the Lot: How Britain Interned and Expelled Its Wartime Refugees* (London: Quartet Books, 1981); Ronald Stent, *A Bespattered Page: The Internment of His Majesty's "Most Loyal Enemy Aliens"* (London: Andre Deutsch, 1980); Tony Kushner and David Cesarani, eds., *The Internment of Aliens in Twentieth Century Britain* (London: Frank Cass, 1993); Richard Dove, ed., *"Totally Un-English"? Britain's Internment of "Enemy Aliens" in Two World Wars, Yearbook of the Research Centre for German and Austrian Exile Studies* 7 (Amsterdam: Rodopi B. V., 2005). For a discussion of the responses of the press, see David Cerarani, "An Alien Concept? The Continuity of Anti-Alienism in British Society Before 1940," in Kushner and Cesarani, *The Internment of Aliens,* pp. 44–45. For an overview of Jewish refugees from Germany and Austria who immigrated to England in the 1930s onward, see Anthony Grenville, *Jewish Refugees from Germany and Austria in Britain, 1933–1970* (London: Vallentine Mitchell, 2010).

*a machine fitter:* As the Wislickis wrote in a letter to Moritz and Else Gans, "We were greatly impressed from the very outset by [Manfred's] will-power, his capability to plan well for himself and his faculty for carrying out his plans whatever the obstacles might have been." Leo and Luise Wislicki to Moritz and Else Gans, July 9, 1945, Gans Family Papers, United States Holocaust Memorial Museum Archives, Washington, DC.

*an engineering degree:* Audio interview with Fred Gray (Manfred Gans) (30192), IWM.

27 *no longer looking:* Multiple emails from Daniel Gans and Aviva Gans Rosenberg to author.

*"You're being interned":* Audio interview with Fred Gray (Manfred Gans) (30192), IWM.

*least known and darkest chapters:* Tony Kushner and David Cesarani point out that the story of the internment was treated as a side note or downplayed until the early 1990s, and their edited volume *The Internment of Aliens in Twentieth Century Britain* was an attempt to revisit this underreported moment in British history.

28 *very worst British internment camps:* Stent, *A Bespattered Page,* p. 152. See also Connery Chappel, *Island of Barbed Wire: The Remarkable Story of World War Two Internment on the Isle of Man* (London: Hale Books, 2005), p. 3. For information on Jewish refugees in

Britain during this time period, see Clare Ungerson, *Four Thousand Lives: The Rescue of German Jewish Men to Britain, 1939* (Cheltenham, UK: History Press, 2014).

*The rats were unafraid:* See Joe Pieri, *Isle of the Displaced: An Italian-Scot's Memoirs of Internment During the Second World War* (London: Neil Wilson, 1977), p. 25.

*They kept kosher:* Gans, *Life Gave Me a Chance,* p. 51.

29  *"lack of food":* Audio interview with Fred Gray (Manfred Gans) (30192), IWM.

*overlooking the Irish Sea:* For the main history of internment on the Isle of Man, see Chappel, *Island of Barbed Wire.*

*pro-Nazi Germans:* Chappel, *Island of Barbed Wire,* p. 43. For a discussion of the Nazis housed there, see Louise Burletson, "The State, Internment and Public Criticism in the Second World War," in Kushner and Cesarani, *The Internment of Aliens,* pp. 104–105.

*"some sleazy harbor town":* Stent, *A Bespattered Page,* p. 159.

*treated as common prisoners:* A partial list of the well-known men who were interned can be found in Gillman and Gillman, *Collar the Lot,* pp. 174–176.

30  *"a no-good city kid":* Masters, *Striking Back,* p. 28.

*"stalking Nazis":* Masters, interview for *About Face.*

31  *two useless mouths to feed:* Masters, *Striking Back,* p. 28.

32  *"Good luck":* Masters, *Striking Back,* p. 28. See also Steven Karras, *The Enemy I Knew: German Jews in the Allied Military in World War II* (Minneapolis: Zenith Books, 2009), p. 236.

*"locked up behind barbed wire":* Masters, *Striking Back,* p. 27.

*"no rights at all":* Masters, *Striking Back,* p. 33.

33  *"let Peter go temporarily":* Audio recording of Peter Masters lecture (20786), IWM.

*the Blitz on London:* Masters, *Striking Back,* p. 37.

*"trying to kill me":* See the first few lines of George Orwell's iconic essay "England Your England."

*the name Paul Streeten:* The information on Paul Streeten comes from his autobiographical essay, Paul Streeten, "Aerial Roots," *PSL Quarterly Review* 39, no. 157 (1986), pp. 135–159; Paul Streeten, unpublished interview with David Simon, November 7, 2006. David Simon shared this interview with me.

34  *no one seemed to care:* Stent, *A Bespattered Page,* p. 110.

*"as an Austrian":* Streeten, "Aerial Roots," p. 145.

35  *the HMT Dunera:* There were nine future X Troopers on the *Dunera,* including Andreas Carlebach, Gotthard Baumwollspinner, Hans Georg Fürth, Egon Vogel, Werner Goldshmidt, Max Lewinsky, Heinz Herman Nell, and Hans Julius Guttmann. The list of internees on the *Dunera* can be found in the excellent sourcebook by Paul R. Bartrop and Gabrielle Eisen, eds., *The Dunera Affair: A Documentary Resource Book* (Melbourne: Jewish Museum of Australia and Schwartz and Wilkinson, 1990), pp. 397–411. The spelling of the names here is from the ship's roster and doesn't necessarily match the spelling I use in this book. The sourcebook is a compilation of a number of personal memoirs and accounts of what unfolded on the ship. Two of the most detailed are "Treatment of the Internees On Board the Dunera," pp. 151–158, and "The Dunera Statement," pp. 206–218.

36  *the instrument was taken:* "Treatment of the Internees On Board the Dunera," p. 152.

*committed suicide:* Gillman and Gillman, *Collar the Lot,* p. 247.

*howled with laughter:* Victor Davies, an X Trooper who was on the *Dunera,* still remembered this treatment at the age of ninety-seven when I interviewed him at his home in 2019. Victor Davies, interview with author, January 2019. "Victor Davies" is a pseudonym, as explained in the afterword.

*common in the United States at the time:* There had been little anti-Semitism in the United States before the 1920s. While there had been instances of prejudice, the country had been largely considered welcoming to Jewish immigrants. In 1924, at a time when America was hit by waves of xenophobia and anti-immigrant sentiment, Congress enacted the Immigration Act (aka the Johnson-Reed Act), which, as a way to stop the massive influx of Jews and Catholics, shut the door to most immigrants from eastern and southern Europe. (This would lead to disastrous results during the Holocaust, when the United States was not an option for Jews trying to escape the Nazis.) Anti-Semitism was at its peak in the United States during the 1930s, when the stock market crash combined with widespread anti-immigrant sentiment and isolationism made Jews a common target.

*different in the UK:* For a history of the Jews in England, see David S. Katz, *The Jews in the History of England, 1495–1850* (New York: Oxford University Press, 1997); Cecil Roth, *A History of the Jews in England* (Oxford: Clarendon Press, 1964). Also see Vivian David Lipman, "England," in *Encyclopedia Judaica,* ed. Fred Skolnik and Michael Berenbaum, 2nd ed., vol. 6 (Detroit: Macmillan Reference, 2007), pp. 410–417.

37 *demagogues and rabble-rousers:* The position of Jews in Britain was complicated by the proposed establishment of a Jewish national home in the British Mandate for Palestine. Although the 1917 Balfour Declaration expressed the government's support for this idea, by 1939 its White Paper instead sought to limit Jewish emigration there.

38 *stabbed in the stomach:* "Treatment of the Internees On Board the Dunera," p. 154.

*"without any special training":* Anthony Firth, "While I Think of It: A Non-biography" (unpublished memoir, n.d.), p. 38. Firth's daughter, Kathryn Firth, shared this with me.

*murdered in an extermination camp:* Letter from Tony Firth to Peter Masters, March 31, 1989, Peter Masters Collection, United States Holocaust Memorial Museum Archives, Washington, DC.

39 *"loading it was not a problem":* Firth, "While I Think of It," p. 38.

*"terrible camp in Hay":* Audio interview with Ron Gilbert (20786), IWM.

*"rabbits, too, at Booligal":* Banjo Paterson, "Hay and Hell and Booligal," in *Complete Poems* (Sydney: HarperCollins, 2014).

40 *"we could live undisturbed":* Anton Walter Freud, unpublished memoir, n.d., p. 15, Major A. W. Freud: Papers Relating to His Internment as an Enemy Alien, 1941 (05/78/1), IWM.

*surprisingly sophisticated fare:* At one point the local farmers were invited to a meal at the camp made by the refugee chefs and were stunned to find "a European gourmet dinner . . . News of this spread like a bushfire and in no time at all the camp had become the hottest restaurant ticket in the outback." Firth, "While I Think of It," p. 52.

*organize their transport:* "Letter of Authority for Major J. D. Layton," in Bartrop and Eisen, *The Dunera Affair,* p. 86.

*transport back to England:* Firth, "While I Think of It," p. 53.

*prepare for war:* Peter Leighton-Langer, *The King's Own Loyal Enemy Aliens: German and Austrian Refugees in Britain's Armed Forces, 1939–1945* (London: Vallentine Mitchell, 2006), p. 8.

41   *"dumping ground of the British army":* Gillman and Gillman, *Collar the Lot,* p. 257.
     *their ship was torpedoed:* "Extract from Layton Interview — Recruitment of Pioneer Corps for U.K.," in Bartrop and Eisen, *The Dunera Affair,* p. 101.

### Chapter 3: The Pioneer Corps

42   *"I joined the Army last week":* Masters, *Striking Back,* p. 40.
43   *"A for Alien" troops:* Leighton-Langer, *The King's Own,* p. 11.
     *"dying to have a go at Hitler":* Hugh Lewis, interview for BBC show on Aberdovey memorial unveiling, May 1999.
     *dull and unchallenging work:* Masters, *Striking Back,* p. 41.
     *"fight the Nazis by unloading freight cars":* Masters, *Striking Back,* p. 42.
44   *would be refused:* Lord Croft, House of Lords, "Aliens in the Pioneer Corps," debate, *Hansard,* July 22, 1941, https://api.parliament.uk/historic-hansard/lords/1941/jul/22 /aliens-in-the-pioneer-corps.
45   *"undoubtedly the most frustrating":* Mans, *Life Gave Me a Chance,* p. 53.
     *"were not being utilized":* Gans, *Life Gave Me a Chance,* p. 64.
     *his acceptance letter:* Manfred Gans, Oral History Interview conducted by Amy Ruben, November 11, 2004, File 2004.563, RG-50.030.0489, United States Holocaust Memorial Museum, Washington, DC.
     *studied advanced math:* Manfred Gans, Oral History Interview conducted by Amy Ruben, November 11, 2004, File 2004.563, RG-50.030.0489, United States Holocaust Memorial Museum, Washington, DC.
     *Penguin paperbacks:* Gans, *Life Gave Me a Chance,* p. 66.
     *Gone with the Wind:* Manfred Gans, diaries, Manfred Gans Collection, United States Holocaust Memorial Museum Archives, Washington, DC.
46   *shooting competitions as well:* Manfred Gans, diary, June 29, 1942, Manfred Gans Collection, United States Holocaust Memorial Museum Archives, Washington, DC.
     *"disassociate oneself":* Audio interview with Colin Anson (484), JML.
     *transformation into being British:* Fry, *German Schoolboy,* p. 57.
     *Colin's confidence:* Audio interview with Colin Anson (484), JML.
47   *to be more efficient:* For an overview of Hitler's campaign of genocide, see David Cesarani, *Final Solution: The Fate of the Jews, 1933–1949* (New York: St. Martin's Press, 2016); Martin Gilbert, *The Holocaust: The Human Tragedy* (New York: HarperCollins, 1987); Raul Hilberg, *The Destruction of the European Jews* (New York: Martino Fine Books, 2019).
49   *Churchill chatted frequently:* For Mountbatten's biography, see Philip Zeigler, *Mountbatten* (London: Smithmark, 1997), and for an extraordinary biography of Churchill, see Andrew Roberts, *Churchill: Walking with Destiny* (New York: Viking, 2018). For an outstanding book that focuses on the leadership qualities of the major figures of the war, including Churchill and Mountbatten, see Andrew Roberts, *Masters and Commanders: The Military Geniuses Who Led the West to Victory in World War Two* (New York: Penguin, 2009).

*see if it was workable:* Churchill often reversed himself like this; after telling his subordinates to "collar the lot" of them, they were now going to try to find likely recruits from the internees for the British Army. Churchill had previously agreed in principle to the idea of using German speakers in the Pioneer Corps to help with the war effort, though he wanted them to be thoroughly vetted: "I presume that this Corps will be most carefully scrubbed and re-scrubbed to make sure no Nazi cells develop in it. I am very much in favor of recruiting friendly Germans and keep them under strict discipline (sic.), instead of remaining useless in concentration camps, but we must be doubly careful we do not get any of the wrong breed." Winston Churchill to Colonel Jacobs, January 3, 1941, CAB 120_243, TNA. For more on Churchill's mercurial nature, see, for example, Erik Larson, *The Splendid and the Vile: A Saga of Churchill, Family, and Defiance During the Blitz* (New York: Crown, 2020), chap. 36.

*swearing was legendary:* Dear, *10 Commando,* p. 13.

50 *"almost impossible to contemplate":* Johnny Coates, interview for BBC show on Aberdovey memorial unveiling, May 1999.

*German-speaking refugees from the Nazis:* "George, Man Who Deceived Rommel," *News Chronicle,* October 25, 1946.

*"let us call them X Troop":* Dear, *10 Commando,* p. 6. A discussion of this is also found in Audio interview with George Lane (13307), IWM.

*highly capable and driven Welshman:* The biographical information on Bryan Hilton-Jones is from his private family archive, held by his daughter in law Ursula Hilton-Jones, who shared it with me.

*X Troop war diary:* Bryan Hilton-Jones, "No. 3 Troop, 10 Commando: A Brief History," appendix to "The History of 46 (RM) Commando August 1943–June 1944 and Activities of No. 10 (Inter-Allied) Commando, June 1942–October 1944," DEFE 2/977, TNA.

### Chapter 4: Joining the Fight

53 *"There was a war on":* Fry, *German Schoolboy,* p. 63.

*serve in the military:* Fry, *German Schoolboy,* p. 63.

54 *"in tropical kit":* Audio interview with Colin Anson (30188), IWM.

55 *killed in a concentration camp:* Audio interview with Colin Anson (30188), IWM.

*"George Lane, a Hungarian":* Firth, "While I Think of It," p. 62.

*"very much in evidence":* Lane, interview for BBC show on Aberdovey memorial.

*"the English are logical":* Firth, "While I Think of It," p. 66. Firth must have assumed that the new mission for which he was being recruited included spying.

56 *held at Leeds Castle:* George Lane, obituary, *Scotsman,* March 31, 2010. In 1944 Lane discovered that his father, who had been helping the Allied cause in Hungary, had disappeared without a trace.

*"Do you play cricket":* Audio interview with George Lane (13307), IWM.

*position in the Grenadiers:* Audio interview with George Lane (28406), IWM. See also Lane, interview for BBC show on Aberdovey memorial.

57 *"making my own decisions":* Lane, interview for BBC show on Aberdovey memorial.

58 *This low acceptance rate:* For an explanation of the number of men who served in X Troop, please refer to the second note for page 3.

*"from the Pioneer Corps to commandos":* Anson, interview for *Churchill's German Army.*

*"What is your name, soldier?":* Firth, "While I Think of It," p. 57.

60 *real names and places of origin:* Hilton-Jones, "No. 3 Troop, 10 Commando," documents the manifold lengths they went to in order to keep the men's real identities secret. See also Fry, *German Schoolboy,* p. 70.
*"a thick Teutonic accent":* Audio interview with Harry Drew (Harry Nomburg) (30198), IWM.

61 *member of the Royal Sussex Regiment:* Fry, *German Schoolboy,* p. 74.

62 *"'I'll think of another name'":* Peter Masters, interview for BBC show on Aberdovey memorial unveiling, May 1999.
*"Royal West Kent Regiment":* Masters, *Striking Back,* p. 54.

63 *to fight Hitler:* Manfred Gans, Oral History Interview conducted by Amy Ruben, November 11, 2004, File 2004.563, RG-50.030.0489, United States Holocaust Memorial Museum, Washington, DC.

64 *return to being Manfred Gans:* Daniel Gans, interview with author.

65 *easier to pronounce:* Lane, interview for BBC show on Aberdovey memorial.
*"a thrilling thing":* Masters, interview for *About Face.*

## Chapter 5: Disaster at Dieppe

67 *1,000 British commandos:* For an overview of Operation Jubilee, see Ronald Atkin, *Dieppe 1942: The Jubilee Disaster* (London: Macmillan, 1980); Ken Ford, *Dieppe: Prelude to D-Day* (Oxford: Osprey, 2003); Robin Neillands, *The Dieppe Raid: The Story of the Disastrous 1942 Expedition* (Bloomington: Indiana University Press, 2005); David O'Keefe, *One Day in August: The Untold Story Behind Canada's Tragedy at Dieppe* (Toronto: Knopf, 2013); "Dieppe Raid," in *The Oxford Companion to World War II,* ed. Ian Dear (Oxford: Oxford University Press, 1995), pp. 298–299.

68 *overlooking White Beach:* Neillands, *The Dieppe Raid,* p. 211.
*"mowed down like flies":* As quoted in Atkin, *Dieppe 1942,* p. 157.
*having lost their minds:* O'Keefe, *One Day in August,* p. 365.

69 *destroyed the papers:* The after-action reports of Latimer and Platt can be found in 10 (1A) War Diary, DEFE 218/40, appendix B (Platt) and appendix C (Latimer), TNA.

70 *"shop windows looked intact":* Lieutenant Herb Prince, as quoted in Atkin, *Dieppe 1942,* p. 153.
*would make it back:* Atkin, *Dieppe 1942,* p. 168; Neillands, *The Dieppe Raid,* p. 218.

71 *"burning with the cause":* Victor Davies, email to author, March 3, 2019.

72 *SS chief Reinhard Heydrich:* Heydrich was in charge of putting Hitler's final solution (the extermination of European Jews) into effect. He oversaw the Nazi protectorates of Bohemia and Moravia and was based in Prague, where he organized the brutal suppression of the Czech Resistance, earning him the nickname "the Butcher of Prague." The SOE, working with the Czechoslovakian government-in-exile, hatched a plot to assassinate Heydrich in Prague on May 27, 1942. The mission was successful, and Heydrich was severely wounded by the mortar attack on his chauffeured car. He died from his injuries on June 4, 1942. As some Czech partisans had cautioned, however, Heydrich's death became an excuse for the Nazis to enact mass murder on Czech civilians. For the full story of the role of the SOE in the Heydrich assassination, see Callum MacDonald, *The Assassination of Reinhard Heydrich* (Edinburgh: Brill, 2007).
*"never let anyone down":* Max Loewy (Maurice Latimer), SOE file, HS9/934/1, TNA.

*"what to do"*: Joseph Smith, naturalization file, "Nationality and Naturalisation: KUGLER, J aka SMITH," HO 405/28718, TNA. I received permission to view this file, which is officially closed until 2073 (one hundred years after he applied for British citizenship).

*particularly in Czechoslovakia*: Smith also had some drawbacks. A couple of times between 1941, when he was recruited, and August 1942 he went missing for a day or two with local women. He mentioned to one of the women on May 30, 1942, that he had "only just come back from France" (Smith, naturalization file). This suggests that he may have been used for advance raids into Vichy France in preparation for the invasion. For an interesting article about the X Troopers from Czechoslovakia, see Jeremy Monk's "Forgotten Heroes? The Czechs of X-Troop," No. 10 Commando, Prague Post, July 30, 2017, https://www.praguepost.com/culture/forgotten-heroes-czech-x-troop-commando.

*Charles Rice, for his part*: H9/H69/5, TNA.

73 *Enigma encryption machines*: Whereas O'Keefe, *One Day in August,* views the Dieppe Raid as being undertaken primarily as a cover for the Enigma pinch, Nicholas Rankin sees the pinch as one aspect of the raid. Nicholas Rankin, *Ian Fleming's Commandos: The Story of 30 Assault Unit in WWII* (London: Faber and Faber, 2011).

*the Hotel Moderne*: O'Keefe, *One Day in August,* pp. 241–243. See also Rankin, *Ian Fleming's Commandos*, p. 3.

*unbreakable Enigmas*: For a history of British attempts to break the Enigma code, see Andrew Hodges, *Alan Turing: The Enigma* (New York: Vintage Books, 2017); B. Jack Copeland, *Colossus: The Secrets of Bletchley Park's Codebreaking Computers* (Oxford: Oxford University Press, 2010).

74 *back to England*: O'Keefe, *One Day in August;* Rankin, *Ian Fleming's Commandos,* chapter 1. In researching this book, I located an intriguing passage in a memoir by the journalist Goronwy Rees, who served under Lord Mountbatten in Combined Operations. Rees helped organize Operation Rutter, and in a voice dripping with condescension he details his interactions with "a small party of Sudeten-German Socialists" who could only have been X Troopers: "But even at this last moment odd and bizarre excrescences added themselves to the plan. In my capacity as odd job man I received instructions, I was not quite clear from whom, that I would be issued with huge numbers of forged French notes in large denominations which would be distributed to a small party of Sudeten-German Socialists in British uniforms who were to be attached to the operation in order to carry out some suicidal mission. The notes were delivered to me by a sergeant of no known regiment in a sealed parcel under the clock at Victoria Station. I gave no receipt for them nor was ever asked for any account of them. The mission was extremely secret and its purpose was not revealed to me. Back on the island, I located the suicide party who spoke no language except their own dialect of German. Room had to be found for them in the boats; they were an embarrassing responsibility. I was unable to distribute all my enormous funds because some members of the party were missing and I had no means of locating them. So I kept those thousands of francs, and I had them in my possession until long after the war, when I finally destroyed them. Nor did I ever know what happened to those bewildered Sudeten-Germans, fighting their own private war in a helpless cause; I imagine they disappeared without a trace on the beaches of Dieppe and that their names, like those mysterious francs, never appeared in any official rec-

ord." Goronwy Rees, *A Bundle of Sensations: Sketches in Autobiography* (New York: Macmillan, 1960), pp. 157–158.

*quest to get an Enigma machine:* When I first learned that X Troop was formed in July 1942 with a handful of Sudeten Germans, I found this strange and illogical. Hilton-Jones always seemed to undertake everything with such care and focus, so why had this initial group been chosen so quickly and then given very little training before being sent on a major amphibious operation? Why did Maurice Latimer, who was so open about discussing his experiences in Czechoslovakia with the others, refuse to discuss Dieppe? Why waste a talented operator like Latimer on such a showy mission when he had already conducted raids, had advanced training, and was being coveted by different agencies that were interested in having him as an asset? Also, why waste fluent German speakers on an operation to a French seaside town? After reading Rankin's *Ian Fleming's Commandos* and O'Keefe's *One Day in August* and speaking with O'Keefe in detail about his findings, I realized that this all made complete sense because the men were likely being used to snatch the Enigma machine.

*"the first raw material":* Hilton-Jones, "No. 3 Troop, 10 Commando." All of the quotes in this section are from this source.

75    *"known as No. 10 Commando":* C. M. Woods to Ian Dear, January 22, 1986, Private Papers of I C B Dear (22991), IWM.

*"a new German respirator":* The after-action reports of Platt and Latimer can be found in 10 (1A) War Diary, DEFE 218/40, appendix B (Platt) and appendix C (Latimer), TNA.

76    *Fleming's men in Naval Intelligence:* O'Keefe, *One Day in August,* pp. 97–98.

*X Troopers were sent to Dieppe:* When I was seeking Miriam Rothschild's file from Bletchley Park, they sent me an email saying, "Unfortunately, Foreign Office personnel files for this period were destroyed many years ago." Museum archivist, Bletchley Park, email to author, February 25, 2019.

*"that's exactly what we did":* Ron Beal, as quoted in O'Keefe, *One Day in August,* p. 360.

77    *"enemy occupied territory":* 10 (1A) War Diary, DEFE 218/40, TNA.

78    *continually attempted to escape:* Joseph Smith and Charles Rice at first were listed as "MIA possibly KIA." It turns out that both of them ended up in the infamous Stalag 344, a large German prisoner of war camp located in the small town of Lamsdorf (now called Lambinowice), in southwest Poland. Many POWs from Dieppe were housed there, and the Germans, in supposed retaliation for British maltreatment of German POWs, tied their hands together for twelve hours a day for weeks on end and sent them out to do grueling work. SOE files reveal several inquiries from SOE to MI5 about the men, asking if they have "passed as Englishmen." The fact that in the POW files Smith is listed as serving with the Buffs (the Royal East Kent Regiment) and Rice is listed as serving with the Royal Sussex Regiment means that during their hellish years in Stalag 344, both men must have convincingly kept up their false personas and effectively hidden that they were in fact German-speaking commandos of X Troop. When the Russians were close to liberating the camp in January 1945, the SS sent most of the prisoners west on a death march through the snowy winter. Smith and Rice survived the march. Smith wrote about his time at Stalag 344 in his debriefing document (August 30, 1945). Upon capture, he was interrogated (likely very brutally) but shared only his name, rank, and serial number and refused to give any other information (which would have included his true name, his true origins, and the real intention of his mission). During his time at Stalag 344 Smith was sent

to four different hard labor camps, where he worked in a stone quarry, laid railroad tracks, and did sandblasting. Remarkably, he made three attempted escapes. On his first try he broke through the bars over a window in his barracks and crawled out, but he was captured by a patrol. The second time he simply walked away from a work site and hid in a house, but he was given away by a Croatian woman. And for his third go he escaped with another prisoner and made it all the way across Germany, only to be captured on the Swiss frontier. After his escape attempts, Smith took on a new persona, calling himself Lance Corporal Krickup. Little did the Germans know that each time they captured Lance Corporal Krickup, he was really Private Joseph Smith of Yorkshire, whose birth name was Josef Kugler. Charles Rice did not attempt any prison escapes, but in his debrief he did note that he undertook sabotage actions against the Germans while "employed on a working party" (debriefing document, August 30, 1945). Smith and Rice both show up in TNA one month later, in September 1945, when Smith, now using his birth name (Josef Kugler), signed the marriage certificate of his sister and Rice in Halifax. Kugler then went to Germany as an interpreter with the British Control Commission and was there until 1947. Bizarrely, Smith doesn't resurface in TNA until December 31, 1972, when he applied for British citizenship. As for Rice, he resurfaces in June 1952, when he applied for naturalization. I also received permission to view his naturalization file, which is officially closed until 2052 (one hundred years after he applied for British citizenship). Smith's and Rice's debriefing documents are found in WO344_294_2, TNA.

## Chapter 6: The Elite of the Elite

79  *twelve other new recruits:* In later recruitments members of X Troop would meet the recruits on the train and oversee the removal of their Pioneer Corps uniforms. Their name changes would take place upon arrival in Aberdovey, Wales, rather than in Bradford.

*forgetting his own nom de guerre:* Audio interview with Colin Anson (30188), IWM.

80  *Ahead lay Aberdovey:* The Welsh spelling of the town is "Aberdyfi." I use "Aberdovey" throughout this book because that is how the men wrote and spoke about it.

*"say the bells of Aberdovey":* "The Bells of Aberdovey," Wikipedia, https://en.wikipedia .org/wiki/The_Bells_of_Aberdovey.

81  *"an end to the Hitler regime":* Gans, interview for BBC show on Aberdovey memorial.

*the middle of the town:* Firth, "While I Think of It," p. 69.

*accepted their green berets:* Fry, *German Schoolboy*, p. 74.

82  *move extremely quietly:* Fry, *German Schoolboy*, p. 82.

*6 shillings and 8 pence:* Fry, *German Schoolboy*, p. 74.

*spoiling their guests:* Firth, "While I Think of It," p. 70.

83  *practiced his new signature:* Masters, *Striking Back*, p. 56.

*"a butterfly at last":* Masters, *Striking Back*, p. 57.

*His tallis and tefillin:* Gans, *Life Gave Me a Chance*, p. 82.

*"the elite of the elites":* Gans, *Life Gave Me a Chance*, p. 84.

*"cold bluish":* Masters, *Striking Back*, p. 59.

84  *vaulted over it:* Masters, *Striking Back*, p. 59.

*"The object was to produce":* Hilton-Jones, "No. 3 Troop, 10 Commando."

*up to forty miles:* Gans, *Life Gave Me a Chance*, p. 91.

85 *Sergeant Lane won:* Audio interview with Miriam Rothschild (30203), IWM.
"*the Hungarian Hunk*": Firth, "While I Think of It," p. 72.
"*a kind of superman*": Peter Terry, as quoted in Karras, *The Enemy I Knew*, p. 85.
"*better than any of us*": Brian Grant, "A Tale of Five Names" (unpublished memoir, 1995), Private Papers of Brian Grant (9287), IWM.
*none of them drowned:* Firth, "While I Think of It," p. 72.
*desperate not to disappoint him:* After the war, the Skipper's letters of recommendation were prized possessions. In fact, the sole document that X Trooper Victor Davies kept from his military service was the letter Hilton-Jones wrote about him, in which Hilton-Jones stated that he was an "excellent soldier due to his intelligence, initiative, and cheerfulness." Bryan Hilton-Jones letter, April 5, 1946, in Davies's possession.

86 "'*simply bring him along*'": Masters, *Striking Back,* pp. 61–62.
*Victor Davies:* "Victor Davies" is a pseudonym, as explained in the afterword.
"*calmly talking me upward*": Letter to Ian Dear, March 23, 1986, Private Papers of I C B Dear (22991), IWM.
"*I am not really British*": Gans, *Life Gave Me a Chance*, p. 93.

87 "*without hesitation*": Lewis, interview for BBC show on Aberdovey memorial.

88 "*I shall call Mr. Churchill*": Masters, *Striking Back,* p. 71.
*even parachuting:* Firth, "While I Think of It," p. 72.
*master lock picker:* Masters, *Striking Back,* p. 62.

89 "*Yes, sir*": Fry, *German Schoolboy,* p. 83.
*murdered in Sachsenhausen concentration camp:* Ken Bartlett letter to Peter Masters, June 17, 1989, Peter Masters Collection, United States Holocaust Memorial Museum Archives, Washington, DC.
"*more about the German army*": Masters, interview for BBC show on Aberdovey memorial.

91 *encourage the prisoner to talk:* There is even an extensive section of one of Masters's diaries that describes in detail, with illustrations, how the men were expected to interrogate captured POWS on the field. This is an extraordinary document that underlines the vital role the X Troopers would play on D-Day and beyond. I present it here in full.

> A: Capture: If he surrenders, only one man approaches him, the others don't disclose their positions because of the possibility of traps.
>
> B: Search: a) weapons, knives, and razors. b) documents c) leave identity discs on prisoners.
>
> C: Treatment: a) separate officers, N.C.Os, men and deserters b) don't fraternize c) give food if only in complete state of exhaustion. Know what to find out! Strength, disposition, intensions.
>
> D: Preliminary Examination: Report: A) 1. What was he doing when captured. 2. Who was with him. 3. What was known of enemy before: Examine and interrogate separately. B) Look at 1. His weapons 2. His documents. 3. Uniform. Result: Identity of POW/Locality of capture/Time and occupation of capture.
>
> E. Main interrogations: What to find out: In defense: 1. Positions of LMGs, fields of fire, dumps. 2. Mortars. 3. S. Mgs 4. Section platoon and Bw. Position 5. Boundaries. 6. HQs 7. 13 and 15 th Coy. 8. Supporting arms, eg. artillery,

projectors, tanks, etc. 9. Casualties 10. Commanders Names 11. Intentions. In Attack: 1. Tasks of section, platoon, 2. Support: how allotted. 3. Special support 4. Boundaries 5. Casualties 6. Commander's name 7. Intentions. 6. How to get it: 1. Prove him lying, ask questions to which an answer is already known. 2. Show of knowledge. 3. Bullying. 4. Let him prove that he knows better. 5. Leave long pauses if no answer comes forth. 6. Don't ask a leading question! 7. Don't ask too many questions too quickly. 8. Don't expect too much 9. Deny spectacular information so as to check it. Result: Strength, Disposition and Intentions of Enemy.

F: Disposal: 1. Make sure that you know the evaluation of POWs before you start. 2. Put documents found in different ranks into different bags and give them to the guards.

G: The Written Report: Should be headed "secret" or "not secret." All names in block letters. Clear heading for every paragraph.

Peter Masters, diary, Alice Masters Collection, United States Holocaust Memorial Museum Archives, Washington, DC.

*the X Troop anthem*: Fry, *German Schoolboy*, p. 83.

*"'we'll all be in big trouble'"*: Ian Harris, interview for BBC show on Aberdovey memorial unveiling, May 1999.

*"Up yours, mate"*: Early in the war Winston Churchill had famously reversed the two-fingered rude salute and told everyone it now meant "V for Victory" over the Nazis, but sometimes he would "forget" to turn his hand around, and rumor had it that every British person knew that he was really saying "Up yours, Hitler."

92   *"ruddy foreigners"*: Grant, "A Tale of Five Names," p. 80.

*"a dozen or more men"*: Fry, *German Schoolboy*, p. 77.

*mere yards away*: Fry, *German Schoolboy*, p. 77.

*"the sound of being shot at"*: Fry, *German Schoolboy*, pp. 77–78.

93   *"frozen solid"*: Fry, *German Schoolboy*, p. 79.

*doze off while they marched*: Fry, *German Schoolboy*, p. 75.

*"'foreigners were fucking fit'"*: Grant, "A Tale of Five Names," p. 80.

*return the cap*: Masters, *Striking Back*, p. 74.

94   *"Colt .45 pistols"*: Masters, *Striking Back*, p. 70.

*murdered his dear father*: Colin Anson, interview for BBC show on Aberdovey memorial unveiling, May 1999.

*new developments in field craft*: Gans, interview for *About Face*.

95   *traitors of the Sudeten German populace*: Masters, *Striking Back*, p. 118.

*loved every minute of it*: Audio interview with George (should be Geoff) Broadman (30190), IWM. Information on Broadman also comes from his son Ladi. Ladi Broadman, interview with author, August 16, 2018.

96   *"superbly self-confident"*: Gans, *Life Gave Me a Chance*, p. 86.

97   *The police had been informed*: In his war diary, Bryan Hilton-Jones writes, "The local constable, P. C. Davies, was let into the secret." Hilton-Jones, "No. 3 Troop, 10 Commando."

*kept quiet about it*: Fry, *German Schoolboy*, p. 74.

*"Teutonic accents"*: Hilton-Jones, "No. 3 Troop, 10 Commando."

*"'Vee are English'"*: Uncredited interview for BBC show on Aberdovey memorial unveiling, May 1999.

*had their birth names in them:* D. V. Wade to Ian Dear, June 22, 1988, Private Papers of I C B Dear (22991), IWM.

*they were likely Jewish as well:* For a history of Jews in Wales, see Cai Parry-Jones, *The Jews of Wales: A History* (Cardiff: University of Wales Press, 2017).

*"had a rough time":* Dylis Jordan, interview for BBC show on Aberdovey memorial unveiling, May 1999.

*spill the beans:* Gans, *Life Gave Me a Chance,* p. 82.

98    *"prosperous and rather snotty":* Hilton-Jones, "No. 3 Troop, 10 Commando."

*"Such good manners":* Uncredited interview for BBC show on Aberdovey memorial unveiling, May 1999.

*"a part of the family":* D. V. Wade to Ian Dear, June 22, 1988, Private Papers of I C B Dear (22991), IWM.

*"handsome bunch of young men":* Uncredited interview for BBC show on Aberdovey memorial unveiling, May 1999.

99    *develop in peace:* Masters, *Striking Back,* p. 66.

*basic survival needs:* Streeten, "Aerial Roots," pp. 148–149.

*philanthropists, naturalists, and conservationists:* Kennedy Fraser's profile of Miriam Rothschild, "Fritillaries and Hairy Violets," *The New Yorker,* October 19, 1987, pp. 45–75. See also Rothschild's book about her uncle Lionel Walter Rothschild, *Dear Lord Rothschild: Birds, Butterflies and History* (Philadelphia: ISI Press, 1983).

100  *"giant tortoises":* Fraser, "Fritillaries and Hairy Violets," p. 45.

*"a rather conceited man":* Fraser, "Fritillaries and Hairy Violets," p. 45.

*"two days off every fortnight":* Fraser, "Fritillaries and Hairy Violets," p. 45.

*Nazi sympathizers in England:* For the biography of Miriam's brother, Victor, see Kenneth Rose, *Elusive Rothschild: The Life of Victor, Third Baron* (London: Weidenfeld and Nicolson, 2003).

101  *create perfect children:* Firth, "While I Think of It," pp. 72–73.

*"They were very intellectual":* Audio interview with Miriam Rothschild (30203), IWM.

*read by her brother, Victor:* Rose, *Elusive Rothschild,* p. 78.

102  *"'the footsteps of true love'":* Audio interview with Miriam Rothschild (30203), IWM.

*betray their fellow commandos:* Gans, *Life Gave Me a Chance,* p. 86.

### Chapter 7: Italy

104  *he was going to die:* For Streeten's account of the campaign, see Streeten, "Aerial Roots," pp. 149–150; Paul Streeten, unpublished interview with David Simon; Paul Streeten, "July 1943: On the Night of the 9th," as quoted in Dear, *10 Commando,* pp. 92–94.

105  *"Let's give the bastards hell":* As quoted in Barbara Brooks Tomblin, *With Utmost Spirit: Allied Naval Operations in the Mediterranean, 1942–1945* (Lexington: University Press of Kentucky, 2004), p. 160.

*"to feel fear":* Paul Streeten, as quoted in Dear, *10 Commando,* p. 93.

*heading to Norway:* For an overview of X Troop in the Italian and Mediterranean campaigns, see Dear, *10 Commando,* chap. 6; Nick van der Bijl, *Commandos in Exile: The Story of 10 (Inter-Allied) Commando, 1942–1945* (Barnsley, UK: Pen and Sword Military, 2008), chap. 7; Nick van der Bijl, *No. 10 (Inter-Allied) Commando, 1942–45: Britain's Secret Commando* (Oxford: Osprey, 2006), pp. 14–18.

*reasons for the invasion:* For a history of the Sicily invasion and Italian campaign, see Rick Atkinson, *The Day of the Battle: The War in Sicily and Italy, 1943–1944* (New York: Henry Holt, 2008); Ian Gooderson, *A Hard Way to Make a War: The Allied Campaign in Italy in the Second World War* (London: Conway, 2009); Gerhard Weinberg, *A World at Arms: A Global History of World War Two* (New York: Cambridge University Press, 2005), pp. 591–601.

106   *planning to invade Greece:* For a history of Operation Mincemeat, see Ben Macintyre, *Operation Mincemeat: How a Dead Man and a Bizarre Plan Fooled the Nazis and Assured an Allied Victory* (New York: Broadway Books, 2010).
*First Canadian Division:* Ian Blackwell, *Battle for Sicily: Stepping Stone to Victory* (Barnsley, UK: Pen and Sword Military, 2008), pp. 93–94.
*The Marines wanted:* It may be anachronistic to call the commandos in the naval units "Marines," as the term didn't really get broad usage until after the war in the UK, but it is technically correct and allows me to use other terms besides "commandos" to describe the men.

107   *"southern leaves and fruits":* Paul Streeten, as quoted in Dear, *10 Commando,* p. 93.

108   *they were all going to drown:* Audio interview with Colin Anson (11883), IWM; Audio interview with Colin Anson, privately recorded, 1988.
*song of the cicadas:* Audio interview with Colin Anson, privately recorded, 1988.
*"coming over the shore":* Fry, *German Schoolboy,* p. 93.
*machine guns using tracer bullets:* Fry, *German Schoolboy,* p. 94.

109   *fifteen taken prisoner:* Audio interview with Colin Anson, privately recorded, 1988.
*"those awful pillboxes":* Audio interview with Colin Anson, privately recorded, 1988.

110   *"everyone laughed":* Fry, *German Schoolboy,* p. 96.
*pears and ripening melons:* 40 (RM) Cdo. War Diary, Records of the Admiralty (hereafter cited as ADM) 202/87, TNA.

111   *his injured comrade's head:* Fry, *German Schoolboy,* p. 99.
*fifty-eight were badly wounded:* 40 (RM) Cdo. War Diary, ADM 202/87, TNA.
*"a bit worse tonight":* Audio interview with Colin Anson (484), JML.

112   *children in the area:* Streeten, "Aerial Roots," p. 150.

113   *no one expected him to survive:* Streeten, "Aerial Roots," p. 150.
*disproportionately on Anson:* While Streeten and Anson were recovering in the hospital, word got back to the War Office that X Troop had performed in an exemplary fashion. New men were thus deployed to take on leadership roles in the Italian campaign, including Brian Grant, who had been snatched from Cambridge University to be shipped to Canada for internment along with Paul Streeten. He was promoted to sergeant major and was put in charge of nine men for Operation Partridge, an amphibious attack behind enemy lines in Italy. The raid was a success, and Grant personally captured some of the twenty-nine Germans. The following night, however, against the protests of Brigadier Tom Churchill, a decision was made to send Grant out to try to locate four commandos who had gone missing. During the mission he stepped on a mine, and this "extremely popular Sergeant" lost his foot and would be out of commission for the rest of the war. The quote is from Hilton-Jones, "No. 3 Troop, 10 Commando." See also Grant, "A Tale of Five Names," p. 498; Masters, *Striking Back,* pp. 134–135; Dear, *10 Commando,* chap. 6; Van der Bijl, *Commandos in Exile,* pp. 52–71.
*"bugles and bullshit":* Audio interview with Colin Anson (484), JML.

114　*the novelist Evelyn Waugh:* Waugh had also been at Freetown around the time that Maurice Latimer was there doing missions for the SOE. It is interesting that X Troop was in close proximity to three of Britain's most important writers, Evelyn Waugh, Graham Greene, and Ian Fleming.

　　*articles for the Vis newspaper:* Fry, *German Schoolboy,* p. 119.

115　*118th Jäger Division:* Operation Flounced War Diary, W0204_7290, TNA.

116　*encounters with the eccentric colonel:* For Anson's discussion of his interactions with Mad Jack Churchill, see Fry, *German Schoolboy,* p. 117.

117　*a huge Allied force had landed:* Operation Flounced War Diary, W0204_7290, TNA.

　　*"coming closer and closer":* Fry, *German Schoolboy,* p. 116.

118　*straight toward the German lines:* 40 (RM) Cdo. War Diary, ADM 202/87, TNA.

　　*attempted to take the ridge:* Fry, *German Schoolboy,* p. 117.

　　*"The Germans were deceived":* Operation Flounced War Diary, W0204_7290, TNA.

　　*a blow to the Nazis' efforts:* Andrew L. Hargreaves, *Special Operations in World War Two: British and American Irregular Warfare* (Norman: University of Oklahoma Press, 2013), p. 192.

　　*captured 160:* Operation Flounced War Diary, W0204_7290, TNA.

　　*knocked unconscious by a mortar shell:* Churchill was flown to Berlin to be interrogated and then taken to Sachsenhausen concentration camp, where he escaped with a fellow officer by crawling through an abandoned drain in September 1944. He was recaptured by the Germans in the Baltic Sea port of Rostock and imprisoned in Tyrol, before escaping again near the end of the war. Walking ninety miles through Italy to Verona, he was picked up by an American patrol. After Germany surrendered in May 1945, Mad Jack volunteered for the war in the Pacific, but on arriving in Burma, he was devastated to learn that the Japanese had signed an armistice. "If it wasn't for those damn Yanks we could have kept the war going another ten years," he was later reputed to have said.

*Chapter 8: The Field Marshal, the Water Polo Star, and the Code Breaker*

120　*flirting with the attendees:* Masters, *Striking Back,* p. 83.

　　*"blowing the cover":* Masters, *Striking Back,* p. 85.

　　*"you lads did very well":* Gans, *Life Gave Me a Chance,* p. 102.

　　*"a separate troop":* Hilton-Jones, "No. 3 Troop, 10 Commando."

121　*"from nothing into sweet fuck-all":* Masters, *Striking Back,* p. 92.

　　*wear a plaster cast for months:* Victor Davies also witnessed the memorable night jump of Maurice Latimer, which he described to me: "The wind drifted him into a group of trees, the parachute got entangled, and he was dangling from a branch and very unhappy. When we got to him, he was in fact just feet from the ground, unable to disentangle himself and totally unaware of how close he was to standing on his feet . . . We had a laugh, shared some drinks, but also thought how much different this would have been in enemy territory." Victor Davies, email to author.

　　*"grass and snails":* Bill Watson, unpublished memoir, September 1979, p. 234, Private Papers of I C B Dear (22991), IWM.

122　*the question was where:* Max Hastings discusses the urgent early desire of the Americans to invade the continent and the ambivalence of the British to do so "right up to the eve of D-Day" in *Overlord: D-Day and the Battle for Normandy* (New York: Vintage Books, 2006). The quote is from p. 19.

*land on the Pas-de-Calais:* There are numerous excellent histories that cover the buildup before D-Day. See, for example, Hastings, *Overlord,* pp. 19–68; John Keegan, *Six Armies in Normandy* (New York: Penguin Books, 1994), pp. 1–20; Andrew Roberts, *The Storm of War: A New History of the Second World War* (New York: Penguin Books, 2010), pp. 461–491; Beevor, *D-Day,* pp. 1–31; Stephen E. Ambrose, *D-Day: June 6, 1944; The Climactic Battle of World War Two* (New York: Simon and Schuster, 1994), pp. 1–195; James Holland, *Normandy '44: D-Day and the Epic 77-Day Battle for France* (New York: Atlantic Monthly Press, 2019), part 1.

123   *strapped to their chests:* Masters, *Striking Back,* p. 101.

    *"capturing a prisoner":* Firth, "While I Think of It," p. 77.

    *the shores of France:* Information on this encounter can be found in Roy Wooldridge letter, DEFE 2/612, TNA; WO 106_4343, TNA. George Lane gave multiple interviews about his experiences, as found in the following sources: Audio interviews with George Lane (13307 and 28406), IWM; Lane, interview for BBC show on Aberdovey memorial; Dear, *10 Commando,* pp. 86–91; Piekalkiewicz, *Secret Agents,* pp. 392–397; Milton, *Soldier, Sailor,* pp. 9–21. For information on Operation Tarbrush and Lane's role in it, see Saunders, *The Green Beret,* pp. 216–217; Owen, *Commando,* pp. 260–270. For Roy Wooldridge's account, see "Rommel Saved Me from Being Shot as a Spy." Information about the operation also comes from my phone interview with Elizabeth Lane, July 28, 2020.

    *men from a range of units:* DEFE 2/612, TNA.

124   *"people who came to land":* Lane, interview for BBC show on Aberdovey memorial.

    *"if we [simply] looked at it":* Bryan Hilton-Jones, as quoted in Saunders, *The Green Beret,* p. 264.

125   *"jeopardized the whole expedition":* DEFE 2/612, TNA.

    *captured by the Germans:* WO 106_4343, TNA.

126   *hills of central Germany:* After his meeting with Lane, Rommel wrote to his wife about his "extraordinary interview with 'a sensible British officer,'" which likely saved Lane's life. Rommel, as quoted in Milton, *Soldier, Sailor,* p. 20.

127   *grow out of ramparts:* Elizabeth Lane, phone interview with author.

    *had not been killed immediately:* Audio interview with Miriam Rothschild (30203), IWM.

128   *"such a successful conclusion":* DEFE 2/612, TNA.

    *"of the highest importance":* DEFE 2/612, TNA.

    *D-Day could go on:* DEFE 2/612, TNA.

### Chapter 9: Southampton, June 4–5, 1944

129   *on a brisk morning:* It is surprising that Lord Lovat addressed the men outdoors (as seen in the photo on page 132), but there surely must have been extreme security in the perimeter around the men to make sure the information on D-Day did not get out.

131   *"prove that tomorrow":* Lord Lovat, *March Past: A Memoir* (London: Weidenfeld and Nicolson, 1978), p. 304.

    *commando units for D-Day:* For the full list, see Van der Bijl, *Commandos in Exile,* p. 201.

*holding the left flank:* Lovat, *March Past,* p. 293.

133  *"would be killed":* Masters, interview for *About Face.*

134  *unaware that he was Jewish:* Audio interview with George Nichols (30200), IWM.

135  *accepted Nichols's invitation:* Masters, *Striking Back,* p. 145.

    *get the hang of it:* Peter Masters, "The French Window: A Scrapbook from Normandy," private family collection.

    *"pretty damn good at that":* Masters, *Striking Back,* p. 154.

    *"as individuals and as a Troop":* Hilton-Jones, "No. 3 Troop, 10 Commando."

    *looked up to them:* Audio interview with Gordon Geiser (Henry Gordon) (30193), IWM.

136  *noted in the X Troop war diary:* Hilton-Jones, "No. 3 Troop, 10 Commando."

    *"finest lot of OCTU applicants":* Hilton-Jones, "No. 3 Troop, 10 Commando."

    *"somebody new now":* Gans, interview for *About Face.*

137  *became exacerbated:* Max Hastings discusses Monty's complicated personality in *Overlord,* 32–33.

    *on several occasions:* The main biography of Montgomery is Nigel Hamilton, *Monty: The Battles of Field Marshal Bernard Montgomery* (New York: Random House, 1994).

    *"I was going to fall into":* Gans, *Life Gave Me a Chance,* p. 134.

138  *played "The Road to the Isles":* Saunders, *The Green Beret,* p. 267.

    *"did not apply to them":* Owen, *Commando,* p. 307.

    *29,000 men land:* Ambrose, *D-Day,* p. 566.

    *pillboxes in the dunes:* Ambrose, *D-Day,* pp. 549–550.

    *followed shortly thereafter by the commandos:* There are numerous excellent histories on D-Day and Normandy. See, for example, Hastings, *Overlord;* Keegan, *Six Armies in Normandy;* Roberts, *The Storm of War,* pp. 461–490; Beevor, *D-Day;* Ambrose, *D-Day;* Milton, *Soldier, Sailor;* Holland, *Normandy '44.*

139  *"likely to encounter":* Masters, *Striking Back,* p. 148.

    *Cold Comfort Farm:* Masters, Oral History of D-Day.

## Chapter 10: Sword Beach, June 6, 1944

140  *greasy sea spray:* Masters's experiences on D-Day are provided in his book *Striking Back;* Audio recording of Peter Masters lecture (20786), IWM; Masters, interview for *About Face;* Peter Masters, Oral History Interview conducted by Esther Finder, August 7, 1998, File 1998.A.0190, RG-50.106.0110, United States Holocaust Memorial Museum, Washington, DC; Peter Masters, Oral History Interview conducted by Joshua Gray, April 19 and 23, 1996, File 996.A.0125, RG-50.106.0024, United States Holocaust Memorial Museum, Washington, DC; Masters, Oral History of D-Day. For more on his experiences, see Ambrose, *D-Day,* pp. 560–564.

142  *heavily defended beach exits:* As Max Hastings points out, in comparison with other beaches where there was massive slaughter, "the Sword landing was a remarkable success." Hastings, *Overlord,* p. 103.

    *fell into the sea:* Beevor, *D-Day,* p. 138.

    *one of Lovat's favorites:* "Piper Bill Millin," Pegasus Archive, http://www.pegasusarchive.org/normandy/bill_millin.htm.

143  *on a Kindertransport train:* Harry Nomburg, life history, n.d., Peter Masters Collection, United States Holocaust Memorial Museum Archives, Washington, DC.

144   *"without a single bullet in my gun"*: Unless otherwise cited, the description of this scene comes from Harry Nomburg, Oral History of D-Day, Eisenhower Center, Peter Kalikow WWII-Era Collection, National WWII Museum, New Orleans; Audio interview with Harry Drew (Harry Nomburg) (30198), IWM.
      *was now playing "The Road to the Isles"*: "Piper Bill Millin."
      *a quarter mile inland*: Angus Konstam, *British Commando: 1940–1945* (Oxford: Osprey, 2016), pp. 55–56; Saunders, *The Green Beret*, p. 266.

145   *heavy, sustained bombardment*: Peter Harclerode and David Reynolds, *Commando: The Illustrated History of Britain's Green Berets from Dieppe to Afghanistan* (Phoenix Mill, UK: Sutton, 2001), p. 44.
      *"cacophony of the devil"*: Gans, *Life Gave Me a Chance*, p. 135.
      *"[The beach] was littered"*: 41 (RM) Cdo. War Diary, DEFE 2/48, TNA.
      *"I've come back"*: Gans, interview for BBC show on Aberdovey memorial.
      *"Good morning, gentlemen"*: Gans, *Life Gave Me a Chance*, p. 136.

146   *"for the want of moving"*: Jim Spearman, as quoted in Owen, *Commando*, p. 301.

147   *take Lion-sur-Mer*: Audio interview with Fred Gray (Manfred Gans) (30192), IWM.

## Chapter 11: Pegasus Bridge, June 6, 1944

148   *Masters wheeled his bike*: Masters's experiences on D-Day are provided in his book *Striking Back*; Audio recording of Peter Masters lecture (20786), IWM; Masters, interview for *About Face*; Peter Masters, Oral History Interview conducted by Esther Finder, August 7, 1998, File 1998.A.0190, RG-50.106.0110, United States Holocaust Memorial Museum, Washington, DC; Peter Masters, Oral History Interview conducted by Joshua Gray, April 19 and 23, 1996, File 996.A.0125, RG-50.106.0024, United States Holocaust Memorial Museum, Washington, DC; Masters, Oral History of D-Day; Masters, "The French Window."

149   *"cannon and machine guns"*: Masters, *Striking Back*, p. 151.
      *"his highly polished shoes"*: Audio interview with George Saunders (13660), IWM.
      *camouflaged machine guns and heavy artillery*: Manfred Gans, Oral History Interview conducted by Amy Ruben, November 11, 2004, File 2004.563, RG-50.030.0489, United States Holocaust Memorial Museum, Washington, DC.

150   *took no casualties*: Gans, interview for *About Face*.
      *"the Franco-Prussian War"*: Audio interview with Fred Gray (Manfred Gans) (30192), IWM.
      *pedal out of the way*: Masters, *Striking Back*, p. 155.
      *"a bicycle was the worst"*: Bryan Samain, *Commando Men: The Story of a Royal Marine Commando in World War Two* (Barnsley, UK: Pen and Sword Military, 2005), p. 6.

151   *"only met that morning"*: Masters, *Striking Back*, p. 154.
      *"had been mortally struck"*: Masters, *Striking Back*, p. 155.
      *"Ah, Corporal Masters"*: Masters, Oral History of D-Day. For more on Masters's terrifying walk, see Masters, *Striking Back*, pp. 155–159; Milton, *Soldier, Sailor*, pp. 321–323.

153   *to reach Pegasus Bridge*: Surprisingly, Stephen E. Ambrose's *Pegasus Bridge: D-Day; The Daring British Airborne Raid* (New York: Simon and Schuster, 2016) fails to mention that members of the Bicycle Troop were the first ones over the bridge (perhaps because he was relying on the myth that Lord Lovat and his piper were the first across). Peter Masters, who was interviewed for Ambrose's *Pegasus Bridge*

and is mentioned in Lovat's memoir, *March Past,* wrote letters to both authors to remind them that the men on the bikes were there first. See Peter Masters to Stephen Ambrose, January 28, 1988, and Peter Masters to Lord Lovat, May 8, 1985, Peter Masters Collection, United States Holocaust Memorial Museum Archives, Washington, DC.

154   *"ever piped across":* "Piper Bill Millin."

     *with three armored cars:* 41 (RM) Cdo. War Diary, DEFE 2/48, TNA.

     *all three vehicles:* 41 (RM) Cdo. War Diary, DEFE 2/48, TNA.

155   *married an Aberdovey woman:* Dear, *10 Commando,* p. 129.

     *say Kaddish:* I want to thank Daniel Gans and Aviva Gans Rosenberg for their gracious help with this passage.

     *west side of the Orne:* Saunders, *The Green Beret,* p. 269.

156   *killed at least twenty-four Germans:* 6 Commando War Diary, ADM 202/87, TNA.

     *Camembert stored there:* Owen, *Commando,* p. 309.

     *tommy gun, knife, and Colt .45:* Audio interview with George Saunders (30201), IWM.

     *camouflage net draped over him:* Audio interview with George Saunders (13660), IWM.

157   *at Sword Beach that day:* 45 (RM) Cdo. War Diary, ADM 202/82, IWM.

     *many others were wounded:* Samain, *Commando Men,* p. 12.

     *"asks the questions here":* Masters, *Striking Back,* p. 163.

158   *"only Allied troops still left alive":* Masters, *Striking Back,* p. 163.

### Chapter 12: Varaville and Beyond, June 7–15, 1944

159   *"Ready, lads":* Masters's experiences on D-Day are provided in his book *Striking Back;* Audio recording of Peter Masters lecture (20786), IWM; Masters, interview for *About Face;* Peter Masters, Oral History Interview conducted by Esther Finder, August 7, 1998, File 1998.A.0190, RG-50.106.0110, United States Holocaust Memorial Museum, Washington, DC; Peter Masters, Oral History Interview conducted by Joshua Gray, April 19 and 23, 1996, File 996.A.0125, RG-50.106.0024, United States Holocaust Memorial Museum, Washington, DC; Masters, Oral History of D-Day; Masters, "The French Window."

     *forced them to retreat:* Masters, *Striking Back;* Masters, Oral History of D-Day.

162   *"and then be withdrawn":* Lord Lovat, as quoted in Owen, *Commando,* p. 313.

     *fill gaps in the line:* Max Hastings discusses the resentment that many in the high command had toward the commando units, which they viewed as a "private army" that "creamed off precious high-quality manpower." Hastings, *Overlord,* pp. 36–37.

     *seaside town of Franceville-Plage:* For more information on 45 (RM) Cdo., see Peter Barnard, *The Story of 45 Royal Marine Commando* (London: McCorquodale, 1994).

     *ahead of the other commandos:* Saunders's and Shelley's actions are described in Audio interviews with George Saunders (13660 and 30201), IWM; Owen, *Commando,* pp. 308–310, 375; Samain, *Commando Men,* pp. 28, 31.

163   *to look like a cravat:* Masters, *Striking Back,* p. 200.

164   *"that ever existed":* Gans, interview for *About Face.*

     *capture the Merville Battery:* The fight for the Merville Battery would continue until mid-August, ending only when the Germans gave it up as part of their general retreat.

165   *"give us a hand":* Captain Douglas Robinson, as quoted in Masters, *Striking Back,* p. 177.

166  *"monkey grease"*: Masters, *Striking Back,* p. 182.

*Colonel Tim Gray was wounded:* 41 (RM) Cdo. War Diary, DEFE 2/48, TNA.

*named Moltke and Hindenburg:* Gans tells the full story of taking the stations in his autobiography, *Life Gave Me a Chance,* pp. 144–162. For more information, see Audio interview with Fred Gray (Manfred Gans) (30192), IWM; Gans, interview for *About Face;* Gans, interview for BBC show on Aberdovey memorial; *One Less Fight;* Manfred Gans, Oral History Interview conducted by Amy Ruben, November 11, 2004, File 2004.563, RG-50.030.0489, United States Holocaust Memorial Museum, Washington, DC.

*most heavily fortified positions:* Saunders, *The Green Beret,* p. 275.

167  *Twenty-First Panzer Division:* Van der Bijl, *Commandos in Exile,* p. 99.

*with four Marines:* 41 (RM) Cdo. War Diary, DEFE 2/48, IWM.

*"too slow to be viable":* Gans, *Life Gave Me a Chance,* p. 146.

*had not been cut through:* For more about the patrols of Gans and the others, and the valuable information they gathered, see 41 (RM) Cdo. War Diary, DEFE 2/48, TNA.

169  *battlefield commissions to second lieutenant:* Van der Bijl, *Commandos in Exile,* p. 119.

170  *"watch them do it":* Masters, *Striking Back,* p. 193. See also Lovat, *March Past,* pp. 350–353.

171  *"a gaggle of noisy geese":* Masters, *Striking Back,* p. 194.

*"give him the last rites":* Bill Millin, as quoted in Owen, *Commando,* pp. 314–315.

*"You are making history":* Lord Lovat, as quoted in Saunders, *The Green Beret,* p. 272.

*be returned to him:* Masters discusses this in a letter to Lovat. Peter Masters to Lord Lovat, July 4, 1979, Peter Masters Collection, United States Holocaust Memorial Museum Archives, Washington, DC.

172  *Everything was on fire:* According to Masters, this is why there are so few photographs and so little film footage of the commandos at D-Day. See Masters, *Striking Back,* p. 197.

*"shell bursts ripped the air":* Masters, *Striking Back,* p. 197.

173  *clutching white flags:* Gans, interview for *About Face.*

*he had gotten to like:* Masters, *Striking Back,* p. 199.

174  *let through the lines:* Masters, *Striking Back,* p. 203.

*loss of their beloved Skipper:* Masters, *Striking Back,* p. 205.

*Chapter 13: Normandy Breakout*

175  *others in their unit:* Masters, "The French Window."

*"marked in such a fashion":* Gans, *Life Gave Me a Chance,* p. 159.

176  *"his great love":* Audio interview with George (should be Geoff) Broadman (30190), IWM.

*"die in the attempt":* Masters, *Striking Back,* p. 65.

*had been shot dead:* For more on Arlen's story, see Samain, *Commando Men,* p. 271. Samain misspells his name. Barnard, *The Story of 45 Royal Marine Commando,* p. 19, also misspells his name.

*"oblivious to fear":* Peter Terry, as quoted in Dear, *10 Commando,* p. 135.

*confiscated their weapons:* Dear, *10 Commando,* p. 135; Van der Bijl, *Commandos in Exile,* p. 124.

177  *avoided these assignments:* Beevor, *D-Day,* p. 257.

178  *"who was allowed to go":* Masters, interview for BBC show on Aberdovey memorial.

*"beating another human being"*: Andrew Turner, interview for BBC show on Aberdovey memorial unveiling, May 1999.

*went on reconnaissance missions*: Manfred Gans, Oral History Interview conducted by Amy Ruben, November 11, 2004, File 2004.563, RG-50.030.0489, United States Holocaust Memorial Museum, Washington, DC.

*preparation, energy, and focus*: Manfred Gans to the Wislickis, July 28, 1944, Manfred Gans Collection, United States Holocaust Memorial Museum Archives, Washington, DC.

*German machine-gun unit*: Gans, *Life Gave Me a Chance*, p. 167.

179    *"Sergeant Gray [Gans] returned"*: 41 (RM) Cdo. War Diary, DEFE 2/48, TNA.

*temporarily put in charge*: Van der Bijl, *Commandos in Exile*, p. 125.

*He immediately promoted*: Masters, *Striking Back*, p. 214.

*"dog biscuits"*: Masters, *Striking Back*, p. 209.

180    *"for many a noisy night"*: Masters, *Striking Back*, p. 212.

*killed or captured*: Masters, *Striking Back*, p. 215.

*hold it for him*: Masters, *Striking Back*, p. 217. Masters also discusses this in Peter Masters to Lord Lovat, July 4, 1979, Peter Masters Collection, United States Holocaust Memorial Museum Archives, Washington, DC.

*"build their reputations again"*: Peter Masters, Oral History Interview conducted by Esther Finder, August 7, 1998, File 1998.A.0190, RG-50.106.0110, United States Holocaust Memorial Museum, Washington, DC.

181    *"parade ground bull-shitter"*: Masters, *Striking Back*, p. 222.

*stuck in the trenches*: Masters, *Striking Back*, p. 251.

*Corporal Ron Gilbert*: I could not understand why X Troopers such as Gilbert and Harris with No. 46 (RM) Cdo. had landed on D-Day plus one rather than on D-Day itself, until I saw this documentary short explaining that 46 (RM) Cdo. had intended to land on a sixth D-Day beach, codename Band, that had been aborted at the last minute. See Mark Felton Productions' *D-Day's Forgotten 6th Beach* (November 1, 2020), https://www.youtube.com/watch?v=5z-CjczAGuM&t=4s.

182    *"staring at each other"*: Audio interview with Ron Gilbert (30194), IWM.

*"I kept that bullet"*: Audio interview with Ron Gilbert (30194), IWM.

*"this little fellow"*: Harris, interview for BBC show on Aberdovey memorial.

183    *"I enjoyed it immensely"*: Audio interview with Ian Harris (30196), IWM.

*"kill as many of the bastards as I could"*: Harris, interview for BBC show on Aberdovey memorial.

184    *"it was like bright daylight"*: Peter Terry, as quoted in Dear, *10 Commando*, p. 144. The attack is also described in 47 (RM) Cdo. War Diary, ADM 202/107, TNA; Karras, *The Enemy I Knew*, pp. 93–94. A letter from the administrative officer of X Troop to Terry's father states that Terry had received a "shotwound" to "the chest." Lieutenant E. R. Langley to Mr. A. Tischler, July 28, 1944, Private Papers of I C B Dear (22991), IWM.

*he eventually recovered*: Lieutenant E. R. Langley to Mr. A. Tischler, July 28, 1944.

185    *east toward the Seine*: Interestingly, among the most effective pathfinders for the US military were the "Ritchie Boys," a large number of whom were German Jewish refugees to America. For information about them, see Bruce Henderson, *Sons and Soldiers: The Untold Story of the Jews Who Escaped the Nazis and Returned with the U.S. Army to Fight Hitler* (New York: HarperLuxe, 2017). In the British sector, it was the X Troopers who were often at the forefront of such endeavors.

*"the Germans on the run":* Audio interview with Fred Gray (Manfred Gans) (30192), IWM.

186  *"not my sin or fault":* Gans, interview for BBC show on Aberdovey memorial.

*no moon to light their way:* For a full report of this mission, see "The History of 46 (RM) Commando." See also Saunders, *The Green Beret*, p. 281.

*the lieutenant ignored him:* Helen Fry, *Churchill's German Army: The Germans Who Fought for Britain in World War Two* (London: Thistle, 2015), pp. 65–66.

*"King's English":* Audio interview with Ian Harris (30196), IWM.

*in close quarters:* "The History of 46 (RM) Commando."

*"Hans, is that you":* Audio interview with Ian Harris (30196), IWM.

187  *"had my cover story [been] blown":* Masters, *Striking Back*, p. 257.

188  *He was sent to:* Audio interview with Gordon Geiser (Henry Gordon) (30193), IWM.

189  *couldn't be moved:* The letters and telegrams relating to Hilton-Jones's hospital stay and injuries are from his private family archive, held by Ursula Hilton-Jones, who shared it with me.

*his recovery at Wolverton hospital:* Hilton-Jones's wife, Edwina, kept a diary, which has the dates of his hospital stay. Edwina Hilton-Jones, diary, private family archive, held by Ursula Hilton-Jones. Bryan Hilton-Jones would eventually intervene on Hartmann's behalf to get him released from British captivity. Ernst Hartmann letter to Bryan Hilton-Jones, June 30, 1947, Bryan Hilton-Jones, private family archive, held by Ursula Hilton-Jones.

*Military Cross in absentia:* The *Gazette* (UK) kept lists of all those awarded medals.

*"It's very simple, chum":* Gans, interview for *About Face.*

190  *"stand in my way":* Gans, interview for *About Face.*

*"a sewage tunnel":* Audio interview with Fred Gray (Manfred Gans) (30192), IWM.

*showered, prayed, and showered again:* Audio interview with Fred Gray (Manfred Gans) (30192), IWM.

*killed, wounded, or taken prisoner:* Dear, *10 Commando*, p. 145.

### Chapter 14: The Adriatic

191  *eleven more X Troopers:* Dear, *10 Commando*, p. 94.

*northern region of the country:* For a history of the Italian and Adriatic campaigns, see Atkinson, *The Day of the Battle;* Gooderson, *A Hard Way;* Weinberg, *A World at Arms,* pp. 591–601; Roberts, *The Storm of War*, pp. 375–406.

192  *Albanian port of Sarandë:* For information on this operation, see Charles Messenger, *Commandos: The Definitive History of Commando Operations in the Second World War* (London: William Collins, 1985), pp. 356–360.

193  *lacerated his skin:* Audio interview with Colin Anson, privately recorded, 1988.

*rain, cold, and wind:* Audio interview with Colin Anson (484), JML.

*"exposure, exhaustion, and trench foot":* 40 (RM) Cdo. War Diary, ADM 202/87, TNA.

*"We were all wet":* Fry, *German Schoolboy*, p. 121.

*"monsoon rain is like":* Tom Churchill, as quoted in Saunders, *The Green Beret*, p. 287.

*"bits of uniform":* Fry, *German Schoolboy*, p. 121.

194  *set meals such as stews:* Fry, *German Schoolboy*, p. 122.

*"German field hospital surrendered":* Fry, *German Schoolboy*, p. 124.

195  *a cache of diesel oil:* 40 (RM) Cdo. War Diary, ADM 202/87, TNA.

*"don't let them get away"*: As quoted in Fry, *German Schoolboy,* p. 127.

*Nothing seemed to bother him:* None of the X Troopers in their interviews or memoirs from the war discussed experiencing post-traumatic stress disorder, although undoubtedly some of them surely struggled with reconciling their personas as warriors with the terrors they must have experienced in battle.

196    *any remaining Germans there:* 2 Special Service Brigade War Diary, p. 16, DEFE 202-85-5, TNA; Audio interview with Colin Anson (484), JML.

*"in four years"*: Fry, *German Schoolboy,* p. 131.

*"bearded sea captains"*: Audio interview with Colin Anson, privately recorded, 1988.

*surrendered the garrison:* Operation Mercerised War Diary, DEFE 2_359, TNA.

*"quite by accident"*: Fry, *German Schoolboy,* p. 131.

### Chapter 15: Walcheren

197    *an enormous convoy:* For information on this operation, see Richard Brooks, *Walcheren 1944: Storming Hitler's Island Fortress* (Oxford: Osprey, 2011), p. 37; "Battle for Scheldt Estuary," in Dear, *The Oxford Companion to World War II,* pp. 978–981; Messenger, *Commandos,* pp. 290–301; Andrew Rawson, *Walcheren: Operation Infatuate* (Barnsley, UK: Leo Cooper, 2003).

*"like D-Day all over again"*: Gans, *Life Gave Me a Chance,* p. 193.

*"battle-hardened and very experienced"*: Gans, *Life Gave Me a Chance,* p. 194.

198    *Hitler intended to fortify it:* "Battle for Scheldt Estuary," p. 978. The entry also points out that this was the sole time information from Ultra regarding a major matter was ignored.

*Allied ships approaching Antwerp:* Messenger, *Commandos,* p. 292.

*behind the German lines:* For a full examination of this campaign, see Anthony Beevor, *Arnhem: The Battle for the Bridges, 1944* (New York: Viking, 2019).

199    *fortified seawalls and dikes:* Operation Infatuate II Westkapelle, ADM 202/407, TNA.

*"rimmed by massive dikes"*: Operation Infatuate II Westkapelle, ADM 202/407, TNA.

*"protected by solid concrete"*: Operation Infatuate II Westkapelle, ADM 202/407, TNA.

200    *seven X Troopers:* Masters, *Striking Back,* p. 270.

*75 mm:* Saunders, *The Green Beret,* p. 295.

*"Morale was high"*: Gans, *Life Gave Me a Chance,* p. 194.

*"far more terrifying than the big one"*: Operation Infatuate II Westkapelle, ADM 202/407, TNA.

201    *the freezing water:* Letter to Ian Dear, March 23, 1986, Private Papers of I C B Dear (22991), IWM.

*hatred of the Nazis:* Bill Watson had one of the most tragic stories of all the X Troopers, which is saying a lot. The information on Watson's life in this chapter comes from Watson, unpublished memoir. See the appendix for a short version of his biography. Bill Watson's private memoir, Private Papers of I C B Dear (22991), IWM.

203    *"Come out and surrender"*: Gans, *Life Gave Me a Chance,* p. 196. Gans also discusses this incident in Audio interview with Fred Gray (Manfred Gans) (30192), IWM; Gans, interview for *About Face;* Gans, interview for BBC show on Aberdovey memorial; Manfred Gans, Oral History Interview conducted by Amy Ruben, November 11, 2004, File 2004.563, RG-50.030.0489, United States Holocaust Memorial Museum, Washington, DC. The incident is also described in Brooks, *Walcheren 1944,* p. 43.

204　*German prisoners of war:* Peter Masters later noted that a photo of Maurice Latimer and his German prisoners with their arms raised (see page 204) was the opposite of the infamous Holocaust photo of the Jewish boy with the yellow star with his arms raised. Audio recording of Peter Masters lecture (20786), IWM. Brooks discusses this photo in his book *Walcheren 1944*, p. 43, but he gets some of the information wrong.
　　　*any of his stupid conditions:* Gans, *Life Gave Me a Chance*, p. 197.
　　　*one of the landing craft, tank:* Brooks, *Walcheren 1944*, p. 50.

205　*"mouth, eyes, and hair":* Operation Infatuate II Westkapelle, ADM 202/407, TNA.
　　　*"like wild fire along the dike":* Operation Infatuate II Westkapelle, ADM 202/407, TNA.
　　　*"Here we go again":* Audio interview with Fred Gray (Manfred Gans) (30192), IWM.

206　*"the most gruesome sight":* Gans, *Life Gave Me a Chance*, pp. 202–203.

207　*ready to continue the battle:* Freddy Gray (Manfred Gans) to Joan Gerry (Anita Lamm), November 14, 1944, Manfred Gans Collection, United States Holocaust Memorial Museum Archives, Washington, DC.
　　　*"jolly Austrian":* Masters, *Striking Back*, p. 271.
　　　*double pneumonia:* Letter to Ian Dear, March 23, 1986.
　　　*"a pitiful lazy crowd of soldiers":* Manfred Gans to the Wislickis, November 14, 1944, Manfred Gans Collection, United States Holocaust Memorial Museum Archives, Washington, DC.

208　*POW camp in Domburg:* Gans, *Life Gave Me a Chance*, p. 212.

209　*and the Shermans:* Brooks, *Walcheren 1944*, p. 87.

210　*"How we felt":* Manfred Gans to the Wislickis, November 14, 1944, Manfred Gans Collection, United States Holocaust Memorial Museum Archives, Washington, DC.
　　　*surrender of Walcheren:* 41 (RM) Cdo. War Diary, DEFE 2/48, TNA; Operation Infatuate II Westkapelle, ADM 202/407, TNA.

211　*"'Good morning, Good morning'":* Operation Infatuate II Westkapelle, ADM 202/407, TNA.
　　　*"one of the most gallant operations":* Merle Miller, *Ike the Soldier: As They Knew Him* (New York: Perigee Trade, 1988), p. 711.
　　　*"the door to Antwerp":* Operation Infatuate II Westkapelle, ADM 202/407, TNA.
　　　*"We have decided":* As discussed in Gans, *Life Gave Me a Chance*, p. 217.

212　*near the border:* Gans, *Life Gave Me a Chance*, p. 217.
　　　*"king's commission in the commandos":* Manfred Gans to the Wislickis, December 4, 1944, Manfred Gans Collection, United States Holocaust Memorial Museum Archives, Washington, DC. He also discusses his commission in Gans, *Life Gave Me a Chance*, p. 218.

214　*"Yours Jo, or rather Anita":* Anita Lamm to Manfred Gans, February 1, 1946, Manfred Gans Collection, United States Holocaust Memorial Museum Archives, Washington, DC.

215　*"Love, Manfred":* Manfred Gans to Anita Lamm, March 6, 1945, Manfred Gans Collection, United States Holocaust Memorial Museum Archives, Washington, DC.
　　　*startling news from New York:* Theo and Manfred Gans received an undated letter from Erna Beihoff in New York City that says, "Dear Theo and Manfred, Yesterday came the good news via Switzerland that your parents are in good health in Th." She adds that hopefully "you will receive one or the other letter now" and closes with "Present address Theresien-Stadt Protectorate." Another letter dated May 22,

1945, states that their parents are in Theresienstadt. Although the signature in this letter is illegible, we can assume it is the "other letter" Erna is referring to above. A May 24, 1945, telegram from Theo to Tel Aviv (presumably to his brother Gershon) says, "Fred with parents but aged send cross [Red Cross] parcels." All of these are in the Manfred Gans Collection, United States Holocaust Memorial Museum Archives, Washington, DC.

*"longer leaves can't be granted"*: Manfred Gans to the Wislickis, December 26, 1944, Manfred Gans Collection, United States Holocaust Memorial Museum Archives, Washington, DC.

216    *the Thousand-Year Reich:* Hitler gave a speech talking about the Thousand-Year Reich as early as December 18, 1919, at the Zumdeutchen Reich hall. Thomas Weber, *Becoming Hitler: The Making of a Nazi* (New York: Basic Books, 2018), p. 138.

### Chapter 16: Crossing the Rhine

218    *part of the action:* Masters, *Striking Back,* p. 273.

*bring them back for interrogation:* Harry Nomburg to Peter Masters, August 21, 1989, Peter Masters Collection, United States Holocaust Memorial Museum Archives, Washington, DC.

219    *strategic river crossings:* For a history of the Rhine crossings, see Roberts, *The Storm of War,* pp. 491–519; Weinberg, *A World at Arms,* pp. 810–819; Ken Ford, *The Rhine Crossings, 1945* (Oxford: Osprey, 2007).

*get some fresh air:* Masters, *Striking Back,* p. 291.

220    *downstream from Wesel:* For information on Operation Plunder, see Messenger, *Commandos,* pp. 305–309; Saunders, *The Green Beret,* pp. 326–329; Samain, *Commando Men,* pp. 135–148.

*back in the Third Reich:* Masters, interview for *About Face.*

221    *"having a tremendous time":* Audio interview with Ian Harris (30196), IWM.

*"Tell us what unit":* Masters, *Striking Back,* p. 298.

*off their feet:* Masters, *Striking Back,* p. 297.

222    *two men from headquarters were killed:* Samain, *Commando Men,* p. 144.

*"a good one for you":* Masters, *Striking Back,* p. 300.

223    *"I just lost my temper":* Masters, *Striking Back,* p. 305.

*a typical response among the X Troopers:* Masters, *Striking Back,* p. 305.

*"up to my ears in pamphlets":* Masters, *Striking Back,* p. 307.

*the war was over — again:* Peter Masters, Oral History Interview conducted by Esther Finder, August 7, 1998, File 1998.A.0190, RG-50.106.0110, United States Holocaust Memorial Museum, Washington, DC.

224    *killing and capturing Nazis:* Masters, *Striking Back,* p. 306.

*used improvised transport:* Samain, *Commando Men,* p. 150.

*"I just saved them":* Audio interview with Ian Harris (30196), IWM.

*an entire SS battalion:* Audio interview with Ian Harris (30196), IWM; Harris, interview for BBC show on Aberdovey memorial.

226    *Twelfth SS Panzer Division Hitlerjugend (Hitler Youth):* Saunders, *The Green Beret,* p. 332.

*entrenched German positions:* Field Marshall Bernard Montgomery, commendation recommendation for Ian Harris from 45 (RM) Cdo., May 14, 1945, Private Papers of I C B Dear (22991), IWM.

*a scene of utter confusion:* For an account of these events, see Audio interview with Ian Harris (30196), IWM; Harris, interview for BBC show on Aberdovey memorial; Masters, *Striking Back,* pp. 309–311.

228 *"an inspiration to all":* Montgomery, commendation recommendation for Ian Harris.
*"There weren't many medals":* Harris, interview for BBC show on Aberdovey memorial.

229 *"a real soldier's funeral":* Brigadier Derek Mills-Roberts, as quoted in Van der Bijl, *Commandos in Exile,* p. 183. After Griffith was killed, the troop was briefly led by Lieutenant James Monahan, X Troop's intelligence officer, who was actually Irish and not one of the refugees. When he was dispatched to work with the SOE, Lieutenant Ken Bartlett took over.
*"bravest soldier":* Firth, "While I Think of It," p. 93. See also Dear, *10 Commando,* p. 184; Masters, *Striking Back,* p. 310.

### Chapter 17: The Final Push

231 *based on Hilton-Jones's principles:* Audio interview with Colin Anson (30188), IWM.
*above their heads:* Fry, *German Schoolboy,* p. 136.

232 *"I'm a general":* As quoted in Fry, *German Schoolboy,* p. 139.

234 *"I need to get to Paris":* Audio interview with Ron Gilbert (20786), IWM.
*"doing just about nothing":* Manfred Gans to Anita Lamm, March 23, 1945, Manfred Gans Collection, United States Holocaust Memorial Museum Archives, Washington, DC.
*"have had their lesson":* Manfred Gans to the Wislickis, April 1944, Manfred Gans Collection, United States Holocaust Memorial Museum Archives, Washington, DC.

235 *cigars, brandy, and cruelty:* The Gans family would never get their home back from the Germans.

### Chapter 18: Into the Abyss

237 *"working properly on this jeep":* Unless otherwise cited, all of the information in this chapter comes from Manfred Gans's diary of his trip to rescue his parents, Manfred Gans Collection, United States Holocaust Memorial Museum Archives, Washington, DC. The diary is reprinted in Gans, *Life Gave Me a Chance,* pp. 238–266. For more information on Gans's trip, see Audio interview with Fred Gray (Manfred Gans) (30192), IWM; Gans, interview for *About Face;* Gans, interview for BBC show on Aberdovey memorial; Manfred Gans, Oral History Interview conducted by Amy Ruben, November 11, 2004, File 2004.563, RG-50.030.0489, United States Holocaust Memorial Museum, Washington, DC; Karras, *The Enemy I Knew,* pp. 294–298.
*"April is the cruellest month":* T. S. Eliot, "The Waste Land," Bartleby.com, https://www.bartleby.com/201/1.html.

240 *sick with typhoid fever:* Information on the concentration camp comes from Ruth Bondy, "Theresienstadt," in *The Holocaust Encyclopedia,* ed. Walter Laqueur (New Haven, CT: Yale University Press, 2001), pp. 631–635; "Theresienstadt," *Holocaust Encyclopedia,* United States Holocaust Memorial Museum, https://encyclopedia.ushmm.org/content/en/article/Theresienstadt.

243 *"under the Nazis":* Gans, interview for *About Face.*

244 *pro-Nazi and anti-Czech:* Frederick Taylor, *Exorcising Hitler: The Occupation and De-nazification of Germany* (New York: Bloomsbury Press, 2011), p. 77.

*untouched by Allied bombers:* "Until 1945 the Sudetenland had been almost a haven of peace surrounded by the horrors of war, where people experienced neither the food shortages nor the bombing that had threatened Germans elsewhere, nor the fighting of the last months of the war which turned much of Germany into a waste-land." Richard Bessel, *Germany 1945: From War to Peace* (New York: HarperCollins, 2009), p. 82.

246    *"I wouldn't have recognized him":* Manfred Gans, Oral History Interview conducted by Amy Ruben, November 11, 2004, File 2004.563, RG-50.030.0489, United States Holocaust Memorial Museum, Washington, DC.

     *have not triumphed everywhere:* Holocaust survivor and poet Paul Celan wrote a poem, "WIE DU dich ausstirbst in mir," about the extraordinary moment when a survivor is discovered. The title is translated by Peter Lach-Newinsky as "How You Die Yourself Out in Me." Lach-Newinsky's translations of the German poem can be found on his website, https://peterln.wordpress.com/2020/04/16/paul-celan-twenty-poems/. The poem can be found in German in Barbara Wiedemann (Hg.), ed., *Paul Celan. Die Gedichte. Kommentierte Gesamtausgabe in einem Band* (Frankfurt: Suhrkamp Verlag, 2005), pp. 283–284.

248    *not hiding any valuables:* Giora Kaddar, *My Grandfather Moritz Gans* (private family film, 2000). The family shared this film with me.

     *in his wooden leg:* As elderly Orthodox Jews, Moritz and Else would likely have been shot out of hand before they even got to Theresienstadt had Moritz not had the wherewithal to hide a letter in his wooden leg detailing his exemplary service in World War One, which he likely showed to low-ranking SS guards. As Manfred Gans told the documentary filmmaker Steven Karras, "My father had special privileges since he was the head of the league for German invalids, orphans, and widows in his town . . . and in 1934 the head of that organization wrote him a complimentary letter . . . He always had this letter — kept in his wooden leg that he had lost in the Tyrol attack in Italy." Gans, interview for *About Face.*

     *two slices of bread a day:* Kaddar, *My Grandfather Moritz Gans.*

     *a British commando officer:* Daniel Gans said that his grandmother Else told him that when they heard there was a British officer outside, they knew immediately it had to be Manfred, because it was his personality to achieve the impossible. Daniel Gans, interview with author.

250    *get the Dutch Jews out:* Manfred Gans to the Wislickis, May 23, 1945, Manfred Gans Collection, United States Holocaust Memorial Museum Archives, Washington, DC.

     *won his own private war:* Gans, interview for BBC show on Aberdovey memorial.

### Chapter 19: Denazification

251    *"a lonely walk":* Fry, *German Schoolboy,* pp. 141–142.

     *eighty-seven men served:* Hilton-Jones, "No. 3 Troop, 10 Commando."

252    *high number for any unit:* Up to 142 men may have gone through the training and served in other theaters or on an ad hoc basis, as in the half troop in Italy formed during the final days of the war. The number of wounded and those who received medals varies slightly in different lists.

     *Allies' denazification campaign:* The full list of where the men were serving as part of this effort is located in DEFE 2/1231, TNA.

*the Nuremberg trials:* For information on denazification, see Richard Bessel, *Germany 1945: From War to Peace* (New York: Harper Perennial, 2010), pp. 169–211; Konrad H. Jarausch, *After Hitler: Recivilizing Germans, 1945–1995* (New York: Oxford University Press), pp. 23–45.

253   *hunting down Nazis:* Fry, *German Schoolboy*, p. 145.
      *"ghost of a German schoolboy":* Fry, *German Schoolboy*, p. 151. For more information on Anson's denazification work, see Helen Fry, *Denazification: Britain's Enemy Aliens, Nazi War Criminals and the Reconstruction of Post-war Europe* (Cheltenham, UK: History Press, 2010).

254   *"What's all this":* Fry, *German Schoolboy*, p. 151.
      *"take another life in revenge":* Fry, *German Schoolboy*, p. 154.
      *"happened to be exceptionally high":* Bryan Hilton-Jones, as quoted in Fry, *German Schoolboy*, p. 155.

255   *the Werewolf movement:* For a discussion of the Werewolf movement, see Taylor, *Exorcising Hitler*, pp. 22–29. Richard Bessel points out that the Werewolf movement turned out to be fairly limited, although it inspired a great deal of fear in Allied occupiers. Bessel, *Germany 1945*, p. 176.
      *the woods near Hildesheim:* Van der Bijl, *Commandos in Exile*, p. 187.

256   *before they received them:* Audio interview with Ron Gilbert (30194), IWM.
      *"like a detective job":* Audio interview with George (should be Geoff) Broadman (30190), IWM.

257   *a number of German Jews:* Fry, *Denazification*, p. 39.
      *"killed my mother":* Fred Jackson, as quoted in Dear, *10 Commando*, p. 186.

258   *previously excluded Jews:* Gans, *Life Gave Me a Chance*, p. 272.
      *to silence them:* Manfred Gans to Anita Lamm, June 1, 1945, Manfred Gans Collection, United States Holocaust Memorial Museum Archives, Washington, DC.
      *"Nazi propaganda":* Manfred Gans to Anita Lamm, June 1, 1945, Manfred Gans Collection, United States Holocaust Memorial Museum Archives, Washington, DC.

259   *"will ever come back":* Manfred Gans to the Wislickis, December 21, 1945, Manfred Gans Collection, United States Holocaust Memorial Museum Archives, Washington, DC.
      *"military government duties":* Commando Group to Chief of Combined Operations, May 22, 1945, DEFE 2/1231, TNA.
      *"never been Nazis at all":* Manfred Gans to Anita Lamm, July 14, 1945, Manfred Gans Collection, United States Holocaust Memorial Museum Archives, Washington, DC.
      *"otherwise they won't know":* Manfred Gans to Anita Lamm, July 14, 1945, Manfred Gans Collection, United States Holocaust Memorial Museum Archives, Washington, DC.
      *encouraged to remain in Germany:* In May 1945 Gans and Andrew Kershaw applied for transfers to the military government. A secret letter in support of their application was sent to Combined Operations stating that Gans and Kershaw were "keen young officers who would do extremely well in this type of work" and it was therefore "strongly recommended" that their request be approved. DEFE 2/1231, TNA.
      *few remaining Jewish survivors:* Manfred Gans to Anita Lamm, November 14, 1945, Manfred Gans Collection, United States Holocaust Memorial Museum Archives, Washington, DC.

*"the soldier from Theresienstadt"*: Manfred Gans to Anita Lamm, December 6, 1946, Manfred Gans Collection, United States Holocaust Memorial Museum Archives, Washington, DC.

260 *Kahn and his wife:* Manfred Gans to the Wislickis, January 1946, Manfred Gans Collection, United States Holocaust Memorial Museum Archives, Washington, DC.

*"German parentage":* Manfred Gans to Anita Lamm, November 30, 1945, Manfred Gans Collection, United States Holocaust Memorial Museum Archives, Washington, DC.

*imprisoned at Paderborn:* Manfred Gans to Anita Lamm, May 13, 1946, Manfred Gans Collection, United States Holocaust Memorial Museum Archives, Washington, DC.

261 *give them a lecture:* Manfred Gans, Oral History Interview conducted by Amy Ruben, November 11, 2004, File 2004.563, RG-50.030.0489, United States Holocaust Memorial Museum, Washington, DC.

*their monstrous behavior:* Gans, *Life Gave Me a Chance,* p. 309.

*"get rid of the war":* Manfred Gans, Oral History Interview conducted by Amy Ruben, November 11, 2004, File 2004.563, RG-50.030.0489, United States Holocaust Memorial Museum, Washington, DC.

262 *naturalization papers during the war:* E. R. Langley, Administrative Officer of X Troop, to Combined Operations HQ, May 7, 1945, DEFE 2/1231, TNA. This file contains documents on the attempts to get X Troop commandos naturalized (e.g., "Naturalization of Members of No. 3 Troop, No. 10 (IA) Commando"), a list of where the men served as part of the denazification efforts, and a list of all the X Troopers.

*"after the war was over":* "Notes on Meeting Held at Home Office on Naturalization of Aliens Who Served in the Forces or in the Merchant Navy," December 7, 1945, DEFE 2/1231, TNA; Brief for CCO "Naturalization of Commandos," August 3, 1946, DEFE 2/1231, TNA.

263 *top secret meeting:* "Notes on Meeting Held at Home Office on Naturalization of Aliens."

*"These men are now":* Hilton-Jones, "No. 3 Troop, 10 Commando."

264 *A detailed memorandum:* The memorandum does not state who the author was.

*"valuable national work":* Brief for CCO "Naturalization of Commandos."

*"preference being given to them":* Brief for CCO "Naturalization of Commandos."

*they were not British citizens:* Gans, *Life Gave Me a Chance,* p. 164.

265 *"had that chance again":* Harris, interview for BBC show on Aberdovey memorial.

*"so proud of these men":* Mountbatten's quotes about the troop appeared in a range of newspapers after the banquet, including the *Times* (UK) and the *Scotsman,* both October 24, 1946. He later told commando John Franklin that the men of X Troop were "the bravest of the brave." As recounted in John Franklin letter to Peter Masters, n.d., Peter Masters Collection, United States Holocaust Memorial Museum Archives, Washington, DC. At the same time Major General Robert Laycock, chief of Combined Operations, was also going public in support of what he labeled this "mostly Jewish troop." "All of the men were of the highest courage and intelligence," Laycock said. As quoted in "George, Man Who Deceived Rommel," *News Chronicle,* October 25, 1946.

266 *"most worth-while":* Hilton-Jones, "No. 3 Troop, 10 Commando."

*Afterword*

273   *fully accepted into society*: For a history of the Jews in England, see David S. Katz, *The Jews in the History of England, 1495–1850* (New York: Oxford University Press, 1997); Cecil Roth, *A History of the Jews in England* (Oxford: Clarendon Press, 1964). Also see Vivian David Lipman, "England," in *Encyclopedia Judaica,* ed. Fred Skolnik and Michael Berenbaum, 2nd ed., vol. 6 (Detroit: Macmillan Reference, 2007), pp. 410–417. For a succinct overview of British Jewish life, see Paul Vallely, "A Short History of Anglo-Jewry: The Jews in Britain, 1656–2006," *Independent,* June 13, 2006, https://www.independent.co.uk/news/uk/this-britain/a-short-history-of-anglo-jewry-the-jews-in-britain-1656-2006-6098403.html.

  *"rub it in the face"*: Richard (Dicky) Tennant to Peter Masters, January 10, 1998, Peter Masters Collection, United States Holocaust Memorial Museum Archives, Washington, DC.

274   *include the word "Jewish"*: Martin Sugarman oversaw the creation of a small bronze Star of David, made by the prominent sculptor Robert Erskine, to rest at the foot of the memorial, as can be seen in the photo on page 275. Martin Kay placed it there in August 2020, with the hope it would remain for years to come as a mark of the Jewish origins of the troop.

  *"eighty-six German-speaking refugees"*: As explained in an earlier note, depending on the source the total number varies between 87 and 142. The X Troop war diary ("The History of 46 [RM] Commando") and most secondary sources put the number at 87, which is the number I use in this book.

275   *"different social and religious backgrounds"*: Neil Storkey, clerk to Aberdyfi Community Council, to Martin Sugarman, March 2018. Martin Sugarman shared this with me.

276   *"the end of the matter"*: Clerk to the Aberdyfi Community Council, email to Martin Sugarman, July 23, 2020. Martin Sugarman shared this with me. The local tourist office never answered Sugarman's repeated requests to update the pamphlet.

  *let the crosses stand*: According to Martin Sugarman, some X Troopers, including the following, still have crosses on their graves at the request of their assimilated relatives or non-Jewish spouses: Peter Wells (Werner Auerhahn), Minturno (Italy); George Franklyn (Günter Max Frank), Hermanville-sur-Mer (France); Didi Fuller (Eugen Kagerer-Stein), Ranville (France); James Griffith (Kurt Glaser), Becklingen (Germany); Kenneth Graham (Kurt Wilhelm), Hermanville-sur-Mer; Max Laddy (Max Lewinsky), Hermanville-sur-Mer; Eric Howarth (Erich Nathan), Reichswald (Germany); Ernest Webster (E. G. Weinberger), Bayeux (France).

  *ask him questions on my behalf*: Tish sent me a series of emails with his responses to my questions.

277   *"unpleasant and unkindly feeling"*: Paul Streeten, unpublished interview with David Simon.

279   *Herman Wouk*: When writing my book *Young Lions,* I was in touch with Wouk, who described the same love of military service and passion for fighting the Nazis that would be evident among the X Troopers.

  *establish a safe life*: Aviva Gans Rosenberg pointed out to me that her father Manfred Gans's service as a commando inspired a generation of family members in Israel, including a cousin who became a paratrooper in the Israeli army.

*Quentin Tarantino's vengeful Jews:* Kim Masters, "My Father, the Inglourious Basterd," Daily Beast, August 9, 2009, updated July 14, 2017, https://www.thedailybeast.com /my-father-the-inglourious-basterd.

280    *"Last Post":* "Last Post" is the British counterpart of America's "Taps."

## Appendix

296    *enjoyed his cherished pastimes:* Streeten, "Aerial Roots," p. 150.

297    *packed together "like sardines":* All of the quotes in this entry come from Watson, unpublished memoir.

# Illustration Credits

170 Group photo of Shelley, Arlen, Saunders, Hepworth, Stewart, 1943.
United States Holocaust Memorial Museum, courtesy of Peter Masters

183 Ian Harris.
Courtesy of the Harris Family

202 Landing of the commandos at Westkapelle, Walcheren, November 1, 1944.
Imperial War Museum

203 Commandos on Walcheren, November 1, 1944.
Imperial War Museum

204 Maurice Latimer with captured prisoners, Walcheren, November 1, 1944.
Imperial War Museum

214 Anita Lamm.
United States Holocaust Memorial Museum, courtesy of Manfred Gans

226 Ian Harris leading captured German prisoners, Osnabrück, April 1945.
Imperial War Museum

228 James Griffith's makeshift grave, Essel, Germany, April 1945.
United States Holocaust Memorial Museum, courtesy of Peter Masters

233 Ron and Lilo Gilbert in Paris.
Courtesy of the Gilbert Family Archive

235 Sherman tank in Borken, March 1945.
Imperial War Museum

268 Peter and Alice Masters on their wedding day, April 6, 1950.
Courtesy of the Masters Family Collection

269 Peter Masters's painting of D-Day with his poem "The Sweet Life."
Courtesy of the Masters Family Collection

275 Memorial to X Troop in Aberdovey, Wales.
Courtesy of Martin Kay

290 Gans family in Israel, 1958.
Permission granted by Daniel Gans and Aviva Gans Rosenberg

# Index

Page numbers in *italics* indicate illustrations; "n" in page numbers indicates a note.